Commissioning Editors: Laurence Hunter and Ellen Green
Project Development Manager: Siân Jarman
Project Manager: Nancy Arnott
Designer: Sarah Russell

THE COMPLETE PLAB

Extended-Matching Questions

M Afzal Mir

Formerly Senior Lecturer and Honorary Consultant Physician
University Hospital of Wales
Cardiff

E Anne Freeman
Consultant Physician
Royal Gwent Hospital
Newport
Gwent

Shu F Ho
Consultant Physician
Royal Shrewsbury Hospital
Shrewsbury

Jacob Easaw
Consultant Cardiologist
Weston General Hospital
Weston-Super-Mare

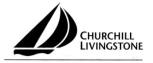

CHURCHILL
LIVINGSTONE

EDINBURGH LONDON NEW YORK OXFORD PHILADELPHIA ST LOUIS SYDNEY TORONTO 2004

CHURCHILL LIVINGSTONE
An imprint of Elsevier Limited

First published 2003

ISBN 0-443-07092-X

British Library Cataloguing in Publication Data
A catalogue record for this book is available from the British Library

Library of Congress Cataloging in Publication Data
A catalog record for this book is available from the Library of Congress

Notice
Medical knowledge is constantly changing. Standard safety precautions must be followed, but as new research and clinical experience broaden our knowledge, changes in treatment and drug therapy may become necessary or appropriate. Readers are advised to check the most current product information provided by the manufacturer of each drug to be administered to verify the recommended dose, the method and duration of administration, and contraindications. It is the responsibility of the practitioner, relying on experience and knowledge of the patient, to determine dosages and the best treatment for each individual patient. Neither the Publisher nor the authors assume any liability for any injury and/or damage to persons or property arising from this publication.
The Publisher

your source for books,
journals and multimedia
in the health sciences
www.elsevierhealth.com

The
publisher's
policy is to use
**paper manufactured
from sustainable forests**

Printed in China

In the part 1 section of the Professional and Linguistic Assessments Board (PLAB) examination, the objective is to test the candidates' clinical knowledge and the application of their knowledge to their everyday practice. Currently, this is accomplished by a three-hour extended-matching question (EMQ) examination that contains 200 questions divided into a number of themes. Each question explores a theme that may be a symptom, sign, investigation, diagnosis or a management decision, with the help of five stems of clinical scenarios that are derived from ordinary clinical practice. With each question there is a list of 11 options from which the examinees have to choose the most likely match, or the correct answer, for each stem, as advised in the lead-in statement.

The emphasis of the examination is on clinical management and includes science as applied to clinical problems. The exam is confined to core knowledge, skills and attitudes relating to conditions commonly seen at the SHO level and does include the generic management of life-threatening situations and some rare, but still important, conditions. This format is now increasingly being used in the final MB examination in various medical colleges.

Unlike the multiple-choice question format an incorrect answer does not attract a negative mark, but to get a positive mark the examinee has to assign the most appropriate answer to each stem. Obviously, the best way to gain competence in assessing these clinical vignettes is by applying oneself assiduously to clinical clerkship during the undergraduate years, and to clinical experience during subsequent house jobs. However, we hope, in producing this book, to help both medical students and postgraduate doctors to embellish their clinical experience, widen their knowledge and learn the art of applying their knowledge to answering extended-matching questions. This book contains approximately 200 questions on the most relevant themes in medicine, surgery and its allied specialities, obstetrics and gynaecology, paediatrics and psychiatry. We hope that the book will help medical students to make the best use of their clerkship and ward work, and that it helps examinees in the final MB and the PLAB part 1 to overcome the EMQ hurdle.

We do encourage all potential PLAB candidates to obtain and read a copy of the GMC guidance document entitled, 'The PLAB test – Part 1 – advice to candidates'. This is obtainable from the GMC central office in London.

Acknowledgements

Some questions in this book, particularly in the surgical specialities, have been contributed by various surgical specialists. Other questions have been reviewed by colleagues in their respective fields all of whom have given us valuable advice and comments. Our grateful thanks go to them all. Their names follow in alphabetical order: Mr Kieron Bahl, Mr William Hart, Mr David Hughes, Dr Dean Jenkins, Mr Anton Joseph, Dr Manzoor Malik, Mr Sujid Mithra, Dr Jamuna Prakash Mysore, Mr Alan Ng, Dr Stephen Nirmal, Mr Geoff Shone, Dr Madhusudan Srinivasan, Mr Sathya Thampiraj, Mr Sunil Vyas and Dr Nerys Weston.

Cardiff
2004

M.A.M.
E.A.F.
S.F.H.
J.E.

Contents

Introduction

The assessment of overseas medical graduates for their eligibility to practise in the UK is carried out by the Professional and Linguistic Assessments Board (PLAB) through a two-part examination. A pass in this test makes a doctor eligible to apply for limited registration if he or she has the offer of an approved training post in the National Health Service (NHS). Part 1 of the PLAB examination is a written examination and Part 2 is a practical test referred to as the Objective Structured Clinical Examination (OSCE).

The chief objective of the written examination is to identify doctors who have achieved an acceptable clinical and academic standard in medicine and surgery, and their subspecialities, obstetrics and gynaecology, paediatrics and psychiatry. The General Medical Council (GMC) has to ensure that doctors who have trained overseas, and whose qualification is not eligible for full registration, have adequate knowledge and ability to practise in this country. The examination has to be constructed in such a way that it covers the depth and breadth of knowledge that the Council considers essential for practising doctors. Theoretically, this could be done by asking candidates to write essays on important clinical subjects. The GMC considered this but gave it up for a variety of reasons. The chief weakness of the long essay answer is that examinees can hide their areas of weakness in the critical areas that they do not know, by writing long chunks of what they do know that is vaguely germane to the question asked. This format is time-consuming to mark and suffers from the inevitable subjectivity of examiners. The test-wise examinee with good handwriting and grammar is likely to score more than the examinee with poor style and vocabulary but with better knowledge of the subject under discussion.

At first, the GMC chose the multiple-choice question (MCQ) format which tests specific areas of an examinee's knowledge without allowing them to insert unsolicited or qualifying information. The answers are easy to mark quickly, with the use of a computer, and thereby the examiners' subjectivity is removed. Candidates have to commit themselves by marking a 'yes' or a 'no' to a given statement and guesses tend to be mostly wrong and score a negative mark.

Unfortunately, the MCQ format also has many drawbacks, the chief one being that it does not test doctors' clerking skills or their application of knowledge to clinical practice, thus defeating the very objective of the GMC for setting this examination. A great deal of expertise and care are required to construct the questions: inexperienced examiners leave technical flaws that are exploited by test-wise examinees. The MCQ format tests isolated, sometimes trivial, facts without exploring core knowledge and clinical application. The true/false dichotomy seldom suits clinical practice, in which most decisions require the thoughtful integration of knowledge and experience to select the best possible option. The GMC came to the conclusion that the written examination had to be designed to test not only knowledge but also its application to a wide range of clinical situations. The originators of the MCQ in North America were already abandoning it and working on a new format in the form of extended-matching questions.

The extended-matching question (EMQ)

This question format, now adopted by the GMC, tests the decision-making ability of candidates in a variety of clinical situations. Each question is set around a theme that may be a symptom, sign, side effect, investigation, diagnosis or management decision. This is followed by a lead-in statement asking the examinee to choose the most appropriate answer, from a list of options, for each of five extended clinical scenarios, referred to as 'stems', such as one might encounter in everyday clinical practice. The questions are designed to test application of knowledge and any relevant experience to clinical assessment and management, by using commonly encountered patient vignettes. These vignettes and the probable decisions are constructed so as to be appropriate for the expected standard being tested. The scenarios give minimum but important details as encountered in clinical practice about the patient's age, gender, past history, relevant symptoms and signs, and sometimes occupation, ethnic origin and one or more key investigations. If occupation or ethnic origin happens to be critical in making a decision in one stem then this information is provided in all five stems, in order not to give unfair advantage to test-wise candidates. Several options tend to be plausible for each stem and the candidate has to choose the most appropriate or likely one for each scenario.

One of the basic requirements of this format is that the options are listed in an alphabetical order so as not to give candidates any unintended advantage. Each correct or most appropriate option should be the 'best' answer for its scenario, and incorrect answers, or distracters, should be plausible and not deceptive or tricks. In choosing the most appropriate diagnosis, investigation, or therapeutic option, candidates have to guard against any personal bias based on epidemiological or ethnic reasons related to their country of origin. In some cases, the 'most likely' option may vary from one country to another. Because of these various constraints, the extended-matching questions are difficult and time-consuming to design; on average each theme takes about two hours to construct. Despite these problems, this format has been adopted by the GMC because it is best suited for testing candidates' clinical knowledge and expertise.

This book

This book contains over 200 key themes spread over all the specialities that are tested in the Part 1 of the PLAB examination. Each theme contains 11 options listed from A to K and candidates have to choose a correct answer for each of over 1000 clinical scenarios. We have given our chosen correct answers over the page after each theme, together with explanations supporting our choices. The themes cover all possible presentations and events and the options consist of a multitude of clinical decisions. The scenarios are based on various contributors' experience and knowledge but they carry a significant influence from the current format used in the PLAB Part 1 examination. The length of the scenarios is variable depending on the complexity of the clinical situations they represent. This structure will broaden candidates' clinical knowledge, hone their discriminatory powers and familiarize them with the different forms of questions they will encounter in the examination. Some scenarios occur more than once but the context or the tasks are different. Additionally, this inevitable repetition allowed us to add some more information about these common conditions.

The complexity varies from very easy to very difficult, with the majority of questions lying in the middle of the knowledge spectrum expected from practising junior doctors. Although this book has been written for candidates taking their PLAB exam, we believe it will be equally useful for undergraduate and other postgraduate students preparing for their exams. It should also provide a valuable learning experience for all undergraduate students in their clerking and the acquisition of clinical knowledge. Of the 1000 or more clinical scenarios given in this book, students of medicine may find many in their everyday practice, and they may have to make many of the decisions explained in this book.

How to use this book

This book was written to serve three objectives. First, it should widen the clinical horizons of students and help them to get the best out of their clinical practice. Secondly, it should help students in decision making at every stage of clinical assessment. Thirdly, it should familiarize them and sharpen their skills for this format of exam. To achieve these objectives, we would suggest that students allow themselves 5 minutes for each theme, read the lead-in statement and consider *carefully* what is required, and then study each stem and select the most appropriate answer for each scenario from the list of options. Students should pick up the correct options that they know and make an educated guess for the others and progress quickly from one question to another. They should consider each scenario carefully and not discard an option simply because it was used once; some options are used more than once. They should progress from one odd-numbered page to another without checking the correct answers and reading our explanations given on the even-numbered pages. It is important that candidates preparing for the exam should keep to the time limits and not take more than 5 minutes for each question. When one section has been completed then they should compare their answers with those given by us on the answer pages, and score 1 for each correct answer and 0 for the incorrect ones (there being no negative scoring in this format). An average candidate should be able to score between 50 and 60%.

Students should read our explanations for all answers, even for the ones they have correctly selected. These answers contain other useful facts that will allow users to increase their knowledge as they work through the questions. This process will broaden their knowledge and improve their reasoning for supporting their decisions. If students mimic the exam style in attempting the questions in this book, as we have suggested above, then they will familiarize themselves with this format, hone their skills in quickly selecting the correct options, and cultivate the ability to answer the questions within the allotted time.

We believe that this book will serve doctors well, even after they have passed the examination hurdle.

Medicine

Cough

A   Angiotensin-converting enzyme (ACE) inhibitor medication
B   Asthma
C   Cardiac failure
D   Inhaled foreign body
E   Middle ear disease
F   Oesophageal reflux
G   Psychogenic
H   Pulmonary embolism
I   Sinusitis
J   Smoker's cough
K   Tuberculosis

For each presentation below, choose the SINGLE most likely cause from the above list of options. Each option may be used once, more than once, or not at all.

1. A 56-year-old man complains of headaches and a troublesome cough associated with a post-nasal drip.

2. A 67-year-old woman with ischaemic heart disease and hypertension complains of a persistent dry cough ever since her medication was altered several weeks ago.

3. A 50-year-old obese woman presents with a two-year history of a dry cough, which is worse at night and which has not responded to various inhalers.

4. A 46-year-old woman presents with nocturnal wheezing and cough. She has orthopnoea and paroxysmal nocturnal dyspnoea. Her peak flow diary has revealed morning dips.

5. A 35-year-old smoker has a productive cough with weight loss and drenching night sweats. A chest X-ray shows a right hilar mass with partial collapse of the right upper lobe.

Answers to **1.1**

1. **I   Sinusitis**

   Sinusitis may present as facial pain, headache and nasal tenderness with a purulent nasal discharge or post-nasal drip and paroxysms of cough, mainly at night.

2. **A   Angiotensin-converting enzyme (ACE) inhibitor medication**

   Cough is common in cardiac failure. However, this patient's cough seems to coincide with the start of ACE inhibitor therapy for control of her blood pressure. It inhibits the breakdown of bradykinin which causes a small but significant increase in the incidence of cough. The cough is usually very troublesome and necessitates withdrawal of the drug.

3. **F   Oesophageal reflux**

   Abnormal oesophageal reflux is defined as significant acid exposure (pH<4.0) to the distal oesophagus for more than 1–2 hours (cumulative time >5%) over a 24-hour period, as established by intraoesophageal pH monitoring. Heartburn is the commonest presenting feature but the respiratory symptoms of hoarseness, persistent cough and wheezing can sometimes predominate. There is often a demonstrable increase in the sensitivity of the cough reflex. Obesity is a predisposing factor for reflux.

4. **B   Asthma**

   Airway tone has a circadian rhythm, being highest at 4 a.m., and lowest in mid-afternoon. This, together with bronchial hyper-responsiveness in asthma, produces symptoms that are worse in the early morning and are associated with diurnal variability in airflow obstruction. Orthopnoea and paroxysmal nocturnal dyspnoea may occur in both heart failure and asthma but the latter is more likely here in view of the morning dips in the peak flow readings.

5. **K   Tuberculosis**

   Primary tuberculosis is asymptomatic in the majority of patients but there may be cough, fever, weight loss, night sweats and haemoptysis in some patients. Nodal hilar enlargement is usually unilateral and may cause bronchial compression. Bronchial carcinoma (not on the list) is less likely in this young patient. Cough should never be dismissed as a smoker's cough without a full clinical assessment. Besides, this patient has other symptoms which suggest a subacute infection.

Abdominal pain

A   Appendicitis
B   Carcinoma of the bowel
C   Carcinoma of the pancreas
D   Chronic cholecystitis
E   Chronic pancreatitis
F   Cystitis
G   Diverticulitis
H   Duodenal ulcer
I   Gastric ulcer
J   Irritable bowel syndrome
K   Munchausen's syndrome

For each presentation below, choose the SINGLE most likely cause from the above list of options. Each option may be used once, more than once, or not at all.

1. A 45-year-old man of no fixed abode presents with severe abdominal pain for the last 3 days. He also complains of having vomited large amounts of fresh blood before his admission. Examination shows that he is well-perfused with several laparotomy scars on his abdomen. His haemoglobin is 15.2 g/dl.

2. A 67-year-old man gives a long history of intermittent abdominal discomfort, distension and nausea. Examination of the abdomen shows a positive Murphy's sign.

3. A 56-year-old woman presents with troublesome abdominal distension and bloating relieved by defaecation. She is often constipated with stools which are ribbon-like in appearance. Her weight remains stable.

4. A 35-year-old man complains of dyspepsia and epigastric pain relieved by antacids. He has had the symptoms on and off for the last year and finds that the pain is worse when he is hungry.

5. A 75-year-old woman presents with a severe pain in the left iliac fossa associated with fever and constipation. There is tenderness and guarding on the left side of the abdomen. The white cell count shows a leucocytosis.

Answers to **1.2**

1.   K   Munchausen's syndrome

Munchausen's syndrome is more common in men than women. Patients repeatedly present with dramatic illnesses which seem to require urgent medical or surgical intervention. They may submit to invasive investigations or even surgery, but then often suddenly discharge themselves before treatment is complete. In this case, the presence of multiple surgical scars together with the absence of anaemia or hypovolaemic shock, in a patient who has apparently brought up a large quantity of blood, should raise some suspicion.

2.   D   Chronic cholecystitis

Chronic cholecystitis is characterized by chronic inflammation and thickening of the gallbladder as a result of gall stones. Symptoms and signs are often vague and non-specific and there may be intolerance to fatty foods. Examination may reveal tenderness over the gallbladder and a positive Murphy's sign (elicited by asking the patient to breathe in when gently palpating the gallbladder area – patient will be in pain and hold his breath on inspiration).

3.   J   Irritable bowel syndrome

The irritable bowel syndrome is a form of functional bowel disorder. It is characterized by abdominal pain relieved by defaecation, or by a change in bowel habit with altered stool frequency/consistency associated with a sensation of abdominal distension. The patient often looks well despite the frequent episodes of pain. In an older patient, the irritable bowel syndrome is a diagnosis of exclusion, and should be made after appropriate gastrointestinal investigations.

4.   H   Duodenal ulcer

Epigastric pain is a characteristic feature of a peptic ulcer. The pain of a duodenal ulcer (DU) occurs at night as well as during the day. The relationship with food is variable, but patients with a DU may complain of hunger pain whereas those with gastric ulcers may find exacerbations of discomfort after meals.

5.   G   Diverticulitis

Diverticulitis is due to inflammation of one or more diverticula, almost always found in the sigmoid colon. There is persistent pain usually in the left iliac fossa or evidence of peritonitis, often accompanied by fever and leucocytosis. Complications include recurrent, periodic inflammation and pain, perforation (leading to peritonitis) or local abscess formation, intestinal obstruction, haemorrhage and fistula formation (vesicocolic, vaginocolic, enterocolic and colocutaneous).

Headache

A   Cervical spondylosis
B   Cluster headache
C   Drugs
D   Meningitis
E   Migraine
F   Raised intracranial pressure
G   Sinusitis
H   Subarachnoid haemorrhage
I   Temporal arteritis
J   Tension headache
K   Thunderclap headache

For each presentation below, choose the SINGLE most likely cause from the above list of options. Each option may be used once, more than once, or not at all.

1. A 64-year-old man presents with a pain in his head associated with tongue and jaw claudication.

2. A 50-year-old woman has a 3-month history of headaches associated with nausea and vomiting. Coughing and bending over exacerbate the severity of the headaches.

3. A 36-year-old man presents with a 5-year history of nocturnal right-sided headaches. They occur for about half an hour every day for several weeks, before recurring again several months later. There is no aura or vomiting but often there is a transient right Horner's syndrome.

4. A 52-year-old woman is admitted with a sudden onset of severe occipital headache associated with vomiting. She is apyrexial. Both a computerized tomography (CT) scan of the head and lumbar puncture are normal.

5. A 45-year-old man complains of a 12-month history of daily episodes of 'tight band' sensations in his head and pressure behind the eyes. He has recently lost his appetite and has early morning waking.

Answers to **1.3**

1.   I   Temporal arteritis

Giant-cell or temporal arteritis is rare in those under the age of 50 years. There may be scalp sensitivity with thickened and tender arteries. Jaw and tongue claudication may also be present. Visual problems include blurred vision, amaurosis fugax, diplopia and blindness (due to ischaemic optic neuropathy).

2.   F   Raised intracranial pressure

The cardinal symptoms of raised intracranial pressure are headaches (exacerbated by coughing, straining or stooping), vomiting and drowsiness. Causes include intracranial tumours, abscess or haematoma. Sinister symptoms include deteriorating vision and level of consciousness. There may be papilloedema (with an enlarged blind spot), 6th nerve palsy (a false localizing sign) and optic atrophy (blindness).

3.   B   Cluster headache

Cluster headaches occur mainly in men between 20–50 years of age. They are usually unilateral, occur in clusters of about 4–16 weeks during which headaches occur daily, lasting 30–120 minutes, and are worse at night. It is different from migraine in that there is no aura or vomiting. Sufferers tend to find relief when getting out of bed and walking around, as opposed to confining themselves to bed as with migraine. The cause is unknown. Autonomic involvement is shown by the presence of a Horner's syndrome.

4.   K   Thunderclap headache

Thunderclap headache is a syndrome of a sudden onset of severe headache with a benign prognosis. It needs to be distinguished from a subarachnoid haemorrhage by the finding of a normal computerized tomography (CT) scan of the head and the absence of blood or xanthochromia in the cerebrospinal fluid.

5.   J   Tension headache

This patient has features of endogenous depression, which is frequently associated with tension headaches. The headache is usually described as a feeling of pressure or tightness over the head, which occurs daily and is worse towards the end of the day. There is no associated photophobia, vomiting or visual disturbances. Treatment consists of reassurance, relaxation therapy and antidepressants.

Dysphagia

A   Achalasia
B   Benign stricture
C   Bulbar palsy
D   Myasthenia gravis
E   Oesophageal candidiasis
F   Oesophageal carcinoma
G   Oesophageal spasm
H   Oesophageal web
I   Pharyngeal pouch
J   Pseudobulbar palsy
K   Systemic sclerosis

For each presentation below, choose the SINGLE most likely cause from the above list of options. Each option may be used once, more than once, or not at all.

1. A 65-year-old man with difficulty in swallowing presents with an aspiration pneumonia. He has a bovine cough and a fasciculating tongue. Sometimes as he swallows food it comes back through his nose.

2. A 45-year-old woman complains of pain in her hands precipitated by exposure to the cold weather. She is breathless on walking and, when eating, she can feel food suddenly sticking in the gullet. It seems to be in the middle of her oesophagus but she cannot localize exactly where it sticks. It is usually relieved with a drink of water.

3. A 55-year-old woman complains of retrosternal chest pain and dysphagia which is intermittent and unpredictable. The food suddenly sticks in the middle of the chest, but she can clear it with a drink of water and then finish the meal without any further problem. A barium meal shows a 'corkscrew oesophagus'.

4. A 60-year-old man presents with dysphagia and pain on swallowing both solids and liquids. A barium meal shows gross dilatation of the oesophagus with a smooth narrowing at the lower end of the oesophagus.

5. A 72-year-old man presents with intermittent difficulty in swallowing with regurgitation of stale food material. Sometimes he wakes at night with a feeling of suffocation.

Answers to **1.4**

1. C Bulbar palsy

Bulbar palsy is a lower motor neurone lesion affecting the muscles supplied by the lower cranial nerves (9–12), the nuclei of which are in the medulla. The tongue is flaccid and fasciculating with a flaccid dysarthria, absent palatal movement and a bovine cough. There is usually dysphagia and nasal regurgitation. Causes include motor neurone disease, syringobulbia, Guillain–Barré syndrome, poliomyelitis and neurosyphilis.

2. K Systemic sclerosis

This patient has Raynaud's phenomenon (the digital arteries have an exaggerated physiological response to the cold with intense vasospasm producing white numb fingers which, on rewarming, go blue, then red and are extremely painful), dysphagia with poor localization (found in more than 90% patients with systemic sclerosis due to the replacement of smooth muscle with fibrous tissue) and breathlessness from cryptogenic fibrosing alveolitis. The underlying condition is systemic sclerosis. It can also cause renal failure, arthritis/myositis, malabsorption from bacterial overgrowth, and pericardial effusion.

3. G Oesophageal spasm

This scenario is characteristic of diffuse spasm of the oesophagus. Oesophageal spasm is due to spontaneous, non-propagated oesophageal contractions producing dysphagia and chest pain. It may show in a barium meal as bizarre and marked oesophageal contractions/rings. Oesophageal manometry may be needed to confirm the diagnosis in less severe cases. It is usually not responsive to treatment but a trial of nitrates or a calcium channel antagonist (e.g. nifedipine) is worthwhile. Patients should be reassured that the chest pain is not angina.

4. A Achalasia

Achalasia is due to degeneration of the ganglion cells of the myenteric plexus or vagal nuclei. It is a chronic, progressive disorder characterized by failure of relaxation of the lower oesophageal sphincter. Dysphagia characteristically starts for both liquids and solids. Its appearance on barium meal (smooth, tapered narrowing with a dilated oesophagus containing food residue) differs from a benign stricture (short, smooth outlines) and oesophageal carcinoma (irregular stricture). Aspiration pneumonia and oesophageal carcinoma are complications of achalasia.

5. I Pharyngeal pouch

A pharyngeal pouch is a protrusion through the posterior pharyngeal wall between the oblique and transverse fibres of the inferior constrictor muscle. It usually affects the elderly and is twice as common in men. Regurgitation of undigested food after a meal, during the next meal or when turning at night is common. The dysphagia worsens with an enlarging pouch. There may be gurgling noises heard in the neck.

Itching

A Atopic eczema
B Dermatitis herpetiformis
C Hyperthyroidism
D Lichen planus
E Lymphoma
F Primary biliary cirrhosis
G Psoriasis
H Psychogenic
I Scabies
J Uraemia
K Urticaria

For each presentation below, choose the SINGLE most likely cause from the above list of options. Each option may be used once, more than once, or not at all.

1. A 60-year-old vagrant presents with generalized itching. There are widespread excoriation marks on his trunk and arms with linear tracts around his wrists and between his fingers.

2. A 45-year-old woman presents with pruritus. On examination, she has skin pigmentation and investigations show a raised serum alkaline phosphatase and the presence of antimitochondrial antibodies.

3. A 29-year-old woman has developed an itchy, scaly rash, particularly over her wrists, with fine white streaks overlying the lesions. Her nails have ridges and her buccal mucosa is lined with a lacy, white pattern.

4. A 20-year-old man complains of a recent onset of itching which has followed a viral infection. There are numerous weals of all sizes on his skin, particularly after he has scratched it. These can last for up to an hour.

5. A 60-year-old man complains of tiredness, lethargy and itching that is severe after a hot bath. He also has nocturia, polyuria, nausea and vomiting. Examination reveals pallor, pigmentation and generalized oedema.

Answers to **1.5**

1. I Scabies

The linear or curved tracts may contain mites, their eggs or faeces.
Typical sites include the finger webs, wrists, elbows, ankles, genitalia and
breasts. It usually occurs in overcrowded and poor hygienic settings.
Treatment is with malathion or permethrin.

2. F **Primary biliary cirrhosis**

The underlying diagnosis is primary biliary cirrhosis. Pruritus is an early
symptom when the liver function tests are still normal except for a
raised alkaline phosphatase. Anti-mitochondrial antibodies are present
in >95% of patients. There is progressive destruction of the bile ducts,
portal tract fibrosis and cirrhosis. Ursodeoxycholate and ciclosporin
(cyclosporin) may be of use in improving symptoms and the serum liver
enzymes. Supplementation of fat-soluble vitamins (A, D, E, K) may be
required. The pruritus is often difficult to control but colestyramine
(cholestyramine) and plasmapheresis may be helpful. Liver
transplantation is needed in patients with end-stage disease.

3. D **Lichen planus**

The clinical picture is of lichen planus which is characterized by flat-
topped (planus) papules in polygonal configuration with fine, white
dots or white reticulated lines (Wickham's striae) on the surface. The
cause is unknown but a similar rash may be caused by drugs (thiazides,
gold, phenothiazines, quinidine, antimalarials, sulphonamides, beta
blockers, penicillamine) or graft-versus-host disease. About 30% of
patients have hepatitis C. The nails may be affected by direct invasion of
lichen planus (ridging, bubbling, pterygium and atrophy) and a white,
lacy pattern on the buccal mucosa is a highly suggestive finding.

4. K Urticaria

Urticaria is a transient swelling of the skin, caused by vasodilatation and
accumulation of tissue fluid in the dermis. Histamine is the main
mediator in simple urticaria but other types of urticaria can involve non-
immunological mechanisms. In most cases the cause is unknown but it
may follow exposure to a variety of allergens such as a viral or parasite
infection, drugs (e.g. penicillin) or seafood.

5. J Uraemia

Uraemic symptoms include fatigue, breathlessness, ankle swelling,
anorexia, vomiting, nocturia and pruritus (particularly after a hot bath).
Examination may reveal pigmentation, pallor and brown nails.

Jugular venous pulse abnormalities

1.6

A Atrial myxoma
B Complete heart block
C Constrictive pericarditis
D Mitral regurgitation
E Pericardial effusion
F Pulmonary regurgitation
G Pulmonary stenosis
H Superior vena caval obstruction
I Tricuspid regurgitation (TR)
J Tricuspid stenosis
K Ventricular ectopics

For each presentation below, choose the SINGLE most likely cause from the above list of options. Each option may be used once, more than once, or not at all.

1. A 75-year-old woman presents with breathlessness and orthopnoea requiring four pillows at night to feel comfortable. Examination reveals an elevated jugular venous pressure with prominent *v* waves.

2. A 54-year-old man complains of stridor and breathlessness. He also has headaches and dizziness. His face and upper limbs are oedematous and cyanosed. His neck veins are notably distended but are not pulsatile.

3. An 82-year-old woman presents with blackouts, tiredness and lethargy. She has been fairly fit and well until 2 months ago. She has a profound bradycardia with cannon *a* waves.

4. A 56-year-old man complains of abdominal swelling, fatigue, cough and dyspnoea. The venous pressure is elevated with exaggerated *x* and *y* descents and a positive Kussmaul's sign.

5. A 45-year-old woman is admitted with pyrexia, arthropathy, breathlessness and syncope. She was recently diagnosed as having pulmonary emboli. There is an early diastolic sound and a mid-diastolic rumble. Her jugular venous pressure is elevated with prominent *a* waves.

Answers to **1.6**

1. **I   Tricuspid regurgitation (TR)**

    Exaggeration of the *v* wave (second venous upstroke during systole from right atrial filling) is the hallmark of tricuspid regurgitation (TR). The commonest cause of TR is dilatation of the right ventricle and the tricuspid valve ring due to right ventricular failure secondary to mitral valve disease, Eisenmenger's syndrome, cor pulmonale, etc. Causes of primary TR include rheumatic heart disease, carcinoid syndrome and infective endocarditis.

2. **H   Superior vena caval obstruction**

    Superior vena caval obstruction is usually caused by bronchogenic carcinoma (especially small-cell carcinoma), lymphoma, aortic aneurysm, mediastinal fibrosis and retrosternal goitre. Physical signs are often subtle. Classically, it causes oedema and cyanosis of the face, upper limbs and neck, and distended, non-pulsatile neck veins with enlarged and tortuous anastomotic veins on the anterior chest wall.

3. **B   Complete heart block**

    Cannon *a* waves are caused by the right atrium contracting against a closed tricuspid valve. This may occur intermittently in complete heart block, ventricular tachycardia and extrasystole, or regularly in junctional rhythms and 2:1 heart block.

4. **C   Constrictive pericarditis**

    Constrictive pericarditis occurs due to scarring of the pericardium, which then compresses the heart and restricts cardiac filling. Causes include post-viral, tuberculous and pyogenic infections, rheumatoid arthritis, post-irradiation, post-cardiac surgery and neoplasia. Kussmaul's sign (a paradoxical rise in venous pressure on inspiration) may be present but it is not specific. Prominent *x* descent (systolic collapse) and *y* descent (diastolic collapse) are suggestive of constrictive pericarditis. Cardiac tamponade causes a high venous pressure with prominent *x* descent and absent *y* descent.

5. **A   Atrial myxoma**

    Atrial myxomas are usually single polypoid lesions found much more commonly in the left atrium attached to the interatrial septum. They obstruct the mitral and tricuspid valves simulating valvular stenosis. They may also cause systemic or pulmonary embolization, heart failure or tachy- or bradyarrhythmias. They may also produce an immunological phenomenon mimicking infective endocarditis or a connective tissue disease. Prominent *a* waves (caused by increased resistance to right atrial emptying) are also seen in tricuspid stenosis and in right ventricular hypertrophy from any cause such as pulmonary hypertension or stenosis.

Proximal muscle weakness

A   Cushing's syndrome
B   Diabetic amyotrophy
C   Duchenne muscular dystrophy
D   Hypocalcaemia
E   Hypokalaemia
F   Hypothyroidism
G   Myasthenia gravis
H   Non-metastatic manifestation of malignancy
I   Polymyalgia rheumatica
J   Polymyositis
K   Thyrotoxicosis

For each presentation below, choose the SINGLE most likely cause from the above list of options. Each option may be used once, more than once, or not at all.

1. A 70-year-old man gives a 2-month history of painful thighs and difficulty in getting up from a chair. Examination reveals wasting of the quadriceps with absent knee reflexes. His plasma glucose is 18 mmol/L and glycosylated haemoglobin A_1c is elevated at 9%.

2. A 45-year-old woman with long-standing asthma has gained weight and complains of weakness on climbing stairs. She requires a maintenance steroid dose of at least 15 mg prednisolone per day.

3. A 45-year-old woman gives a 3-month history of palpitations and weight loss of 5 kg despite a good dietary intake. Although she cannot stay still she has difficulty getting off the chair and in climbing stairs. Her resting pulse rate is 90/minute. She has hyperreflexia with proximal muscle weakness.

4. A 56-year-old man with recently diagnosed chronic renal failure complains of paraesthesia, cramps, difficulty in getting up from a chair and muscle spasms. Both Chvostek's and Trousseau's signs are positive.

5. A 47-year-old woman presents with symmetrical proximal muscle weakness and wasting. Her muscles are tender with reduced tendon reflexes. Her serum creatinine phosphokinase (CPK) is elevated.

Answers to **1.7**

1. **B   Diabetic amyotrophy**

   This multifocal neuropathy usually affects elderly, obese diabetics. It presents as a painful, asymmetrical wasting of the quadriceps with depressed or absent knee reflexes. It is associated with poor glycaemic control and may be present at the time of diagnosis. It usually resolves with good diabetic control that often requires insulin.

2. **A   Cushing's syndrome**

   Iatrogenic Cushing's syndrome due to the long-term use of steroids is commoner than other forms of this disease. Other causes include pituitary-dependent bilateral adrenocortical hyperplasia (Cushing's disease), adrenal tumour and ectopic adrenocorticotrophic hormone (ACTH) secretion (small-cell bronchial carcinoma).

3. **K   Thyrotoxicosis**

   The history of weight loss despite a good appetite, palpitations and a resting tachycardia are all features of thyrotoxicosis. Most patients have some degree of proximal muscle weakness and muscle atrophy. The tendon reflexes are often exaggerated but there is no hypertonia or clonus.

4. **D   Hypocalcaemia**

   Proximal muscle weakness occurs in renal failure (not on the list) both as a result of hypocalcaemia and osteomalacia. Hypocalcaemia causes muscular irritability which is demonstrable by the two signs mentioned. Chvostek's sign is twitching of the facial muscles on tapping the facial nerve, and Trousseau's sign is the induction of carpopedal spasm (painful flexion of the metacarpal joints and adduction of the thumb across the palm) after inflation of the sphygmomanometer cuff above the systolic blood pressure for 5 minutes. The spasm relaxes approximately 5 seconds after the cuff is deflated (not instantly).

5. **J   Polymyositis**

   Polymyositis is associated with muscle tenderness and weakness/ wasting. There may also be arthralgia, dysphagia and Raynaud's phenomenon. Creatinine phosphokinase is raised, electromyography shows short, polyphasic motor potentials and muscle biopsy shows necrosis of the muscle fibres with regeneration and inflammation.

Visual defects

A   Amaurosis fugax
B   Bitemporal hemianopia
C   Central scotoma
D   Cortical blindness
E   Hysteria
F   Increased size of the blind spot
G   Left homonymous hemianopia
H   Night glare
I   Right homonymous hemianopia
J   Tunnel vision
K   Uniocular visual loss

For each presentation below, choose the SINGLE most appropriate sign from the above list of options. Each option may be used once, more than once, or not at all.

1. A 27-year-old woman complains of blurring of vision and weakness of both legs. She had weakness of her left arm 3 months ago which resolved spontaneously. On testing her central vision, there is a circular area of deficit about 5 mm in diameter adjacent to her blind spot. Fundoscopy reveals optic atrophy.

2. A 54-year-old woman complains of coarsening of her facial features, sweats and headaches. She also has a bilateral visual field defect and tends to bump against the door frame when she enters a room.

3. A 70-year-old man presents with sudden onset of a mild, right-sided weakness and has noticed that he has been bumping into things on his right side.

4. A 65-year-old woman has been bumping into things while walking. On testing she is unable to read or recognize objects but she denies that there is a problem with her eyesight.

5. A 75-year-old woman presents with deteriorating peripheral vision. She has been on various eyedrops for a number of years. Her pupils are small and non-reactive to light.

Answers to **1.8**

1. C   Central scotoma

The history is suggestive of demyelinating disease with lesions
disseminated in time and place within the central nervous system. It
causes optic neuritis (disc swelling associated with early visual loss)
which leads to optic atrophy. In the early stages the patient complains of
blurring of vision, as if seeing through frosted glass. Central scotoma is
associated with optic neuritis/atrophy.

2. B   Bitemporal hemianopia

Acromegaly is due to a primary pituitary adenoma in 99% of cases. This
can cause compression of the optic chiasma and hence bitemporal
hemianopia. Features of active disease include headaches, sweats and
changing head or hand/feet size. The best screening test is the serum
IGF-1 (insulin growth factor-1) concentration.

3. I   Right homonymous hemianopia

The patient has had a left-sided stroke causing right-sided weakness. The
left optic radiation is affected and thus he may have a right
homonymous hemianopia (same side as the weakness).

4. D   Cortical blindness

Cortical blindness with denial (Anton's syndrome) is due to bilateral
occipital lobe damage by infarction, trauma or tumour. There is little or
no insight into the visual loss despite being blind so there is often
denial of the visual impairment. A homonymous visual field defect is
frequently seen.

5. J   Tunnel vision

This patient is on meiotic eyedrops for glaucoma which is usually
associated with a high intraocular pressure. The nerve fibres within the
rim of the optic nerve head are damaged by the high pressure and
impaired blood supply. There is optic cupping and tunnel vision in
long-standing cases. It is almost always due to reduced outflow of
aqueous humour.

Dysarthria

A   Amyloidosis
B   Bulbar palsy
C   General paresis of the insane
D   Huntington's chorea
E   Hypothyroidism
F   Multiple sclerosis
G   Myasthenia gravis
H   Myotonic dystrophy
I   Parkinson's disease
J   Pseudobulbar palsy
K   Temporomandibular arthritis

For each scenario below, choose the SINGLE most likely cause from the above list of options. Each option may be used once, more than once, or not at all.

1. A 28-year-old woman with clumsy hand movements is noted to have jerky and explosive speech. In the past she has had episodes of diplopia.

2. A 67-year-old man has a monotonous, slurred speech. He has an expressionless face and a festinant gait.

3. A 52-year-old man has slurred and suppressed speech. Examination reveals bilateral partial ptosis and frontal balding with difficulty in releasing his grip after shaking hands.

4. A 70-year-old man with a past history of strokes has a high-pitched, indistinct and unmodulated so-called 'Donald Duck' speech.

5. A 55-year-old woman has a hoarse, croaking voice. She also has a slow relaxing phase of the tendon reflexes particularly noticeable at the ankles.

Answers to **1.9**

1.   F   Multiple sclerosis

This lady has a speech pattern characteristic of the cerebellar syndrome. The clumsiness suggests cerebellar dysfunction and the past history of diplopia points to the diagnosis of multiple sclerosis.

2.   I   Parkinson's disease

Parkinson's disease is characterized by the triad of bradykinesia, tremor and rigidity. The speech may be slurred and monotonous without any accents or emphases due to rigidity of the speech-articulating muscles.

3.   H   Myotonic dystrophy

Myotonic dystrophy is an autosomal dominant condition. Its features include ptosis, frontal balding, cataracts, cardiomyopathy, impaired intellect, testicular atrophy, diabetes mellitus and slurred speech (from tongue and pharyngeal myotonia). There is no treatment for the weakness which is the main cause of disability but phenytoin, quinine or procainamide may be useful for the myotonia.

4.   J   Pseudobulbar palsy

The spasticity of the tongue is the main cause of an unmodulated speech. The tongue, larynx and pharynx have bilateral cortical representation. Causes of bilateral supranuclear lesions include a cerebrovascular accident of the bilateral internal capsules (commonest cause), multiple sclerosis, motor neurone disease and high brainstem tumours.

5.   E   Hypothyroidism

She has the features of hypothyroidism. In advanced cases, speech is slow and the voice is low-pitched and hoarse. Other features include carpal tunnel syndrome, cerebellar syndrome, anaemia, peripheral neuropathy, pseudodementia, coma, hypothermia and psychosis.

Purpura/spontaneous bruising

A   Cushing's syndrome
B   Ehlers–Danlos syndrome
C   Haemophilia
D   Henoch–Schönlein purpura
E   Infective endocarditis
F   Meningitis
G   Polyarteritis nodosa
H   Scurvy
I   Senile purpura
J   Thrombocytopenic purpura
K   Von Willebrand's disease

For each patient below, choose the SINGLE most likely cause from the above list of options. Each option may be used once, more than once, or not at all.

1. A 79-year-old woman complains of being easily bruised. She is otherwise well and remains active and independent.

2. A 45-year-old man is noted to have purpura with very thin and elastic skin. His joints are hyperextensible.

3. A 67-year-old woman presents with tiredness and malaise. She has a mild spiking temperature, a purpuric rash over her shins and splenomegaly. She has microscopic haematuria.

4. A 16-year-old boy presents with a long history of bleeding and bruising following minor trauma. His platelet count and bleeding time are normal, but his activated partial thromboplastin time (APTT) is prolonged.

5. A 75-year-old widower is noted to have spontaneous bruising, perifollicular purpura and bleeding from his gums. He lives alone with little social contact.

Answers to **1.10**

1. **I** **Senile purpura**

Senile purpura is due to atrophy of the supporting tissues of the cutaneous blood vessels commonly occurring in the elderly and affecting the dorsal aspects of the hand and forearm.

2. **B** **Ehlers–Danlos syndrome**

Ehlers–Danlos syndrome is one of a heterogeneous group of inherited collagen diseases. Clinical features include easy bruising, the presence of abnormal, velvety, hyperelastic skin which heals poorly, hyperextensible joints and lax ligaments with recurrent dislocations of the patella, shoulders and hips. Other features may include recurrent hydroarthrosis, pneumothorax, dissecting aneurysm and mitral valve prolapse. Pseudotumours over the knees and elbows may be present following organization of haematomas caused by minor trauma.

3. **E** **Infective endocarditis**

Patients with subacute endocarditis may present with a low-grade fever, malaise and weight loss, and there may be the symptoms associated with heart failure or embolism. Small petechial or mucosal haemorrhages result from vasculitis. Microscopic haematuria, as a result of emboli or focal glomerulonephritis, occurs in over 50% of patients. The extent of any splenomegaly depends on the duration of the illness.

4. **C** **Haemophilia**

Spontaneous bruising with haematomas in muscles and joints occurs after minimal trauma in haemophilia. The inheritance is X-linked recessive, with a deficiency or abnormality of factor VIII in haemophilia A, and of factor IX in haemophilia B. The bleeding time is prolonged in Von Willebrand's disease (low levels of factor VIII-related antigen), but it is normal in haemophilia. The activated partial thromboplastin time (APTT) is prolonged in haemophilia, but may be normal or prolonged in Von Willebrand's disease.

5. **H** **Scurvy**

A dietary history should be obtained in older people especially if they live alone. Fruit and vegetables are good sources of vitamin C. Perifollicular purpura and excessive bleeding from multiple sites are common in scurvy. The diagnosis may be confirmed by measuring the leucocyte vitamin C concentration. Treatment is with vitamin C supplements.

Erythema nodosum

A   Coccidioidomycosis
B   Crohn's disease
C   Leprosy
D   Oral contraceptive pill
E   Rheumatic fever
F   Sarcoidosis
G   Streptococcal infection
H   Sulphonamides
I   Toxoplasmosis
J   Tuberculosis
K   Ulcerative colitis

For each presentation below, choose the SINGLE most likely cause from the above list of options. Each option may be used once, more than once, or not at all.

1. A 46-year-old Scottish woman with a history of rheumatoid arthritis, controlled on treatment, presents with erythema nodosum.

2. A 55-year-old man from the Middle East presents with facial coarsening with 'leonine facies' and gross thickening of the ear lobes. He has recently developed erythema nodosum.

3. A 19-year-old Welsh woman presents with erythema nodosum shortly after developing a sore throat and fever.

4. A 42-year-old Afro-Caribbean woman presents with a recent onset of painless, smooth and mobile cervical lymphadenopathy and erythema nodosum. There is evidence of lymphocytosis with 5% atypical lymphocytes on the blood film.

5. A 35-year-old Irishman is admitted with bilateral hilar lymphadenopathy, erythema nodosum and arthralgia.

Answers to **1.11**

1. **H** **Sulphonamides**

Sulfasalazine (sulphasalazine) is a combination of 5-aminosalicylic acid and sulfapyridine (sulphapyridine) and is used as a disease-modifying drug in rheumatoid arthritis, in mild/moderate ulcerative colitis for the maintenance of remission, and in active Crohn's disease. The side effects of sulphonamides consist of rashes (including erythema nodosum), Stevens–Johnson syndrome, renal failure, blood dyscrasia (bone marrow suppression and agranulocytosis) and oligospermia.

2. **C** **Leprosy**

Leprosy is caused by the acid-fast bacillus *Mycobacterium leprae*. The two extreme ends of the spectrum are tuberculoid leprosy (localized disease because of marked immunological response) and lepromatous leprosy (generalized disease because of impaired cell-mediated immunity). Two forms of lepra reactions (immunological mediated reactions) are recognized. Type II lepra reaction (erythema nodosum leprosum) is a type III hypersensitivity reaction seen in the lepromatous end of the spectrum (50% with treated lepromatous leprosy (LL) and occasionally in untreated LL or treated borderline LL). It is characterized by fever, arthralgia, painful neuritis, erythema nodosum, iridocyclitis, acute lymphadenitis and epididymo-orchitis. Type I reaction occurs frequently in treated borderline tuberculoid leprosy, borderline leprosy, and borderline lepromatous leprosy. It is a type IV hypersensitivity reaction characterized by acute swelling and inflammation of existing lesions. Painful neuritis may also occur.

3. **G** **Streptococcal infection**

This patient has a streptococcal throat infection causing erythema nodosum.

4. **I** **Toxoplasmosis**

Toxoplasmosis is caused by an intracellular protozoon (*Toxoplasma gondii*) and occurs in only about 10% of immunocompetent individuals. It can be difficult to distinguish from infectious mononucleosis (not on the list), except that there are only a small number (<10%) of atypical lymphocytes. Serological tests can be used to confirm acquired infection. The Paul–Bunnell (monospot) test is negative.

5. **F** **Sarcoidosis**

He has acute sarcoidosis. This has a good prognosis; 80% settle spontaneously and have a normal chest X-ray after 1 year.

Interpretation of cardiovascular clinical signs

A Aortic regurgitation
B Aortic stenosis
C Bacterial endocarditis
D Constrictive pericarditis
E Hypertrophic cardiomyopathy
F Mitral regurgitation
G Mitral stenosis
H Pericardial tamponade
I Pulmonary regurgitation
J Pulmonary stenosis
K Tricuspid regurgitation

For each scenario below, choose the SINGLE most likely cause from the above list of options. Each option may be used once, more than once, or not at all.

1. A 45-year-old woman is found to have a mid-diastolic rumbling murmur localized to the apex and best heard on expiration in the left lateral position.

2. A 35-year-old man has a double apical pulsation and a jerky carotid pulse. He complains of breathlessness and intermittent dizziness.

3. A 56-year-old man with known bronchogenic carcinoma complains of worsening breathlessness. Examination reveals pulsus paradoxus and also Kussmaul's sign with soft heart sounds.

4. A 45-year-old woman has a collapsing pulse with evidence of Corrigan's sign and Quincke's sign.

5. A 68-year-old woman has a loud pansystolic murmur heard over the sternum and the adjacent left third interspace. It becomes louder during inspiration and is loudest with her breath held in inspiration. Her jugular venous pressure is elevated with large v waves.

Answers to **1.12**

1.   **G   Mitral stenosis**

This patient has mitral stenosis. Murmurs originating from the left heart (mitral and aortic) are louder in expiration, whilst right-sided (tricuspid, pulmonary) ones are louder on inspiration.

2.   **E   Hypertrophic cardiomyopathy**

Hypertrophic cardiomyopathy is characterized by hypertrophy of the ventricle (left, right or both) and especially of the interventricular septum (asymmetrical septal hypertrophy) in the absence of any cardiac or systemic cause. It is usually familial with an autosomal dominant transmission and typically presents between the ages of 20 and 40 years. Outflow obstruction is present in about a quarter of patients. A double apical impulse (palpable 4th heart sound) is caused by atrial systole. Presenting symptoms may be exertional dyspnoea, chest pain, palpitations or syncope.

3.   **H   Pericardial tamponade**

A large pericardial effusion can be caused by malignant infiltration, as in this case, which may require pericardiocentesis. Reaccumulation may require pericardial fenestration. The clinical features include tachycardia, a low pulse volume, pulsus paradoxus (an exaggerated arterial pressure fall with inspiration, indicating severe circulatory impairment), Kussmaul's sign (a paradoxical rise in jugular venous pressure with inspiration) and soft heart sounds. The chest X-ray will show a globular heart. The diagnosis can be confirmed with an echocardiogram.

4.   **A   Aortic regurgitation**

Aortic regurgitation may be associated with Corrigan's sign (vigorous arterial pulsations in the neck), de Musset's sign (head-nodding with each pulse), Quincke's sign (capillary pulsation in the nail beds), Duroziez's sign (diastolic murmur when the femoral artery is compressed and auscultated proximally) and the Austin Flint murmur (functional mid-diastolic murmur – a regurgitant jet that interferes with the opening of the anterior mitral valve leaflet). This murmur in early diastole is best heard over the lower left sternal edge with the breath held in deep expiration.

5.   **K   Tricuspid regurgitation**

The murmur of tricuspid regurgitation (TR) is louder with inspiration (Cavallo's sign), whilst that of mitral regurgitation is louder with expiration. An elevated jugular venous pressure with giant *v* waves is diagnostic of TR. The commonest cause is functional, i.e. dilatation of the right ventricle and the tricuspid valve ring due to right ventricular failure from any cause.

Pyrexia of undetermined origin

A   Blood cultures
B   Bronchoscopy
C   Chest X-ray
D   Echocardiography
E   Lumbar puncture
F   Lymph node biopsy
G   Mid-stream specimen of urine
H   Serum ferritin
I   Stool culture
J   Thick and thin blood films
K   Ultrasound scan of the abdomen

For each presentation below, choose the SINGLE most discriminating investigation from the above list of options. Each option may be used once, more than once, or not at all.

1. A 20-year-old student presents with malaise, fever, rigors and sweats occurring several days after returning from a fortnight's holiday in Tanzania. Examination is normal apart from a temperature of 39°C.

2. A 45-year-old man gives a 3-month history of weight loss, night sweats and fever. He has pruritus and has experienced alcohol-induced pain in his left axilla where there are a number of enlarged lymph nodes.

3. A 67-year-old woman presents with a 3-month history of malaise and worsening breathlessness. Examination reveals splinter haemorrhages, finger clubbing and an early diastolic murmur audible over the left sternal edge. She also has a low-grade pyrexia. Blood cultures are negative.

4. A 20-year-old man has a 2-day history of a flu-like illness with neck stiffness and photophobia. He is pyrexial and has a purpuric rash.

5. A 30-year-old woman presents with a 2-month history of feeling unwell together with a spiking temperature, arthralgia and a maculopapular rash which is worse at the peaks of the pyrexia.

Answers to **1.13**

1. J Thick and thin blood films

Plasmodium falciparum causes the predominant type of malaria in Africa and the most severe form of the disease. Case fatality is 1% (or 1–3 million deaths/year) globally. Malaria can present with a number of symptoms and signs none of which are specific or diagnostic. It must be excluded by repeated thick and thin blood films in any patient with an acute fever and history of possible exposure (i.e. recent travel to an endemic country). About 98% of patients with falciparum malaria present within the first 3 months but some can present up to 1 year later. Cerebral malaria (due to mechanical obstruction of the cerebral microcirculation) causes 80% of the deaths from falciparum malaria.

2. F Lymph node biopsy

This patient has the symptoms of lymphoma (the triad of fever, weight loss of >10% body weight and night sweats). Lymphadenopathy is usually painless but alcohol-induced pain at the site of lymph nodes is very suggestive of lymphoma. Lymph node biopsy, or bone marrow biopsy in advanced disease, is essential for diagnosis. Sternberg–Reed cells are present in Hodgkin's lymphoma.

3. D Echocardiography

There is evidence of aortic regurgitation probably secondary to bacterial endocarditis. Clinical features include haematuria, new or changing murmurs, splinter haemorrhages, Osler's nodes, clubbing, Janeway lesions, arthralgia, Roth spots, conjunctival haemorrhages, splenomegaly, cerebral emboli and mycotic aneurysms. The commonest organisms include *Streptococcus viridans* (50% of cases), *Enterococcus faecalis* and *Staphylococcus aureus*. Echocardiography, especially transoesophageal, is useful for identifying the vegetations.

4. E Lumbar puncture

He has meningism, fever and purpura which indicate a probable diagnosis of meningococcal meningitis caused by *Neisseria meningitidis*. A CSF examination showing an abundance of neutrophils, high protein, low sugar and meningococci on Gram staining will establish the diagnosis.

5. H Serum ferritin

Adult-onset Still's disease is a febrile syndrome in young adults (usually 16–35 years) and affecting multiple organs. Diagnosis is mainly one of exclusion but hyperferritinaemia (>5 times normal) is present in 90% of cases. Clinical features include a high, spiking fever (with return of the temperature to normal), arthralgia/arthritis, sore throat, transient maculopapular rash (mildly pruritic in one-third of cases), lymphadenopathy, hepatosplenomegaly and pleuritis/pericarditis. Rarely, there may be aseptic meningitis, cranial nerve palsies, iritis and peripheral neuropathy.

Suspected intra-abdominal pathology

A   Abdominal X-ray
B   Angiography
C   Chest X-ray
D   Colonoscopy
E   Computerized tomography (CT) scan of the abdomen
F   Electrocardiogram
G   Gastroscopy
H   Magnetic resonance imaging (MRI) of the abdomen
I   Radionuclide studies
J   Sigmoidoscopy
K   Ultrasound scan of the abdomen

For each presentation below, choose the SINGLE most discriminating investigation from the above list of options. Each option may be used once, more than once, or not at all.

1. A 16-year-old boy presents with recurrent, painless, bright-red rectal haemorrhage. He is otherwise well and examination is unremarkable.

2. A 65-year-old woman is admitted with severe abdominal pain and nausea. She takes regular diclofenac for her arthritis. Her abdomen is rigid with rebound tenderness in the epigastrium.

3. A 60-year-old woman presents with a 2-stone weight loss over the last 4 months and jaundice with vague abdominal discomfort. She has smoked 20 cigarettes/day for many years. On examination, she is cachectic and a distended gallbladder is palpable.

4. A 78-year-old lady is found to have a microcytic anaemia and a mass in the left lower quadrant of her abdomen. Rectal examination is normal.

5. A 65-year-old man is admitted to the surgical unit with a massive haematemesis which has not settled. His haemoglobin is falling despite a blood transfusion of five units. Gastroscopy on admission showed blood in the stomach with no obvious source of bleeding.

Answers to **1.14**

1. I   Radionuclide studies

A Meckel's diverticulum is the commonest congenital abnormality of the gastrointestinal tract. It is mainly asymptomatic, but in children complications can arise due to ectopic gastric mucosa in the diverticulum. Rectal bleeding is the main symptom – any child with a massive, painless haemorrhage per rectum has a Meckel's diverticulum unless proven otherwise (other presentation is small bowel obstruction). The most important test is a technetium (Tc) scan which localizes the ectopic gastric mucosa, for the gastric mucosa concentrates sodium pertechnetate. Treatment is by surgical resection.

2. A   Abdominal X-ray

This patient has a probable perforated peptic ulcer with acute chemical peritonitis. An abdominal X-ray may reveal air under the diaphragms.

3. E   Computerized tomography (CT) scan of the abdomen

Painless, obstructive jaundice with weight loss is highly suggestive of pancreatic carcinoma. Some patients may complain of a dull ache in the epigastrium radiating to the back, aggravated by lying supine and relieved by sitting up. A distended gallbladder is palpable in 60% of cases. CT scanning of the abdomen will reveal a pancreatic lesion and show any metastatic spread to the liver.

4. D   Colonoscopy

This patient has a colonic carcinoma which is causing occult blood loss and anaemia. A colonoscopy or double-contrast barium enema is needed to confirm the diagnosis.

5. B   Angiography

In patients with an acute gastrointestinal haemorrhage, angiography is useful to locate the source of bleeding when it is unknown. It also allows the bleeding to be stopped by the selective infusion of drugs or embolic material. The likely lesions include angiomatous malformations, small neoplasms, a Meckel's diverticulum or small ulcers.

Haemoptysis

A   Blood cultures
B   Blood gases
C   Bronchoscopy
D   Chest X-ray
E   Computerized tomography (CT) scan of the chest
F   Echocardiogram
G   Electrocardiogram
H   Full blood count
I   Lower limb venogram
J   Sputum culture and sensitivity
K   Ventilation and perfusion scan

For each presentation, choose the SINGLE most discriminating investigation from the above list of options. Each option may be used once, more than once, or not at all.

1. A 46-year-old man presents with a 1-week history of breathlessness and orthopnoea. He has a cough productive of pinkish, frothy sputum. Auscultation reveals a gallop rhythm.

2. A previously well 35-year-old man presents with a 3-day history of haemoptysis, fever and a cough productive of purulent sputum.

3. A 23-year-old man is admitted with a 6-month history of intermittent haemoptysis, wheezing and diarrhoea. His chest examination is normal.

4. A 52-year-old woman had numerous chest infections during childhood. She now presents with a chronic, productive cough and, more recently, haemoptysis. She has clubbing of the fingers and bilateral, coarse crackles in her chest.

5. An elderly man developed sudden left-sided pleuritic chest pain and breathlessness 3 days ago following a trip to America. He presents with one episode of haemoptysis. He has been a life-long smoker.

Answers to **1.15**

1. F Echocardiogram

Pulmonary oedema is associated with a cough, often productive of frothy, blood-stained sputum. A gallop rhythm (combination of a left ventricular third heart sound and tachycardia) is a clinical sign of heart failure. Echocardiography is an essential non-invasive test of left ventricular (LV) function. Treating LV systolic dysfunction with angiotensin-converting enzyme inhibitors and beta blockers reduces morbidity, mortality and hospitalization rates.

2. D Chest X-ray

The history is suggestive of pneumonia. A chest X-ray is needed to confirm pneumonic consolidation and to exclude other lesions.

3. C Bronchoscopy

Bronchial carcinoid is a highly vascular 'cherry-like' tumour causing recurrent haemoptysis and bronchial obstruction. It may rarely (in about 5% of cases) metastasize to the liver producing the classic symptoms of the carcinoid syndrome, i.e. cyanotic flushing, intestinal cramps and diarrhoea. Bronchoscopy identifies up to 80% of carcinoid tumours in the main bronchi although biopsy may be followed by brisk haemorrhage.

4. E Computerized tomography (CT) scan of the chest

Childhood respiratory infection (especially measles and whooping cough) can cause bronchiectasis. The bronchial walls are damaged with an impaired mucociliary transport mechanism resulting in frequent bacterial infections. Computerized tomography (CT) is the imaging method of choice for the detection of bronchiectasis.

5. K Ventilation and perfusion scan

A long-haul flight has resulted in a long period of immobility and the sudden onset of pleuritic pain and haemoptysis is highly suggestive of a pulmonary embolism.

Anaemia

A Barium enema
B Bone marrow biopsy
C Coombs' test
D Erythrocyte sedimentation rate (ESR)
E Faecal occult blood
F Ferritin level
G Folate level
H Gastroscopy
I Haemoglobin electrophoresis
J Ham test
K Vitamin B_{12} level

For each presentation below, choose the SINGLE most discriminating investigation from the above list of options. Each option may be used once, more than once, or not at all.

1. A 65-year-old English woman presents with sudden onset of back pain (collapsed T12 vertebra on X-ray) and anaemia (Hb 9.4 g/dl). A peripheral blood film has shown rouleaux formation and her ESR is 90 mm/h.

2. A 40-year-old Chinese man is incidentally found to have a severely hypochromic, microcytic blood picture (Hb 11.2 g/dl). He is asymptomatic.

3. A 45-year-old Welshman is admitted with a recent onset of tiredness and passing black, tarry stools. His weight has been stable. On examination, he is pale and his Hb is 10.5 g/dl.

4. A 37-year-old Afro-British woman presents with a 2-week history of tiredness and mild jaundice following a severe chest infection 1 month previously. She is normally fit and well. On examination, she is found to be mildly anaemic (Hb 11.1 g/dl) and icteric with an enlarged spleen.

5. A 78-year-old Englishman presents with lethargy and bruising for the past 6 months. Examination reveals purpura. He has a normochromic, normocytic anaemia (Hb 10.4 g/dl), thrombocytopenia and a low white cell count.

Answers to **1.16**

1. B   Bone marrow biopsy

The presence of rouleaux formation (rolls of red cells resembling piles of coins) on a blood film and the high ESR are commonly seen in multiple myeloma. Clinical features include bone pain, pathological fractures, anaemia, repeated infections, bleeding tendency (thrombocytopenia and interference of coagulation by myeloma protein), renal failure and hypercalcaemia. A bone marrow biopsy shows increased plasma cells.

2. I   Haemoglobin electrophoresis

The β-thalassaemia trait is a common and usually asymptomatic abnormality. Red cells are hypochromic and microcytic but the iron and ferritin stores are normal. Haemoglobin electrophoresis shows raised HbA_2 (>3.5%) and a raised HbF (blood normally consists predominantly of HbA with a trace of HbF and HbA_2).

3. H   Gastroscopy

Melaena is the passing of black, tarry stools (altered blood) per rectum due to haemorrhage into the upper gastrointestinal tract. Gastroscopy demonstrates the cause of the bleeding in the majority of cases. During the procedure, interventions such as injection of oesophageal varices or bleeding ulcers may be performed.

4. C   Coombs' test

A positive Coombs' test (agglutination of red cells when purified animal anti-human globulin reacts with human red cells coated with antibody or complement) occurs in haemolytic disease of the newborn, autoimmune haemolytic anaemia, drug-induced immune haemolytic anaemia and haemolytic transfusion reactions. In this case, infection with *Mycoplasma pneumoniae* has caused cold-acquired autoimmune haemolytic anaemia (AIHA). The antibody is usually IgM and binds to red cells best at 4°C. Intravascular haemolysis occurs 10–14 days after the onset of respiratory symptoms. Rarely, it can be severe and life threatening.

5. B   Bone marrow biopsy

A peripheral blood film and bone marrow biopsy are essential for diagnosis in the presence of pancytopenia. The cause in this patient is the myelodysplastic syndrome. Other causes of pancytopenia include aplastic anaemia, bone marrow infiltration (carcinoma, lymphoma), acute leukaemia, hypersplenism, megaloblastic anaemia and paroxysmal nocturnal haemoglobinuria.

Back pain

A   Computerized tomography (CT) scan of the chest
B   Electrocardiogram
C   Gastroscopy
D   Isotope bone scan
E   Magnetic resonance imaging (MRI) of the spine
F   Myeloma screen
G   Prostatic specific antigen
H   Transthoracic echocardiogram
I   Ultrasound scan of the abdomen
J   Ventilation perfusion scan
K   X-ray spine

For each presentation below, choose the SINGLE most discriminating
investigation from the above list of options. Each option may be used
once, more than once, or not at all.

1.   A 56-year-old woman presents with a sudden onset of bilateral lower
     limb weakness and central back pain. Examination reveals a spastic
     paraparesis with a sensory level at the umbilicus.

2.   A 70-year-old woman has lost 2 stone in weight over the last 6 months.
     She complains of central back pain. On examination, she is mildly
     icteric.

3.   A 45-year-old man is admitted with a sudden onset of left-sided tearing
     chest and back pain 2 hours previously. He has signs of aortic
     regurgitation and radiofemoral delay.

4.   A 27-year-old woman presents with sudden onset of left-sided back pain
     which is worse on inspiration. She has been on the oral contraceptive
     pill for the last 5 years. Clinical examination is normal.

5.   A 72-year-old man with a 12-month history of urinary symptoms of
     dribbling and hesitancy presents with recent onset of back pain. He is
     found to have hypercalcaemia (serum calcium of 3.2 mmol/L). His
     erythrocyte sedimentation rate (ESR) is 13 mm/h.

Answers to **1.17**

1. E   Magnetic resonance imaging (MRI) of the spine

Spinal cord compression is indicated by the presence of a sensory level on the trunk. It may be caused by spinal cord neoplasms, metastases, epidural abscess/haemorrhage, disc lesions and arteriovenous malformations. An MRI scan can identify most lesions. Lumbar puncture should be avoided as it can precipitate severe paralysis.

2. I   Ultrasound scan of the abdomen

Carcinoma of the head of the pancreas presents with pain (which may be mild and often ignored by the patient and the doctor), jaundice and weight loss. If there is jaundice with a carcinoma of the body or tail of the pancreas (rare) then the lesion has already metastasized to the porta hepatis lymph nodes. Ultrasonography can detect lesions as small as 2 cm.

3. A   Computerized tomography (CT) scan of the chest

The history and examination are suggestive of a dissecting aortic aneurysm. There is usually mediastinal widening visible on the plain chest X-ray. Definitive diagnosis depends on a transoesophageal echocardiogram (not transthoracic echocardiogram), MRI or CT scan of the chest.

4. J   Ventilation perfusion scan

A pulmonary embolus needs to be excluded with a ventilation/perfusion scan in view of the sudden onset of pleuritic pain and the use of oral contraceptive medication.

5. G   Prostatic specific antigen (PSA)

Hypercalcaemia suggests metastatic carcinoma or myeloma, but the latter is less likely in the presence of a normal ESR. The PSA is a good screening tool for prostatic carcinoma particularly as this patient has prostatic symptoms. It is preferable to a bone scan as it will indicate the origin of any possible bony metastases. Treatment for disease confined to the prostate gland is radical prostatectomy or radiotherapy. Metastatic disease may be treated with orchidectomy, or an LHRH (luteinizing hormone releasing hormone) analogue such as buserelin or goserelin, with an antiandrogen such as flutamide or cyproterone.

Weight loss

A Barium enema
B Barium meal
C Blood glucose
D Bronchoscopy
E Faecal occult blood
F Gastroscopy
G Lateral chest X-ray
H Prostatic specific antigen
I Thyroid function tests
J Ultrasound of the abdomen
K Ziehl–Nielsen (ZN) stain of the sputum for acid-fast bacilli

For each presentation below, choose the SINGLE most discriminating
investigation from the above list of options. Each option may be used
once, more than once, or not at all.

1. A 78-year-old Caucasian woman complains of being restless and losing
weight despite having a good appetite. Examination reveals a thin and
anxious patient with atrial fibrillation.

2. A 38-year-old Indian man presents with a troublesome productive cough
with weight loss and night sweats. His chest X-ray shows some
shadowing in the left upper zone.

3. A 76-year-old Welsh woman complains of a 6-month history of
dysphagia and weight loss. It has been gradual in onset and mainly
affects solids which seem to stick retrosternally.

4. A 30-year-old man of West Indian origin presents with a 4-week history
of weight loss, polyuria and polydipsia.

5. A 67-year-old Englishman complains of tiredness and weight loss. He
has an iron deficiency anaemia (Hb 7.2 g/dl). His recent gastroscopy
had revealed gastric erosions.

Answers to **1.18**

1. **I   Thyroid function tests**

   She has features of thyrotoxicosis, i.e. being restless and fidgety with atrial fibrillation. Other classic features include weight loss, tremor, palpitations and hyperactivity. Apathy, weight loss and depression may be the predominant symptoms in the elderly. The commonest cause of thyrotoxicosis is Graves' disease, followed by toxic nodular goitre (often in older people with goitre).

2. **K   ZN stain of the sputum for acid-fast bacilli**

   Tiredness, anorexia, weight loss, fever and cough are features of pulmonary tuberculosis (TB). In the UK, the incidence of TB in immigrants from the Asian subcontinent is 40 times higher than in the local Caucasian population. Pulmonary TB is highly likely in the presence of shadowing in the upper zone on his chest X-ray. Bronchoscopy, with bronchial lavage, may be needed if sputum is not available for ZN staining.

3. **F   Gastroscopy**

   A gastroscopy is probably the best investigation because it is possible to visualize any oesophageal lesions, perform biopsies and also to treat with laser, stenting or dilatation of a stricture as necessary.

4. **C   Blood glucose**

   Diabetes mellitus, hypercalcaemia and hypokalaemia are common causes of polyuria and polydipsia. In diabetes mellitus, there is an osmotic diuresis due to glycosuria which results in dehydration and thirst (hypertonic extracellular fluid). Weight loss may be due to dehydration and the accelerated breakdown of fat and muscle due to insulin deficiency. Diabetic ketoacidosis may be the presenting feature if early symptoms are missed.

5. **A   Barium enema**

   The gastric erosions found may not account for the weight loss, i.e. they may be a red herring. It is important to exclude pathology of the large bowel with either a colonoscopy or barium enema. Blood loss of >20 ml/day will result in iron deficiency anaemia (0.5–1.2 ml/day in a normal person). If these investigations still do not provide a diagnosis (having excluded haematuria) in the presence of persistent bleeding, consider a barium meal and follow-through to study the small bowel. Also consider coeliac or superior mesenteric angiography.

Investigation of tiredness and lethargy

A   Autoimmune screen
B   Blood glucose
C   Hepatitis screen
D   Mantoux test
E   Serum insulin growth factor (IGF)-1
F   Short Synacthen test
G   Sleep study (polysomnography)
H   Tensilon test
I   Thyroid function test
J   24-hour urinary cortisol
K   Ultrasound scan of the abdomen

For each presentation below, choose the SINGLE most discriminating investigation from the above list of options. Each option may be used once, more than once, or not at all.

1. A 45-year-old man complains of tiredness, headaches, sweats and difficulty in getting up from a chair and climbing stairs. His wife feels that his facial features have coarsened over the last 5 years.

2. A 45-year-old woman presents with weakness and lethargy. For the last 6 months she has found it difficult to finish a meal and sometimes food regurgitates into her nasal passage. She also has intermittent diplopia.

3. A 54-year-old obese gentleman is worried about his tiredness. He has even fallen asleep whilst eating or driving. His wife has forced him to sleep in a separate bedroom because of his snoring.

4. A 48-year-old man presents with tiredness and pruritus. He has noticed dark discoloration of his urine, whilst his stools have been paler than usual. He has also developed an intolerance to fatty foods.

5. A 38-year-old man presents with tiredness and dizziness. He also complains of difficulty in getting to sleep at night. He has increased pigmentation which is more marked in the skin creases and around the nipples.

Answers to 1.19

1. E Serum insulin growth factor (IGF)-1

In the vast majority of cases, acromegaly is the result of a primary pituitary adenoma. Before presentation, symptoms can include headaches, excessive sweating, increasing size of hands and feet, visual field defect (bitemporal hemianopia), paraesthesiae and arthralgia.

2. H Tensilon test

Myasthenia gravis is due to a loss of post-synaptic acetylcholine receptors (AChR) caused by IgG anti-AChR antibodies. It is characterized by skeletal muscle weakness that worsens with exercise. Common symptoms include diplopia, ptosis, nasal speech and nasal regurgitation of food. A raised level of serum anti-AChR antibodies is specific for myasthenia gravis, but the titres may be normal. Clinically, intravenous edrophonium (Tensilon), a simple bedside test is used to confirm the diagnosis.

3. G Sleep study (polysomnography)

Obstructive sleep apnoea may be associated with marked obesity, retrognathia, a short neck and enlarged tonsils. Sleep disruption can cause daytime hypersomnolence which can be disabling and dangerous. Other common symptoms include loud snoring, unrefreshing sleep and witnessed episodes of apnoea. Sleep studies can document sleep fragmentation and dips in oxygen saturation with apnoea.

4. K Ultrasound scan of the abdomen

His symptoms suggest obstructive jaundice. The ultrasound scan of the abdomen is useful in determining the diameter of the bile ducts. If there is no dilatation, then a liver biopsy or endoscopic retrograde cholangiopancreatography (ERCP) may be required for diagnosis.

5. F Short Synacthen test

He has Addison's disease, probably secondary to an autoimmune adrenalitis. Skin pigmentation is nearly always present in primary hypoadrenalism but is absent in secondary hypoadrenalism (e.g. long-term steroid therapy, inadequate adrenocorticotrophic hormone (ACTH) production due to hypothalamic-pituitary disease). There may be hypotension, nausea, vomiting and diarrhoea. A short Synacthen test involves giving intramuscular tetracosactide (tetracosactrin) (a synthetic polypeptide identical with the first 24 aminoacids of ACTH). Normally, the plasma cortisol rise at 30 minutes is at least 550 nm/L.

The unconscious patient

A Blood cultures
B Blood gases
C Blood glucose
D Brainstem death tests
E Carboxyhaemoglobin level
F Cardiac monitor
G Computerized tomography (CT) of the head
H Lumbar puncture
I Thyroid function tests
J Toxicology screen
K Urea and electrolytes

For each scenario below, choose the SINGLE most discriminating investigation from the above list of options. Each option may be used once, more than once, or not at all.

1. A 47-year-old woman is found collapsed in her home. Examination reveals meningism and bilateral extensor plantars. Fundal haemorrhages are seen.

2. A 67-year-old man with severe chronic obstructive pulmonary disease is brought to the A&E department by ambulance. His breathing and conscious level have both deteriorated with oxygen given during the journey. However, his oxygen saturation on pulse oximetry is only 90%.

3. A middle-aged couple are found semi-conscious in their caravan by their teenage son, who had woken in the middle of the night with nausea and vomiting. All three of them had been well the previous evening.

4. A 45-year-old man collapses on the ward. It is immediately obvious that he has had a cardiorespiratory arrest.

5. A 56-year-old diabetic lady is found unresponsive at home by her neighbour. She is currently being treated for a urinary tract infection. There is no focal neurological deficit on examination.

Answers to 1.20

1. G   Computerized tomography (CT) of the head

Subarachnoid haemorrhage is invariably due to rupture of an
intracranial saccular aneurysm. The patient may be comatose if the
bleeding is extensive. A rapid rise in intracranial pressure is responsible
for subhyaloid haemorrhages that are sometimes seen in the fundi.
Meningism is common but may not be present for the first few hours.
There may not be any focal neurological deficit unless there is bleeding
within the brain substance or pressure on the 3rd cranial nerve from an
aneurysm of the posterior communicating artery. Computerized
tomography (CT) of the head will show blood in the CSF pathways, a
collection of blood or an arteriovenous malformation. In 10% of cases,
the scan may be normal in which case a lumbar puncture is necessary.
The CSF will be blood-stained or, if the haemorrhage is more than
12 hours old, the CSF will be xanthochromic.

2. B   Blood gases

This patient has type 2 respiratory failure (PO_2<8 kPa/60 mmHg and
PCO_2>7 kPa/55 mmHg). Causes include ventilatory failure e.g. chronic
obstructive pulmonary disease, chest wall deformities, respiratory muscle
weakness (Guillain–Barré syndrome) and depression of the respiratory
centre. These patients rely on hypoxia for respiratory drive and there is a
high chance that this man had received high-flow oxygen in the
ambulance. This leads to hypercapnia and risk of a respiratory arrest.
Blood gases are essential for assessing blood pH and PCO_2 levels.

3. E   Carboxyhaemoglobin level

Combustion of any fuel in the absence of adequate oxygen will cause
carbon monoxide poisoning. Caravans rely on propane or butane gas
for heating/cooking/refrigeration that, if not properly maintained, can
cause carbon monoxide poisoning. Carboxyhaemoglobin is formed by
the combination of oxygen and carbon monoxide and this prevents the
formation of oxyhaemoglobin. Headache, nausea and vomiting are
common symptoms with mental impairment and coma in severe cases.

4. F   Cardiac monitor

It is important to ascertain whether he is in VF (ventricular fibrillation)
or non-VF arrest, the former being best treated with immediate DC
(direct current) cardioversion.

5. C   Blood glucose

It is essential to exclude hypoglycaemia, diabetic ketoacidosis or
hyperosmolar non-ketotic hyperglycaemia in any ill, diabetic patient.

Investigations using serum antibodies

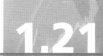

A Anticentromere antibodies
B Antimitochondrial antibodies
C Antinuclear factor antibodies
D Antiphospholipid antibodies
E Antismooth muscle antibodies
F Cytoplasmic antineutrophil cytoplasmic antibodies (cANCA)
G Double-stranded DNA antibodies
H Extractable nuclear antigen antibodies
I Perinuclear antineutrophil cytoplasmic antibodies (pANCA)
J Rheumatoid factor
K Scl-70 (scleroderma) antibodies

For each presentation, choose the SINGLE most discriminating investigation from the above list of options. Each option may be used once, more than once, or not at all.

1. A 45-year-old woman is incidentally found to have a raised serum alkaline phosphatase level from base-line blood tests done during a routine medical examination. Examination reveals mild generalized pigmentation.

2. A 45-year-old woman presents with a thrombotic stroke with right-sided weakness. There is a history of three previous miscarriages. She has a mild thrombocytopenia.

3. A 50-year-old woman presents with a 6-month history of difficulty in swallowing and painful hands particularly when exposed to the cold. Examination reveals telangiectasia on her face and shiny, tight skin over her fingers with atrophy of the finger pulps.

4. A 38-year-old man gives a 3-month history of early morning pain and stiffness in his joints mainly affecting both hands. X-rays of his hands show soft tissue swelling and bony erosions.

5. A 35-year-old woman presents with central chest pain relieved by sitting forward. She also complains of arthralgia, myalgia and malaise. Examination reveals facial erythema and a pericardial rub.

Answers to 1.21

1. **B   Antimitochondrial antibodies**

   Primary biliary cirrhosis (PBC) usually affects middle-aged women, is often asymptomatic in the early stages and may be discovered on routine examination. It causes progressive destruction of the bile ducts and eventually cirrhosis. Serum anti-mitochondrial antibodies are found in 95–99% of patients with PBC. One of the earliest symptoms is pruritus which can precede the jaundice and hepatomegaly by several years. It is associated with skin pigmentation and hypercholesterolaemia. Patients are at risk of oesophageal varices, malabsorption (especially of the fat-soluble vitamins A, D, E and K) and osteomalacia.

2. **D   Antiphospholipid antibodies**

   Primary antiphospholipid syndrome is characterized by thromboses (arterial and venous) and/or recurrent (more than two) miscarriages in the absence of systemic lupus erythematosus. Other features include chorea, thrombocytopenia (autoimmune), livedo reticularis, thrombotic stroke and heart valve abnormalities (sometimes with non-infective vegetations).

3. **A   Anticentromere antibodies**

   CREST (calcinosis, Raynaud's phenomenon, oesophageal involvement, sclerodactyly and telangiectasia) syndrome is a more benign variant of systemic sclerosis. Anticentromere antibodies are specifically raised in about 80% cases.

4. **J   Rheumatoid factor**

   Rheumatoid factors are autoantibodies usually IgM class and directed against IgG. The American College of Rheumatology criteria for the diagnosis of rheumatoid arthritis include morning stiffness of at least 1 hour duration, arthritis of three or more joint areas including the hand joints, symmetrical arthritis, rheumatoid nodules, positive rheumatoid factor and radiological changes in the hands and wrists (osteoporosis, joint space narrowing, periarticular erosions and angular deformity).

5. **G   Double-stranded DNA antibodies**

   Systemic lupus erythematosus is a multi-system, connective tissue disease affecting the joints (small joint arthritis, aseptic necrosis of the hip), skin (livedo reticularis, vasculitis, butterfly facial rash, alopecia), lungs (pleurisy/effusion, pulmonary fibrosis), Raynaud's phenomenon, heart (pericarditis, endocarditis), abdomen (vasculitis causing mesenteric ischaemia/infarct), nervous system (fits, stroke, mononeuritis multiplex, peripheral neuropathy) and blood (anaemia, leucopenia and thrombocytopenia). Ds-DNA antibodies are specific for this condition.

Interpretation of respiratory function tests

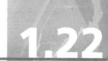

A Asthma
B Chronic bronchitis
C Emphysema
D Goodpasture's syndrome
E Hyperventilation syndrome
F Kyphoscoliosis
G Pleural plaques
H Pneumonectomy
I Polycythaemia
J Pulmonary fibrosis
K Tracheal stenosis

For each presentation below, choose the SINGLE most likely cause from the above list of options. Each option may be used once, more than once, or not at all.

1. A 56-year-old man presents with cough, breathlessness and haemoptysis. His pulmonary function tests show a restrictive pattern with a carbon monoxide K_{CO} (transfer coefficient) at 227% of the predicted normal. He has a mild microcytic anaemia.

2. A 57-year-old woman recently had lung function tests which have shown D_LCO (diffusing capacity for CO) 60%, K_{CO} (rate of uptake/min) 124% and VA (alveolar distribution volume) 55% of the predicted normal.

3. A 63-year-old man presents with a 1-year history of breathlessness. His lung function tests reveal a raised FEV_1/FVC ratio of 89% with a low transfer coefficient of 57% of the predicted normal.

4. A 65-year-old man is investigated for wheezing. His flow volume loop has a square appearance.

5. A 55-year-old man with long-standing breathlessness has an FEV_1 of 1.3 L and FVC of 2.4 L. His blood gases on air show a P_{O_2} of 8.9 kPa and P_{CO_2} of 4.7 kPa.

Answers to **1.22**

1. D Goodpasture's syndrome

Goodpasture's syndrome is an autoimmune disorder (type 2 cytotoxic reaction) characterized by pulmonary haemorrhage and renal disease (crescentic nephritis). Anti-glomerular basement membrane antibodies against antigens of the glomerular and alveolar basement membranes are detected. Typically there is an elevated Kco because of extravasated blood in the alveoli combining with inhaled carbon monoxide. An increase in the transfer factor is also seen in polycythaemia and occasionally in asthma.

2. H Pneumonectomy

$D_L$co (diffusing capacity for CO) = V_A (alveolar distribution volume) × Kco (rate of uptake/min). This patient has had a pneumonectomy. The effective alveolar volume falls but the Kco is elevated, as the remaining alveolar units are normal.

3. J Pulmonary fibrosis

This patient has a restrictive lung disorder which has adversely affected gas exchange. It is probably caused by pulmonary fibrosis.

4. K Tracheal stenosis

The expiratory flow volume loop is obtained when the subject exhales with maximum effort from a total lung capacity to the residual volume. It normally has a triangular appearance, i.e. the maximum flow achieved early on and with a decrease in maximal flow rate with falling lung volume (volume depending on the flow in normal subjects). With tracheal stenosis, the maximal flow rate is independent of lung volume with squaring of the flow loop. The common cause of tracheal stenosis is a stricture following tracheal intubation or tracheostomy.

5. C Emphysema

He has obstructive airways disease. It is likely that he is a pink puffer (emphysema) in view of his hypocapnia. Typical features include nicotine-stained fingers, tachypnoea, pursing of the lips (to increase airway pressure and outward gradient thereby preventing collapse of the peripheral airways), hyperinflated chest, use of accessory muscles with indrawing of the intercostal spaces during inspiration, and reduced breath sounds. In contrast, chronic bronchitics are classically cyanosed and hypercapnic with the so-called blue-bloater appearance.

Clinical presentations of sarcoidosis

A   Anterior uveitis
B   Cardiomyopathy
C   Diabetes insipidus
D   Erythema nodosum
E   Hypercalcaemia
F   Lupus pernio
G   Mikulicz's syndrome
H   Mononeuritis multiplex
I   Peripheral neuropathy
J   Posterior uveitis
K   Pulmonary fibrosis

For each scenario below, choose the SINGLE most likely clinical manifestation of sarcoidosis from the above list of options. Each option may be used once, more than once, or not at all.

1. A 36-year-old woman with known sarcoidosis presents with bilateral, red, painful eyes and photophobia. She is otherwise fairly fit and well. Slit-lamp examination shows precipitates on the internal surface of the cornea.

2. A 50-year-old woman has a diffuse, purplish infiltration of the nose, cheek and lips. She has a long history of sarcoidosis and keloid formation.

3. A 47-year-old man with chronic sarcoidosis complains of severe polyuria (10 L/24 h) and polydipsia. Plasma osmolality and serum sodium are essentially normal.

4. A 55-year-old woman with sarcoidosis complains of dry, gritty eyes. There is diffuse swelling of both lacrimal and salivary glands.

5. A 43-year-old man with sarcoidosis presents with dizziness and incipient syncope. His electrocardiogram shows low-voltage complexes and left bundle branch block. A 24-hour ECG tape reveals runs of supraventricular and ventricular tachycardia.

Answers to **1.23**

1. **A** **Anterior uveitis**

Uveitis is common in sarcoidosis affecting about one-third of patients. Acute anterior uveitis presents as a sudden onset of blurred vision with a painful red eye; posterior uveitis presents with progressive visual loss. It may be part of uveoparotid fever which consists of parotid gland enlargement, uveitis, fever and cranial nerve palsies (especially the facial nerve). Recurrent episodes of anterior uveitis may be associated with cataract, glaucoma or calcified corneal band keratopathy.

2. **F** **Lupus pernio**

Lupus pernio is a chronic, violaceous skin lesion (cutaneous granuloma), particularly affecting the nose, cheeks and ears. It seldom resolves completely and is usually associated with pulmonary sarcoidosis, uveitis, phalangeal bone cysts and nasal bone involvement. Other features of late, chronic fibrotic disease are skin plaques and subcutaneous nodules. Erythema nodosum is the commonest early lesion and often occurs with bilateral hilar lymphadenopathy and uveitis.

3. **C** **Diabetes insipidus**

The hypothalamus and the posterior pituitary gland may be affected by sarcoidosis, disturbing the hypothalamic–pituitary axis and causing cranial diabetes insipidus (deficiency of vasopressin). Plasma osmolality and serum sodium are normal when the osmoregulatory thirst centre is intact. Hypercalcaemia would be unlikely here as the urinary volume is excessive.

4. **G** **Mikulicz's syndrome**

Mikulicz's syndrome is the combination of enlarged lacrimal and parotid glands due to infiltration with sarcoid granulomas. It may be associated with keratoconjunctivitis sicca (reduced tear secretion which is detected using the Schirmer's test).

5. **B** **Cardiomyopathy**

Cardiac involvement in sarcoidosis may cause restrictive or congestive features due to increased stiffness of the myocardium and impaired systolic function. There may be arrhythmias, heart block, pericarditis and sudden death. A ventricular aneurysm, in the absence of significant ischaemic heart disease, is highly suggestive of sarcoidosis. The response to steroids is poor. Steroids cause resolution of the granulomas but increase the risk of ventricular aneurysm formation. Some patients need a permanent pacemaker and some with intractable cardiac failure will need heart transplantation.

Clinical presentation of cancer

A Acute myeloid leukaemia
B Adenocarcinoma of the caecum
C Apical cancer of the lung
D Brain tumour
E Carcinoma of the head of the pancreas
F Gastric carcinoma
G Laryngeal carcinoma
H Liver metastases
I Multiple myeloma
J Ovarian carcinoma
K Prostatic carcinoma

For each of the following patients choose the SINGLE most likely diagnosis from the list of options. Each option may be used once, more than once, or not at all.

1. A 72-year-old lady presents to her GP with a 10 kg loss of weight over the last 6 months. She has also become slightly yellow in colour. She has lost her appetite and has an aching sensation in the abdomen that is aggravated by lying and eating and wakes her in the night. CA Pan

2. A 65-year-old man complains of back pain following a minor fall. He has been unwell for 4 months with a decreased exercise tolerance and malaise. He looks pale, has difficulty with micturition especially at night and is becoming unable to live alone. An X-ray of his lumbosacral spine shows sclerotic changes in the lumbar vertebrae and pelvis.

3. An 83-year-old man presents to his GP with a weight loss of 8 kg over the last 6 months and has felt anxious and depressed. He has difficulty in sleeping but says his appetite is good. Apart from some constipation he feels well and wonders if sleeping tablets might help. He has a hypochromic anaemia.

4. A 60-year-old lady presents with fits and weakness of her left arm. She has had several episodes where her left arm has become suddenly stiff and clumsy, followed by a heavy feeling. The arm has not fully recovered from the first episode and now she cannot hold objects in her left hand.

5. A 70-year-old man presents to the A&E department with confusion and falls. He is pyrexial and pale with bruises, purpura and gingival hypertrophy. He has been recently unwell, has lost weight and has become very frail.

Answers to **1.24**

1. E   Carcinoma of the head of the pancreas

Classically, carcinoma of the head of the pancreas presents in older people with weight loss, abdominal pain (the contention that painless jaundice is the first manifestation of carcinoma of the pancreas is erroneous) and jaundice. The latter is due to progressive compression of the bile duct as it passes through the head of the pancreas. Liver metastases can also present with jaundice. However, the marked weight loss, the lack of bowel or chest symptoms, jaundice and vague pain excacerbated by a supine posture make pancreatic carcinoma the most likely diagnosis.

2. K   Prostatic carcinoma

Prostatic carcinoma often presents insidiously, as in this case. Minor prostatic symptoms (such as nocturia) may be ignored as a 'natural part of ageing'. This gentleman presents late with spread to the bones causing sclerotic changes and back pain. Anaemia may be an associated feature due to myelofibrosis or marrow infiltration. The diagnosis is confirmed by the serum prostatic specific antigen (PSA) and a prostatic biopsy.

3. B   Adenocarcinoma of the caecum

A change in bowel habit is a cardinal feature of colorectal carcinoma. Caecal carcinoma usually presents with anaemia from occult blood loss and is less likely to cause constipation. However, given the weight loss, hypochromic anaemia (a well-known complication of the right colonic neoplasm) and lower gastrointestinal symptoms, caecal carcinoma is the most likely diagnosis for this case.

4. D   Brain tumour

This patient is describing focal seizures followed by paralysis of the arm (Todd's paralysis), which can be due to a slow-growing brain tumour that has caused inflammation/irritable focus in the cerebral cortex.

5. A   Acute myeloid leukaemia

The pallor (anaemia) and widespread bruising (thrombocytopenia) suggest a haematological malignancy. Of the two, acute myeloid leukaemia and multiple myeloma, the former is a more probable diagnosis because gingival hypertrophy, together with anaemia and thrombocytopenia, is usually associated with acute myelomonocytic leukaemia.

Causes of chest pain

A   Bornholm disease
B   Dissecting aortic aneurysm
C   Myocardial infarction
D   Oesophagitis
E   Pancoast's tumour
F   Pericarditis
G   Pneumonia
H   Pneumothorax
I   Pulmonary embolism
J   Ruptured oesophagus
K   Tietze's syndrome

For each presentation below, choose the SINGLE most likely cause from the above list of options. Each option may be used once, more than once, or not at all.

1. A 76-year-old man presents with weight loss and a 4-week history of a constant pain in the left side of his chest. There is evidence of a left Horner's syndrome.

2. A 55-year-old woman complains of sudden onset of a severe, searing chest pain radiating to the back. There is radiological evidence of mediastinal widening.

3. A 20-year-old man develops sudden onset of chest pain associated with fever, headache and a mild sore throat. Examination is normal apart from localized chest wall tenderness.

4. A 60-year-old man complains of a cough, productive of mucopurulent sputum, and sudden onset of severe left-sided pleuritic chest pain. Examination of the chest reveals bronchial breath sounds at the left lung base.

5. A 65-year-old man presents to the A&E department with left-sided chest pain with localized tenderness anteriorly. His electrocardiogram is normal.

Answers to **1.25**

1. E   Pancoast's tumour

Carcinoma at the apex of the lung can involve the ribs and affect the
lower part of the brachial plexus (C8, T1, T2), causing shoulder pain
and wasting of the inner aspect of the arm. There may be a Horner's
syndrome (meiosis, enophthalmos, anhydrosis and partial ptosis) due to
involvement of the sympathetic ganglia.

2. B   Dissecting aortic aneurysm

The history and X-ray findings are suggestive of a dissecting aortic
aneurysm which ideally needs confirmation with transoesophageal
echocardiography or MRI/CT scan of the thorax. Dissection of the
ascending aorta should be treated surgically (as there is a risk of cardiac
tamponade), whilst that involving the descending aorta can be treated
medically (reduce the systolic arterial pressure to 100 mmHg). Failure of
perfusion to the limbs or the major organs is an indication for surgery.

3. A   Bornholm disease

Bornholm disease, or epidemic myalgia, is usually caused by coxsackie B
virus and rarely by echovirus. It mainly affects children (pain is
commonly abdominal with superficial muscle tenderness) and young
adults. Pericarditis, aseptic meningitis and orchitis are possible
complications. There is usually a full recovery within 1 week.

4. G   Pneumonia

The presence of a chest infection with clinical evidence of consolidation
is highly suggestive of pneumonia being the cause of the pleurisy (sharp,
localized chest pain exacerbated by deep inspiration or coughing). Other
causes of pleuritic chest pain include pulmonary infarction, carcinoma
and connective tissue diseases (e.g. rheumatoid arthritis, systemic lupus
erythematosus).

5. K   Tietze's syndrome

Pain associated with local tenderness over the costochondral junctions is
known as Tietze's syndrome and is self-limiting and benign. It is usually
unilateral and often affects up to three joints.

Causes of hypertension

A   Acromegaly
B   Adult onset polycystic kidney disease
C   Chronic glomerulonephritis
D   Coarctation of the aorta
E   Conn's syndrome
F   Cushing's syndrome
G   Essential hypertension
H   Hypernephroma (renal-cell carcinoma)
I   Phaeochromocytoma
J   Pre-eclampsia
K   Renal artery stenosis

For each presentation below, choose the SINGLE most likely cause from the above list of options. Each option may be used once, more than once, or not at all.

1.   A 56-year-old woman presents with headache, sweating and palpitations. Examination is unremarkable apart from hypertension (BP 190/105 mmHg). A 24-hour urinary vanillylmandelic acid (VMA) level is elevated.

2.   A 73-year-old man presents with rapidly deteriorating renal function after being started on an angiotensin-converting enzyme (ACE) inhibitor for hypertension. He is known to have peripheral vascular disease.

3.   A 24-year-old woman with severe hypertension presents with malaise, muscle weakness and hypokalaemia. The plasma aldosterone level is elevated but renin activity is undetectable.

4.   A 35-year-old woman presents with headaches and hypertension. There is clinical evidence of radiofemoral delay. The chest X-ray shows cardiomegaly with scalloping of the lower margins of the 5th, 6th and 7th ribs.

5.   A 57-year-old man presents with fever, weight loss, sweating and haematuria. He has a palpable mass in his right flank and is hypertensive.

Answers to **1.26**

1. **I** Phaeochromocytoma

Phaeochromocytomas release both adrenaline and noradrenaline; 90% of the tumours are benign and 90% are located in the adrenal gland. They may be associated with other disorders such as multiple endocrine neoplasia (MEN) type 2 syndrome, or von Hippel Lindau syndrome. Patients may present with hypertension (not always intermittent), heart failure, headache, palpitations and sweating. Screening involves measuring urinary VMA or metanephrines.

2. **K** Renal artery stenosis

In renovascular disease, ACE inhibitors can cause renal deterioration especially in the presence of volume depletion. ACE inhibitors cause a marked fall in glomerular filtration rate by efferent glomerular arteriolar dilatation and hence reducing glomerular filtration pressure. The two commonest causes of renovascular hypertension are atheromatous disease and fibromuscular dysplasia (mainly between 30–50 years of age and occurring more commonly in women).

3. **E** Conn's syndrome

Conn's syndrome (adrenal adenoma) accounts for about 60% of cases of primary hyperaldosteronism. Renin activity is suppressed in primary and is elevated in secondary hyperaldosteronism. The majority of patients with primary hyperaldosteronism are asymptomatic, but some may have muscle weakness, nephrogenic diabetes insipidus (insensitivity to antidiuretic hormone, causing polyuria and polydipsia), paraesthesiae and tetany from hypokalaemic alkalosis causing a decrease in ionized calcium.

4. **D** Coarctation of the aorta

Coarctation of the aorta is narrowing at, or just distal to, the insertion of the ductus arteriosus. Patients may be asymptomatic for many years and discovered incidentally from a routine chest X-ray (bilateral rib notching from a collateral arterial circulation involving the periscapular and intercostal arteries). Complications include infective endocarditis (on the coincident bicuspid aortic valve), uncontrolled hypertension and cerebral haemorrhage from rupture of a cerebral artery aneurysm.

5. **H** Hypernephroma (renal-cell carcinoma)

A renal-cell carcinoma may secrete renin and so cause secondary hypertension and hypokalaemic alkalosis. Symptoms include weight loss, haematuria, loin pain and pyrexia. There may be secondary polycythaemia from the secretion of erythropoietin.

Causes of electrocardiographic (ECG) abnormalities

A Hypercalcaemia
B Hypocalcaemia
C Hypokalaemia
D Hypothermia
E Hypothyroidism
F Jervell–Lange–Nielson syndrome
G Lown–Ganong–Levine syndrome
H Pulmonary embolism
I Romano–Ward syndrome
J Sick sinus syndrome
K Wolff–Parkinson–White syndrome

For each scenario below, choose the SINGLE most likely cause from the above list of options. Each option may be used once, more than once, or not at all.

1. A 77-year-old woman is found unconscious in her garden and taken by ambulance to the A&E department. She is normally fit and well and has been looking forward to her Christmas family reunion. Her electrocardiogram shows sinus bradycardia with broad, slurred J waves adjacent to the QRS complex.

2. A 40-year-old woman collapses on the gynaecology ward. Her electrocardiogram shows right axis deviation, right bundle branch block and Q waves with T wave inversion in lead III.

3. A 17-year-old man is incidentally found to have a prolonged QT interval of 500 ms. He has been profoundly deaf since early childhood and has a strong family history of sudden death.

4. A 68-year-old woman presents with dizziness, palpitations and blackouts. Her 24-hour ECG tape shows a combination of brady- and tachyarrhythmias with pauses of up to 3 to 4 seconds.

5. An 82-year-old woman presents with generalized muscle weakness and dizziness. She has a history of controlled hypertension. Her electrocardiogram shows small T waves and prominent U waves.

Answers to **1.27**

1.   D   Hypothermia

This patient collapsed outdoors on a winter's day and has been exposed
to the cold. The classic Osborne, or J wave (extra deflection at the end of
the QRS complex), appears when the core body temperature drops to
32°C, although it may also be seen in other conditions such as trauma
and cerebral haemorrhage. Hypothermia is also associated with sinus
bradycardia, atrial fibrillation and prolonged PR and QT intervals.

2.   H   Pulmonary embolism

Electrocardiographic changes occur in 80% of cases of *major* pulmonary
embolism, including the classic S deflection in lead I and a Q and
inverted T wave in lead III (S1, Q3, T3 pattern) which reflect right
ventricular strain. Other changes suggestive of acute cor pulmonale
include right axis deviation, partial or complete right bundle branch
block, T wave inversion in anterior chest leads and ST depression in
inferior leads.

3.   F   Jervell–Lange–Nielson syndrome

Congenital causes of the long QT syndrome include the
Jervell–Lange–Nielson (autosomal recessive with coexisting congenital
deafness) and the Romano–Ward (autosomal dominant without
deafness) syndromes. There is a strong history of sudden death in infancy
and patients present with dizzy spells, syncope or sudden death. All first-
degree relatives should be screened for the condition.

4.   J   Sick sinus syndrome

Sinus node disease (sick sinus syndrome) is caused by degenerative
disease, ischaemia or infarction of the sinus node. Subsequently there is
failure of the sinus node to generate or conduct impulses. It commonly
presents as persistent sinus bradycardia, intermittent sinus arrest or the
bradycardia–tachycardia syndrome (usually paroxysmal atrial fibrillation
and sinus arrest).

5.   C   Hypokalaemia

Although hypokalaemia is usually asymptomatic, there may be muscle
weakness and cramps in more severe cases. The most likely cause for
hypokalaemia in this case is thiazide therapy for hypertension.
Associated electrocardiographic changes include small T waves (other
causes – pericardial effusion and hypothroidism), ST segment
depression and prominent U waves. The U wave follows the T wave and
may be seen in normal electrocardiographs. Prominent U waves may be
associated with hypokalaemia, hypercalcaemia and hyperthyroidism.

Causes of pericarditis

A Coxsackie virus group B
B Dressler's syndrome
C Neoplastic
D Post-cardiotomy syndrome
E Post-radiotherapy
F Rheumatic fever
G Scleroderma
H Toxoplasmosis
I Tuberculous (constrictive) pericarditis
J Uraemia
K Wegener's granulomatosis

For each presentation below, choose the SINGLE most likely cause from
the above list of options. Each option may be used once, more than once,
or not at all.

1. A 57-year-old man develops fever, a pericardial effusion and a left
    pleural effusion 4 months after being discharged from hospital with an
    acute myocardial infarction.

2. A 48-year-old man complains of weight loss, night sweats and anorexia.
    He has a history of alcohol abuse. He is peripherally vasoconstricted and
    has Kussmaul's sign and pulsus paradoxus. His heart size is normal on
    an X-ray.

3. A 46-year-old man with hypertension and polycystic kidneys, who is
    recovering from a respiratory infection, presents with pericardial pain
    and breathlessness. He is on regular haemodialysis. Investigations for a
    myocardial infarction are negative and his urea and electrolytes are near
    normal.

4. A 76-year-old man has a globular-shaped heart shadow on his chest
    X-ray together with cannon ball lesions in his lung fields. Clinically, he
    has evidence of cardiac tamponade.

5. A 16-year-old boy presents with a migratory polyarthritis, carditis,
    pericarditis and erythema marginatum several weeks after developing a
    sore throat.

Answers to **1.28**

1. **B** **Dressler's syndrome**

It is estimated that Dressler's syndrome (post-myocardial infarction syndrome) affects up to 4% of patients weeks or months after an acute myocardial infarction. It is probably due to an immunological response to damaged cardiac muscle. The syndrome is self-limiting but can recur. There is usually a good response to anti-inflammatory agents.

2. **I** **Tuberculous (constrictive) pericarditis**

He has evidence of constrictive pericarditis or cardiac tamponade with an exaggerated drop in blood pressure on inspiration (pulsus paradoxus), and a paradoxical rise in the JVP on inspiration (Kussmaul's sign). The heart is usually of normal size in constrictive pericarditis and is enlarged in cardiac tamponade, although a normal heart shadow does not exclude tamponade. Tuberculous pericarditis should be suspected with the history of constitutional symptoms in a patient with alcohol abuse. In both effusion and constriction, the addition of steroids to the antituberculous therapy for the first 11 weeks of treatment reduces the need for a pericardectomy.

3. **J** **Uraemia**

The incidence of pericarditis is significantly reduced by adequately treating renal failure with dialysis or renal transplantation. Uraemic pericarditis may develop, as a result of an intercurrent infection or surgery, even if the creatinine and electrolytes are close to normal. There may be fibrinous pericarditis with bloody effusion, or adhesions with constriction.

4. **C** **Neoplastic**

Metastatic carcinoma is the commonest cause of malignant pericarditis, the most common being from the lung, breast, stomach and colon. Pericardectomy or creating a pericardial window into the pleural cavity may prevent recurrence.

5. **F** **Rheumatic fever**

Rheumatic fever mainly occurs between the ages of 6 and 16 years as a result of an abnormal immune reaction to group A beta-haemolytic streptococcus infection. The major criteria for the diagnosis of rheumatic fever are carditis, polyarthritis, chorea, erythema marginatum and subcutaneous nodules. Clinical pericarditis is uncommon in acute rheumatic fever but signifies profound pancarditis.

Causes of pleural effusion

A Cardiac failure
B Chylothorax
C Cirrhosis
D Dressler's syndrome
E Lung carcinoma
F Mesothelioma
G Nephrotic syndrome
H Pulmonary embolism
I Rheumatoid arthritis
J Systemic lupus erythematosus
K Yellow nail syndrome

For each presentation below, choose the SINGLE most likely cause from the above list of options. Each option may be used once, more than once, or not at all.

1. A 65-year-old man is found to have a left pleural effusion. There is also radiological evidence of irregular pleural thickening.

2. A 30-year-old woman is incidentally found to have a small, right pleural effusion. She also has a red, papular facial rash with scarring and follicular plugging.

3. A 57-year-old man is readmitted, 4 weeks after a myocardial infarction, with a febrile illness. There is a pericardial rub and radiological evidence of a small left pleural effusion.

4. A 65-year-old man presents with worsening breathlessness over the last 6 months. A chest X-ray shows small bilateral pleural effusions and cardiomegaly.

5. A 50-year-old man presents with a right pleural effusion after an oesophagectomy for carcinoma. Pleural aspiration produces a milky-coloured fluid.

Answers to **1.29**

1. **F** Mesothelioma

Mesothelioma (occurs after exposure to asbestos) is most frequently diagnosed between 50 and 70 years of age. Other clinical features include dull chest pain, breathlessness, weight loss and cough. A pleural effusion is common. As the tumour progresses, irregular lobulated pleural thickening develops and is best seen on a computerized tomography (CT) scan of the chest. The average latent period between first exposure to asbestos and death from mesothelioma is 20–40 years. Blue asbestos (crocidolite) is much more potent than white asbestos (chrysolite) in causing mesothelioma. Other effects of asbestos on the lung include pleural plaques, pleural thickening and bronchogenic carcinoma.

2. **J** Systemic lupus erythematosus

This patient has the typical butterfly rash on her face (and other sun-exposed areas of skin) of lupus erythematosus. Other skin lesions can include vasculitis, purpura, photosensitivity, urticaria, Raynaud's phenomenon and scarring alopecia. There seems to be pulmonary involvement (cryptogenic pulmonary fibrosis/effusion).

3. **D** Dressler's syndrome

The postmyocardial infarction syndrome (Dressler's syndrome) occurs weeks to months after a myocardial infarction. The onset is sudden consisting of pericarditis, fever and a pericardial effusion. There may also be a pleural effusion. The syndrome is due to an autoimmune response to damaged heart muscle. It is usually self-limiting but treatment with NSAIDs and steroids may be required.

4. **A** Cardiac failure

This patient has congestive cardiac failure probably due to ischaemic heart disease. An echocardiogram is required to assess cardiac function.

5. **B** Chylothorax

A chylothorax is due to a leakage of chylous fluid (fat, transported as chylomicrons, reaches the blood stream through this route) from the thoracic duct. Most cases are acquired through trauma, surgery (e.g. oesophageal resection or those requiring mobilization of the aortic arch), a blunt or penetrating injury and malignant infiltration. The fluid is classically milky-coloured. It is important to distinguish this from an empyema. The presence of chyle is confirmed by examining the fluid microscopically and detecting positive staining of the fat globules.

Causes of pulmonary fibrosis

A Amiodarone
B Ankylosing spondylitis
C Asbestosis
D Cryptogenic fibrosing alveolitis (CFA)
E Extrinsic allergic alveolitis
F Histiocytosis X (Langerhans' cell granulomatosis)
G Methotrexate
H Progressive massive fibrosis
I Sarcoidosis
J Silicosis
K Systemic sclerosis

For each presentation below, choose the SINGLE most likely cause from
the above list of options. Each option may be used once, more than once,
or not at all.

1. A 40-year-old smoker presents with malaise, a non-productive cough,
   haemoptysis and breathlessness. The chest X-ray shows reticulonodular
   shadowing and multiple ring shadows mainly in the upper and mid-
   zones.

2. A 57-year-old woman with a history of treated paroxysmal atrial
   fibrillation and ischaemic heart disease presents with breathlessness,
   cough, fever, malaise and weight loss. The chest X-ray shows
   reticulonodular shadows in the upper zones of both lung fields.

3. A 45-year-old man presents with worsening breathlessness over the last
   4 years. He keeps a number of budgerigars in the house. His chest
   X-ray mainly shows upper lobe contraction and fibrosis.

4. A 60-year-old woman with systemic lupus erythematosus presents with
   breathlessness and a dry cough. She has finger clubbing and bilateral
   basal crackles in her chest. Her chest X-ray shows bilateral basal
   shadows.

5. A 52-year-old man has radiological evidence of bilateral apical fibrosis.
   Examination reveals a 'question mark' posture and the Schober's test is
   abnormal.

Answers to **1.30**

1. F Histiocytosis X (Langerhans' cell granulomatosis)

Pulmonary histiocytosis X is a granulomatous disease of unknown cause which is characterized by Langerhans' cells mixed with eosinophils. It mainly affects young and middle-aged smokers. Up to one quarter of patients are asymptomatic whilst others may complain of cough, breathlessness, chest pain, fever and weight loss. Radiological changes are a combination of cystic structures and interstitial nodules in the upper and mid-zones. Open lung biopsy is usually needed for the diagnosis.

2. A Amiodarone

Amiodarone is a class III antiarrythmic drug that prolongs the action potential, hence prolonging the refractory period of the atria, ventricles, AV node and accessory pathways. It is useful in treating supraventricular and ventricular arrhythmias including those associated with the Wolff–Parkinson–White syndrome. Amiodarone pneumonitis affects up to 10% of those on treatment but is uncommon in those taking 200 mg or less per day. The most common radiological changes are bilateral asymmetrical interstitial or alveolar shadows.

3. E Extrinsic allergic alveolitis

Bird fancier's lung is a form of extrinsic allergic alveolitis caused by the inhalation of avian serum proteins (especially IgA) from the feathers, saliva and excreta. Patients often present with an insidious onset of breathlessness after being chronically exposed to low levels of antigenic dust. Finger clubbing is unusual and there is fibrosis particularly of the upper lobes.

4. D Cryptogenic fibrosing alveolitis (CFA)

There is no specific cause found for cryptogenic fibrosing alveolitis although it may be associated with systemic lupus erythematosus (SLE), rheumatoid arthritis, systemic sclerosis, polymyositis and chronic active hepatitis. Finger clubbing is present in up to 70% of patients with CFA though it is less common in SLE. The fibrosis is mainly confined to the lung bases.

5. B Ankylosing spondylitis

Ankylosing spondylitis is a seronegative spondarthropathy, associated with HLA-B27. In severe cases, there is loss of the lumbar lordosis, fixed kyphosis and compensatory cervical hyperextension producing the 'question mark' posture. An abnormal Schober's test is based on less than the normal 10 cm excursion from the 5th lumbar vertebra upwards when the patient leans forward. Apical fibrosis is found in less than 1% of patients with advanced disease.

Causes of bronchiectasis

A   Allergic bronchopulmonary aspergillosis
B   Cystic fibrosis
C   Hypogammaglobulinaemia
D   Intraluminal foreign body
E   Kartagener's syndrome
F   Malignancy
G   Marfan's syndrome
H   Pulmonary sequestration
I   Sarcoidosis
J   Tuberculosis
K   Yellow nail syndrome

For each presentation below, choose the SINGLE most likely cause from the above list of options. Each option may be used once, more than once, or not at all.

1. A 25-year-old man presents with a worsening productive cough and breathlessness. He has a past history of recurrent infections.

2. A 19-year-old man presents with recurrent chest infections with a cough productive of mucopurulent sputum. He passes fatty, offensive stools which are difficult to flush away.

3. A 45-year-old asthmatic lady is found to have bronchiectasis in the right upper lobe. A full blood count shows eosinophilia.

4. A 35-year-old man presents with otitis media. He has situs inversus, bronchiectasis and infertility.

5. A 56-year-old ex-smoker presents with recurrent right basal bronchopneumonia, persistent purulent sputum and weight loss. Computerized tomography (CT) has shown localized bronchiectasis in the right lower lobe.

Answers to **1.31**

1. **C** Hypogammaglobulinaemia

Patients with hypogammaglobulinaemia (common variable immunodeficiency) often have a long history of sinopulmonary infections leading to bronchiectasis. The diagnosis of humoral immunodeficiency is important, because gammaglobulin replacement can prevent, or at least diminish, further infections.

2. **B** Cystic fibrosis

Cystic fibrosis is an autosomal recessive disorder with a gene mutation on the long arm of chromosome 7. The result is a defective cystic fibrosis transmembrane conductance regulator (CFTR), which reduces chloride excretion into the lumen and increases sodium reabsorption into the epithelial cells. The exocrine gland secretions are thus viscid from the low water content and this can block ducts and airways. The patient has steatorrhoea due to pancreatic insufficiency and bronchiectasis from airway plugging and infections.

3. **A** Allergic bronchopulmonary aspergillosis

The combination of asthma, eosinophilia and chest X-ray abnormalities is suggestive of allergic bronchopulmonary aspergillosis, which is caused by a hypersensitivity reaction to the colonization of the bronchi by *Aspergillus fumigatus*. Occlusion of the airways by mucous plugs causes lobar collapse and bronchiectasis. There is also eosinophilic infiltration of the lungs causing fleeting radiological shadows.

4. **E** Kartagener's syndrome

Kartagener's syndrome is the association of primary ciliary dyskinesia with situs inversus or dextrocardia. Other features include infertility, dysplasia of the frontal sinuses, sinusitis, otitis media and bronchiectasis.

5. **F** Malignancy

Malignancy is likely in this case especially in view of his smoking history, weight loss and age (over 40 years). There may be bronchial obstruction from an endobronchial tumour. Granulomatous diseases such as tuberculosis and sarcoidosis may also cause bronchial stenosis and obstruction. Bronchoscopy is essential to assess the presence of a mechanical obstruction, to take biopsies and to remove a foreign body or a mucous plug if necessary.

Causes of chronic liver disease

A   Alcohol
B   Alpha 1-antitrypsin deficiency
C   Autoimmune hepatitis
D   Cardiac failure
E   Cryptogenic cirrhosis
F   Galactosaemia
G   Haemochromatosis
H   Primary biliary cirrhosis
I   Secondary biliary cirrhosis
J   Viral hepatitis
K   Wilson's disease

For each presentation below, choose the SINGLE most likely cause from
the above list of options. Each option may be used once, more than once,
or not at all.

1. A 60-year-old man presents with liver failure, diabetes mellitus and heart
    failure. There is also evidence of skin pigmentation.

2. A 30-year-old woman complains of lethargy and arthralgia. Examination
    reveals spider naevi, striae, acne, hirsutism and hepatosplenomegaly.

3. A 61-year-old man has the features of chronic liver disease. He does not
    feel he has a problem with drinking. Two days after admission he had
    an episode of delirium tremens.

4. A 57-year-old man has chronic liver disease and severe irreversible
    airways obstruction. He neither drinks alcohol nor smokes.

5. A 36-year-old drug abuser presents with a haematemesis from bleeding
    oesophageal varices.

Answers to **1.32**

1. **G** **Haemochromatosis**

Idiopathic haemochromatosis is inherited as an autosomal recessive condition, and is associated with HLA-A3. It is a multisystem disease with the total body iron being increased. There is hepatomegaly with liver dysfunction, diabetes mellitus, heart failure, pseudogout and skin pigmentation.

2. **C** **Autoimmune hepatitis**

Autoimmune hepatitis (Type 1) typically affects young and middle-aged women. The onset is insidious but may be acute in about a quarter of cases. Amenorrhoea is common. Most patients have smooth muscle autoantibodies and the majority have antinuclear antibodies and high levels of serum immunoglobulins. Type 2 autoimmune hepatitis presents mainly in childhood and tends to be more aggressive.

3. **A** **Alcohol**

This man has a history of alcohol abuse confirmed by his withdrawal symptoms. One should ask the CAGE questions, i.e. 'Have you ever tried to Cut down?', 'Are you Annoyed about people asking about your drinking habit?', 'Do you ever feel Guilty about your drinking?', and 'Do you have an Eye-opener drink in the morning?' A 'yes' in answer to two of these questions is suggestive of an alcohol problem.

4. **B** **Alpha 1-antitrypsin deficiency**

Alpha 1-antitrypsin's main role is to inhibit neutrophil elastase. If the plasma concentration is less than 40%, then connective tissue destruction occurs. The normal allele is M and the common abnormal alleles are S and Z. Alpha 1-antitrypsin deficiency is associated with panlobular emphysema. Normal FEV_1 loss after the age of 30 years is 35 ml/year, but in a non-smoking PiZZ (ZZ homozygote) individual the loss is 80 ml/year. All PiZZ subjects have slowly progressive hepatic damage, with up to 50% developing cirrhosis.

5. **J** **Viral hepatitis**

The majority of patients recover fully from an acute hepatitis B virus (HBV) infection, with up to 95% of adults clearing the virus and its antigens within 3 months of the acute HBV hepatitis. Some will develop chronic active liver disease, leading slowly in most cases to cirrhosis. This patient is likely to have been exposed to hepatitis B virus when sharing needles/equipment for injection.

Causes of ascites

A Budd–Chiari syndrome
B Carcinoma
C Cardiac failure
D Cirrhosis
E Constrictive pericarditis
F Meigs' syndrome
G Myxoedema
H Nephrotic syndrome
I Ovarian overstimulation syndrome
J Pancreatitis
K Tuberculous peritonitis

For each presentation below, choose the SINGLE most likely cause from the above list of options. Each option may be used once, more than once, or not at all.

1. A 52-year-old woman presents with malaise, chest pain, ascites and a right-sided pleural effusion. Examination reveals an ovarian mass. Both the ascitic and pleural fluids have a protein content of 36 g/L.

2. A 56-year-old man has developed ascites and abdominal pain over the last 3 months. There is evidence of tender hepatomegaly but no signs of chronic liver disease. He has a history of polycythaemia rubra vera.

3. A 65-year-old man, with underlying chronic obstructive pulmonary disease, presents with both ascites and severe lower limb oedema. His jugular venous pressure is elevated with v waves. An ultrasound scan of the abdomen shows distended intrahepatic veins and a dilated inferior vena cava.

4. A 51-year-old vagrant is admitted with fever, weight loss and malabsorption. He has ascites with a protein content of 40 g/L, lymphocytes and a negative Ziehl–Nielson (ZN) stain of the fluid. A computerized tomography (CT) scan of the abdomen shows enlarged retroperitoneal lymph nodes.

5. A 47-year-old diabetic presents with pleural effusions, ascites and leg oedema. Her heart size is normal on the chest X-ray. She is found to have hypoalbuminaemia (albumin 23 g/L).

Answers to 1.33

1. **F   Meigs' syndrome**

   Meigs' syndrome is the triad of a benign fibroma or other benign
   ovarian tumour with ascites and a large pleural effusion (usually on the
   right side). The fluid is usually an exudate and contains a few
   mononuclear cells. It is most commonly seen after the menopause. It
   resolves on surgical removal of the tumour.

2. **A   Budd–Chiari syndrome**

   The Budd–Chiari syndrome is due to hepatic vein obstruction usually
   from thrombosis. Most commonly, ascites develops over a few months
   with tender hepatomegaly and dependent oedema. About a quarter
   present with a more rapid onset of ascites, abdominal pain and jaundice
   over about a month whilst some present with fulminant hepatic failure.
   It depends on the speed and extent of the hepatic vein occlusion. Causes
   include inflammatory bowel disease, pregnancy, paroxysmal nocturnal
   haemoglobinuria, polycythaemia rubra vera, oral contraceptives, severe
   dehydration and malignancy.

3. **C   Cardiac failure**

   The ultrasound findings are consistent with cardiac failure, possibly cor
   pulmonale (right heart failure from pulmonary hypertension caused by
   diseases of the lung, thoracic cage or respiratory control mechanisms).
   An echocardiogram is needed to assess cardiac and valvular function.

4. **K   Tuberculous peritonitis**

   Tuberculous peritonitis is rare. It affects debilitated alcoholics and may
   occur in ascites associated with chronic liver disease. It results from local
   spread (blood-borne) from infected mesenteric lymph nodes. Ascites is
   common with, or without, fever and abdominal pain. Investigation of
   the ascitic fluid shows an exudate with lymphocytes. Laparoscopy, which
   can show the peritoneum studded with tuberculomas, is the most
   expeditious method of making the diagnosis.

5. **H   Nephrotic syndrome**

   Causes of transudates include cardiac failure and hypoalbuminaemic
   states (nephrotic syndrome and liver disease). This patient is likely to
   have developed proteinuria/nephrotic syndrome from her diabetes
   mellitus. The hallmark renal lesion is glomerulosclerosis associated
   with arteriolar hyalinosis and interstitial fibrosis. This can progress to
   renal failure. The evolution of diabetic nephropathy can be reduced by
   tight diabetic control, control of arterial pressure, and the use of
   angiotensin-converting enzyme (ACE) inhibitors which have a
   renoprotective effect even in the absence of hypertension.

Causes of malabsorption

A Abetalipoproteinaemia
B Bacterial overgrowth
C Chronic pancreatitis
D Coeliac disease
E Crohn's disease
F Intestinal lymphoma
G Parasitic infestation
H Primary biliary cirrhosis
I Tropical sprue
J Ulcerative colitis
K Whipple's disease

For each presentation below, choose the SINGLE most likely cause from
the above list of options. Each option may be used once, more than once,
or not at all.

1. A 47-year-old man presents with diarrhoea 6 months after he returns
    from India after a 4-week holiday. His diarrhoea is now persistent and
    he has lost 1 stone in weight despite an adequate dietary intake. His
    stools are negative for ova and parasites.

2. A 71-year-old man presents with unexplained weight loss and anaemia.
    The serum ferritin and folate levels are low. A jejunal biopsy shows
    subtotal villous atrophy.

3. A 45-year-old woman complains of pruritus, steatorrhoea, easy bruising
    and weight loss. On examination, she is jaundiced and pigmented with
    excoriation marks.

4. A 40-year-old diabetic is found to have evidence of malabsorption
    together with diarrhoea and weight loss. He has profound postural
    hypotension and requires percutaneous endoscopic gastrostomy (PEG)
    feeding.

5. A 50-year-old man complains of malaise, fever, weight loss, arthralgia
    and diarrhoea. A jejunal biopsy reveals a flattened mucosa containing
    periodic acid-Schiff (PAS) positive macrophages.

Answers to 1.34

1. **G   Parasitic infestation**

    This patient most probably has *Giardia lamblia* infection of his intestine which he probably acquired, from drinking unboiled water, during his holiday in India. *Giardia lamblia* can cause malabsorption in individuals infected with a large number of trophozoites, especially in immunocompromised or IgA-deficient subjects. Large numbers of organisms cover the epithelium of the small intestine causing inflammation and villous flattening. At this stage there are no ova or parasites to be found in stool.

2. **D   Coeliac disease**

    Coeliac disease is an inflammatory disorder of the small intestine induced by dietary gluten in wheat, barley, rye and possibly oats. There is loss of villous height and hypertrophy of the crypts (total mucosal thickness is normal) leading to malabsorption. It may present in infants but should not be overlooked in older patients, who have either always been thin or have lost weight without an obvious reason. In these patients serum folate and ferritin levels are often low.

3. **H   Primary biliary cirrhosis**

    Primary biliary cirrhosis is a chronic cholestatic inflammatory liver disease, the aetiology of which is probably autoimmune. It most commonly affects middle-aged women. There is jaundice with skin pigmentation, a risk of developing oesophageal varices and fat malabsorption leading to deficiency of vitamins A, D, E and K (hence osteomalacia and bruising).

4. **B   Bacterial overgrowth**

    Small bowel bacterial overgrowth may be due to reduced gastric acid secretion (e.g. achlorhydria from pernicious anaemia or chronic atrophic gastritis), intestinal dysmotility (e.g. diabetic autonomic neuropathy, systemic sclerosis) or anatomical disorders (e.g. blind loop syndrome from a Bilroth II gastrectomy, diverticula or enteric fistulae). In this case, both postural hypotension and gastroparesis are features of diabetic autonomic neuropathy.

5. **K   Whipple's disease**

    Whipple's disease is a rare cause of malabsorption and most commonly affects middle-aged males. It can affect any organ (e.g. nervous system, eyes, joints, etc.), but commonly manifests with gastrointestinal involvement causing malabsorption. The organism (*Tropheryma whippleii*) can be identified both between and within abnormal macrophages which stain magenta with periodic acid-Schiff (PAS).

Causes of constipation

A   Acute diverticulitis
B   Colorectal carcinoma
C   Crohn's disease
D   Drug therapy
E   Functional constipation
F   Hirschsprung's disease
G   Hypercalcaemia
H   Hypothyroidism
I   Irritable bowel syndrome
J   Simple constipation
K   Systemic sclerosis

For each presentation below, choose the SINGLE most likely cause from the above list of options. Each option may be used once, more than once, or not at all.

1. A 40-year-old man gives a long history of abdominal discomfort, distension relieved by defecation, and constipation. Examination reveals tenderness in the left iliac fossa.

2. A 62-year-old woman complains of weight loss with severe constipation and occasional diarrhoea. Clinical examination is normal.

3. A 50-year-old woman presents with constipation, straining at defecation and also tenesmus. Clinical examination and sigmoidoscopy are normal.

4. A 56-year-old woman complains of constipation with worsening breathlessness and dysphagia. She also suffers from painful fingers when exposed to the cold.

5. A 70-year-old man with Parkinson's disease has been troubled by constipation. He is on L-dopa replacement therapy and trihexyphenidyl (benzhexol). Examination reveals bradykinesia and cogwheel rigidity.

Answers to **1.35**

1.   I   Irritable bowel syndrome

The irritable bowel syndrome is a functional disorder characterized by constipation, diarrhoea and abdominal pain often relieved by defecation, and is associated with a change in frequency of defecation and/or stool consistency. Examination is unremarkable, but insufflation of air during sigmoidoscopy reproduces the abdominal discomfort. Excessive investigations should be avoided; the patient should be reassured and advised to have a high-fibre diet. Antispasmodics such as mebeverine may be used.

2.   B   Colorectal carcinoma

A change of bowel habit in a previously fit individual is a serious symptom especially if accompanied by weight loss. Carcinoma of the bowel needs to be excluded. The overall 5-year survival for colorectal carcinoma is 30%, but if the tumour is localized to the bowel wall (Duke's A – not breaching serosa) the survival is >95%.

3.   E   Functional constipation

Functional constipation is characterized by persistently difficult and infrequent bowel movement or the sensation of incomplete defecation. Unlike the irritable bowel syndrome, abdominal pain is not part of the diagnostic criteria. It is important to exclude organic obstruction of the lower colon and faecal impaction.

4.   K   Systemic sclerosis

Systemic sclerosis is a connective tissue disease which may cause Raynaud's phenomenon (an exaggerated physiological response to the cold with intense vasospasm and painful rebound hyperaemia), dysphagia, renal failure, pulmonary fibrosis and bowel hypomotility. Sigmoid and rectal involvement is associated with constipation which may alternate with diarrhoea.

5.   D   Drug therapy

Opiates, anticholinergics such as trihexyphenidyl (benzhexol) (to reduce the tremor and rigidity of Parkinson's disease) and iron therapy can all cause constipation, as can poor mobility. Other adverse side effects of anticholinergic drugs include urinary retention, confusion, dry mouth, dizziness and blurred vision.

Causes of haematuria

A Diabetes mellitus
B Factitious
C Goodpasture's syndrome
D IgA nephropathy
E Renal calculi
F Renal-cell carcinoma
G Systemic lupus erythematosus
H Transitional cell carcinoma of the bladder
I Tuberculosis
J Urinary tract infection
K Wegener's granulomatosis

For each presentation below, choose the SINGLE most likely cause from the above list of options. Each option may be used once, more than once, or not at all.

1. A 46-year-old man presents with tiredness, intermittent haemoptysis and macroscopic haematuria. Serum antiglomerular basement antibodies and pANCA (perinuclear antineutrophil cytoplasmic antibodies) are detected.

2. A 54-year-old man presents with anorexia, weight loss, haematuria, pyrexia and left loin pain with an underlying mass. He has a secondary polycythaemia and the urine cytology is negative for malignant cells.

3. A 60-year-old woman is admitted with severe, right loin pain radiating to the groin, and haematuria. Excretion urography shows absence of a pyelogram on the left side 15 minutes after the contrast injection.

4. A 78-year-old woman is admitted with confusion and pyrexia. She has urinary frequency and is sometimes incontinent. Urine dipstick reveals the presence of blood and protein. She is otherwise fit and well.

5. A 46-year-old man presents with nasal mucosal ulceration, cough, pleuritic chest pain and haematuria. A biopsy reveals a necrotizing granulomatous disease. The test for cANCA (cytoplasmic antineutrophil cytoplasmic antibodies) is positive.

Answers to **1.36**

1.   C   Goodpasture's syndrome

Goodpasture's syndrome is a combination of rapidly progressive glomerulonephritis and pulmonary haemorrhage mediated by anti-GBM (glomerular basement membrane) antibodies. Corrected carbon monoxide uptake (KCO) is increased due to free haemoglobin in the alveoli. Outcome without treatment is very poor, most dying within 6 months. Treatment is with plasma exchange and immunosuppressive (prednisolone, cyclophosphamide, azathioprine) therapy. Recovery of renal function is much less likely in the presence of an elevated serum creatinine of >600 µM, especially if oliguric, when treatment is started.

2.   F   Renal-cell carcinoma

Renal-cell carcinoma may produce pyrexia in 20% of patients, and inappropriate erythropoietin in 2% causing erythrocytosis. Rarely, it can cause a left varicocele by invasion of the left renal vein causing impaired drainage of the left testicular vein. Urine cytology is unhelpful. A CT or MRI scan of the abdomen can identify the lesion and stage the tumour.

3.   E   Renal calculi

The excretion urogram showed an acute ureteric obstruction which is usually due to a renal stone. This produces ureteric colic which is very painful as the stone obstructs, or causes spasm of, the ureter. The most common type of renal stone is a calcium oxalate stone. Other types include calcium phosphate, magnesium ammonium phosphate, uric acid and cystine. Stones may be removed endoscopically, by percutaneous ureterolithotomy or extracorporeal shock-wave lithotripsy.

4.   J   Urinary tract infection

It is important to differentiate a simple urinary tract infection from that occurring in the presence of conditions such as diabetes mellitus, or with a structural abnormality of the urinary tract (e.g. obstruction). Excretion urography is not warranted in isolated episodes of urinary tract infection. Infection is usually due to *Escherichia coli* and other coliforms.

5.   K   Wegener's granulomatosis

Classically, Wegener's granulomatosis is a granulomatous, inflammatory and vasculitic condition usually affecting the upper and lower airways, associated with a necrotizing glomerulonephritis and sometimes a disseminated vasculitis. The presence of renal disease confers a worse prognosis. Anticytoplasmic IgG antibodies are specific for neutrophil granules and monocyte lysosomes. Cytoplasmic cANCA is positive in 90% of active Wegener's granulomatosis, and is useful in monitoring disease activity. Treatment is with oral cyclophosphamide. Mean survival with treatment is about 8 years (5 months without treatment).

Causes of urinary incontinence

A   Acute spinal cord compression
B   Behavioural disorder
C   Bladder outflow obstruction
D   Cauda equina compression
E   Epilepsy
F   Fistula
G   Functional
H   Infection
I   Normal pressure hydrocephalus
J   Stress incontinence
K   Urge incontinence

For each scenario below, choose the SINGLE most likely cause from the above list of options. Each option may be used once, more than once, or not at all.

1.   A 76-year-old man is admitted with sudden onset of back pain and bilateral lower limb weakness. He has also been incontinent of urine. Examination reveals a sensory loss over the buttocks and perineum.

2.   A 78-year-old woman presents with increasing confusion and unsteadiness which has resulted in a number of falls. Her husband has noticed that she is frequently incontinent of urine. Examination reveals a gait apraxia (magnetic gait) and a modest memory impairment.

3.   A 36-year-old multiparous, obese woman complains of urinary incontinence when she sneezes or coughs. Physical examination is normal.

4.   A 92-year-old woman presents with abdominal discomfort and urinary incontinence. Examination reveals a distended bladder and there is evidence of faecal impaction on rectal examination.

5.   A 65-year-old woman complains of having to urinate frequently with an urgency to void. Often she is not able to get to the toilet in time.

Answers to **1.37**

1.   D   Cauda equina compression

The commonest causes of cauda equina compression are a central lumbar disc compression (as in this case with sudden onset), tumour, or infection with cytomegalovirus, lymphomatous meningitis and toxoplasma in AIDS patients. It causes lower limb weakness and numbness, impotence and loss of sphincter control (patulous anus and an atonic bladder). Sensory loss is most marked in the saddle-area of the buttocks and perineum. Urgent surgical intervention is required to ensure reasonable neurological recovery. Cord compression produces a spastic paraparesis with urinary retention and overflow incontinence. The sensory level corresponds to the level of the compression.

2.   I   Normal pressure hydrocephalus

The classic presentation of normal pressure hydrocephalus is the triad of gait disturbance ('glued-to-the-floor' sign), incontinence and dementia. A CT scan of the head shows disproportionate ventricular enlargement compared with the degree of cortical atrophy. Ventricular shunting is the definitive treatment but needs to be done early.

3.   J   Stress incontinence

Stress incontinence is probably the commonest cause of incontinence and mainly affects women and predominantly those who have had children. It is associated with an increase in intra-abdominal pressure, weak pelvic floor muscles or pelvic organ prolapse (e.g. cystocele or rectocele).

4.   C   Bladder outflow obstruction

Severe constipation can cause temporary urinary incontinence due to a faecal mass compressing the bladder neck and causing outflow obstruction. Other causes of urinary tract obstruction include causes within the lumen (calculus, renal pelvis/ureteric tumour, blood clot), within the wall (ureteric stricture, urethral stricture, congenital urethral valve) and extrinsic pressure (retroperitoneal fibrosis or tumours, prostatic obstruction).

5.   K   Urge incontinence

Urge incontinence is mainly due to instability of the detrusor muscle of the bladder. Treatment is with bladder retraining and anticholinergic drugs such as oxybutynin and tolterodine.

Causes of hyponatraemia

A   Addison's disease
B   Artefactual
C   Chronic liver disease
D   Diuretics
E   Excessive sweating
F   Hypothyroidism
G   Nephrotic syndrome
H   Oliguric renal failure
I   Pseudohyponatraemia
J   Psychogenic polydipsia
K   Syndrome of inappropriate antidiuretic hormone (ADH) secretion

For each presentation below, choose the SINGLE most likely cause from
the above list of options. Each option may be used once, more than once,
or not at all.

1. A 45-year-old man is recovering from bowel surgery and still requires
    supplementary intravenous fluids as he is being kept on a nil-by-mouth
    regime. He is otherwise well. His serum sodium level is 105 mmol/L
    (normal range 135–145 mmol/L).

2. A 28-year-old diabetic woman complains of dizziness when she stands
    from a sitting or lying position. She is pigmented with significant
    postural hypotension. Her serum sodium is 128 mmol/L.

3. A 32-year-old man is brought into the A&E department in a coma. He
    has severe hyperglycaemia and large amounts of urinary ketones. His
    serum sodium is 115 mmol/L.

4. A 45-year-old man presents with a collapse towards the end of a
    marathon run. He is hypotensive with a tachycardia and reduced skin
    turgor. His serum sodium is 129 mmol/L.

5. A 55-year-old woman, with a history of membranous
    glomerulonephritis, is found to have oedema of her legs extending up to
    the thighs, and a serum sodium level of 125 mmol/L. Her recent
    echocardiogram is normal.

Answers to **1.38**

1. **B   Artefactual**

    The blood sample has probably been taken from the drip arm thus showing a spurious result. It is unlikely that he would have remained so well otherwise. The test for serum urea and electrolytes needs to be repeated. If the hyponatraemia is real then the urinary sodium and serum osmolalities should be determined to investigate the syndrome of inappropriate antidiuretic hormone (ADH) secretion.

2. **A   Addison's disease**

    Autoimmune adrenalitis is the commonest cause of Addison's disease. The history of diabetes, pigmentation and postural hypotension suggests this condition. There is increased renal loss of sodium due to mineralocorticoid deficiency.

3. **I   Pseudohyponatraemia**

    This patient has diabetic ketoacidosis. The high blood glucose causes intracellular fluid to move into the extracellular space causing a pseudohyponatraemia.

4. **E   Excessive sweating**

    The history and signs of volume depletion suggest salt-deficient hyponatraemia due to excessive sweating and an inadequate fluid and salt replacement.

5. **G   Nephrotic syndrome**

    Membranous glomerulonephritis is a cause of the nephrotic syndrome. There is thickening of the capillary basement membrane due to deposition of immune complexes although the antigenic component is often unknown. There is an association with systemic lupus erythematosus, *Plasmodium malariae* infection, malignancy (particularly of the lung and bowel) and the use of penicillamine. There is hypervolaemic/dilutional hyponatraemia with excess total body water and extracellular sodium. Spontaneous recovery occurs in one third of patients, especially in younger subjects, females and those with only mild/moderate asymptomatic proteinuria at the time of presentation. Otherwise, treatment may involve corticosteroids and immunosuppressive drugs.

Causes of hypercalcaemia

A   Familial hypocalciuric hypercalcaemia
B   Hyperparathyroidism
C   Immobility
D   Milk-alkali syndrome
E   Multiple myeloma
F   Sarcoidosis
G   Small-cell carcinoma of the lung
H   Squamous-cell carcinoma of the lung
I   Thiazide diuretics
J   Thyrotoxicosis
K   Vitamin D toxicity

For each presentation below, choose the SINGLE most likely cause from the above list of options. Each option may be used once, more than once, or not at all.

1. A 35-year-old health and fitness instructor complains of nausea over the last 2 months. She is normally fit and well. Although she does not take any prescribed medication she does take overfortified milk and various dietary and mineral supplements. Her serum calcium level is 2.8 mmol/L (normal range 2.15–2.50 mmol/L).

2. A 50-year-old ex-smoker presents with weight loss and increased thirst. He has clubbing of his fingers. His serum calcium is 3.1 mmol/L and there is a right middle lobe consolidation seen on his chest X-ray.

3. A 56-year-old woman has had gradually worsening breathlessness over the last year. Her weight has been stable. There is reticulonodular shadowing on her chest X-ray and she was incidentally found to have a raised calcium level of 2.97 mmol/L.

4. A 76-year-old lady with deafness and frontal bossing presents with a stroke. She was found to have a slightly raised calcium level of 2.65 mmol/L.

5. A 67-year-old man presents with backache and is found to have hypercalcaemia (2.7 mmol/L) and several osteolytic lesions on a skeletal survey. His erythrocyte sedimentation rate (ESR) is elevated at 85 mm/h.

Answers to **1.39**

1.   **K   Vitamin D toxicity**

Vitamin D toxicity is usually iatrogenic. There is increased intestinal calcium absorption and also, in addition to the overfortified milk, this patient probably gets additional vitamin D through other supplements. The homeostatic regulation of alpha$_1$-hydroxylase is sometimes overridden by the substrate 25(OH)D. Treatment is by restricting calcium intake and rehydration. Corticosteroids are rarely needed.

2.   **H   Squamous-cell carcinoma of the lung**

Hypercalcaemia in the absence of bony metastases occurs in about 15% of patients with squamous-cell carcinoma of the lung due to the production of a parathyroid hormone related protein (PTHrP). This is one of the features of the non-metastatic manifestations of malignancy and a common cause of hypercalcaemia. Clubbing is predominantly associated with squamous-cell cancers and occasionally with adenocarcinoma.

3.   **F   Sarcoidosis**

Sarcoidosis is a multisystem non-caseating granulomatous disease. Stage 3 intrathoracic sarcoidosis (pulmonary infiltration without hilar adenopathy) is associated with a poor prognosis. Only one-third of cases remit by 2 years compared with over two-thirds of those with hilar lymphadenopathy alone (Stage 1). It can lead to pulmonary fibrosis and eventually cor pulmonale and death. Hypercalcaemia occurs in less than 10% of patients and is thought to be due to elevated levels of 1,25-dihydroxyvitamin D which is produced by macrophages within the granulomas.

4.   **C   Immobility**

Deafness and frontal bossing (also bowing of the tibia/femur) are suggestive of Paget's disease. It is characterized by uncontrolled bone turnover with excessive local bone resorption and impaired osteoblastic activity, leading to abundant new bone formation which is structurally abnormal and weak. Hypercalcaemia is associated with immobility in Paget's disease which in this case is caused by the stroke. Other complications include high-output cardiac failure, pathological fractures, platybasia (basilar impression of the skull) causing brain stem signs, and osteogenic sarcoma (rare).

5.   **E   Multiple myeloma**

The raised ESR and osteolytic lesions suggest multiple myeloma. Hypercalcaemia is present in about 20% of patients. Pathological fractures are common.

Causes of falls

A   Acute labyrinthitis
B   Aortic stenosis
C   Carotid sinus hypersensitivity
D   Cerebellar syndrome
E   Impaired vision
F   Ménières's disease
G   Parkinson's disease
H   Postural hypotension
I   Sensory ataxia
J   Sick sinus syndrome
K   Vasovagal episode

For each presentation below, choose the SINGLE most likely cause from
the above list of options. Each option may be used once, more than once,
or not at all.

1. A 65-year-old woman presents with several falls associated with
    dizziness over the last 3 months. Examination reveals a slow rising pulse
    and a low systolic blood pressure of 90 mmHg.

2. A 70-year-old man is found lying on the floor at home by his neighbour.
    His balance has been poor for some time and he walks with a stamping
    gait. His Romberg's test is positive.

3. A 60-year-old man has had recurrent falls over the past year. He has
    slowed down considerably and has difficulty turning in bed at night.
    Examination reveals cogwheel rigidity.

4. A 56-year-old woman presents having had several falls associated with
    giddiness particularly when she gets up in the mornings. She has
    underlying ischaemic heart disease and her anti-anginal treatment was
    recently increased.

5. A 70-year-old lady complains of vertigo and vomiting for the last 2 days.
    She has just recovered from a flu-like illness. Since then she has needed
    to hold on to the furniture to prevent herself from falling.

Answers to **1.40**

1. **B** Aortic stenosis

Symptoms of severe aortic stenosis are breathlessness, angina and syncope. The signs of severe disease include a slow rising pulse, low systolic pressure and a quiet or absent second heart sound. In severe stenosis there may be no murmur due to reduced cardiac output. An echocardiogram is required to measure the gradient across the aortic valve. In adults, an aortic valve replacement is indicated for significant symptoms or if there is a gradient of 50 mmHg or more across the valve.

2. **I** Sensory ataxia

A high-steppage or stamping gait (walks with wide-based gait, continuously looking at the ground, raising feet high in the air before stamping them to the ground) indicates dorsal column (conveys touch, vibration and proprioception) loss. It may be due to tabes dorsalis (syphilis infection) or subacute combined degeneration of the cord (B_{12} deficiency).

3. **G** Parkinson's disease

Parkinson's disease is characterized by bradykinesia, rigidity and a resting tremor. Cogwheel rigidity is the combination of rigidity and tremor. It is associated with a loss of the pigmented neurones in the pars compacta of the substantia nigra (80% loss occurs before symptoms arise). The pathological hallmark of the disease is the presence of Lewy bodies (eosinophilic inclusion bodies) in the degenerating neurones of the substantia nigra and selected brain stem nuclei. Oxidative stress and generation of cytotoxic free radicals are implicated in the pathogenesis of Parkinson's disease.

4. **H** Postural hypotension

Although the names of the drugs are not given, it is probable that she is on a beta blocker, calcium channel antagonist and a nitrate, all of which have a hypotensive effect. In combination these drugs can cause significant postural hypotension.

5. **A** Acute labyrinthitis

Vestibular neuronitis/viral labyrinthitis is an acute attack of severe vertigo with nystagmus and vomiting. It accompanies or follows viral infections, is self-limiting and rarely recurs. Ménière's disease, on the other hand, is characterized by deafness, vertigo and tinnitus. The scenario given favours the diagnosis of viral labyrinthitis.

Causes of a spastic paraparesis

A   AIDS myelopathy
B   Anterior spinal artery thrombosis
C   Cord compression
D   Friedreich's ataxia
E   General paralysis of the insane
F   Motor neurone disease
G   Multiple sclerosis
H   Parasagittal meningioma
I   Subacute combined degeneration of the cord
J   Syringomyelia
K   Taboparesis

For each presentation below, choose the SINGLE most likely cause from the above list of options. Each option may be used once, more than once, or not at all.

1. A 69-year-old woman presents with difficulty in articulating her speech and with weight loss of 1 stone over the last 6 months. Examination shows weakness and muscle wasting with fasciculation and increased tone in the legs.

2. A 20-year-old man is seen in clinic with worsening ataxia and paraparesis over the last 12 months. He has kyphoscoliosis, pes cavus and cerebellar signs. Both his knee and ankle jerks are absent but he has extensor plantar responses.

3. A 56-year-old woman complains of sudden loss of power in her legs 12 hours ago. She has a past history of breast carcinoma. Examination reveals increased tone and reflexes in her lower limbs and an impaired sensory level at T10 segment.

4. A 35-year-old man presents with wasting and weakness of the small muscles of the hands. Examination reveals loss of pain and temperature sensations in the upper limbs and a spastic paraparesis.

5. A 60-year-old woman presents with numbness in her hands and feet. On examination, she looks pale. She has evidence of loss of proprioception especially in her lower limbs with absent ankle jerks and extensor plantars.

Answers to 1.41

1. F   Motor neurone disease

Motor neurone disease involves both the upper and lower motor neurones supplying the voluntary muscles of the bulbar region and limbs. There are three patterns which may overlap during the course of the disease: progressive muscular atrophy, amyotrophic lateral sclerosis with spastic para- or tetraparesis, and progressive bulbar palsy. In amyotrophic lateral sclerosis (which this patient has) there is a combination of wasted, fasciculating muscles with clonus or hyper-reflexia. Glutamate toxicity may be a factor causing neuronal damage. The antiglutamate drug, riluzole, may delay progression of the disease.

2. D   Friedreich's ataxia

Friedreich's ataxia is a hereditary spinocerebellar degenerative disorder, inherited as an autosomal recessive trait. The onset is usually before the age of 15 years. Signs include cerebellar ataxia, loss of proprioception, touch and vibration (from loss of dorsal root ganglion cells) and limb weakness (from corticospinal tract involvement). Associated skeletal deformities include pes cavus, pes equinovarus and kyphoscoliosis.

3. C   Cord compression

The cause of acute spinal cord compression in this lady is most likely to be a metastatic tumour. There is usually rapidly advancing weakness of the lower limbs with urinary retention and loss of sensation below the lesion. An MRI scan of the spine is the investigation of choice.

4. J   Syringomyelia

Syringomyelia is a CSF-filled syrinx or cavity within the spinal cord potentially extending over many segments. Surrounding structures including the anterior horn cells, corticospinal tracts and decussating fibres carrying pain and temperature sensation may be destroyed. There is dissociated sensory loss, i.e. the loss of pain and thermal sensation with the preservation of touch and proprioception. There may be scars visible from previous painless burns or cuts.

5. I   Subacute combined degeneration of the spinal cord

Subacute combined degeneration of the spinal cord is due to vitamin B_{12} deficiency. It mainly affects middle-aged or older subjects. There is degeneration of the lateral and posterior columns of the cord resulting in a loss of postural sense in the lower limbs (sensory ataxia) and paraplegia. Peripheral nerve involvement causes peripheral neuropathy. There may be overt anaemia, and visual impairment (scotoma) that may progress to optic atrophy.

Causes of nystagmus

A Acoustic neuroma
B Arnold–Chiari malformation
C Brain stem glioma
D Cerebellar infarction
E Congenital
F Ménière's syndrome
G Middle ear disease
H Multiple sclerosis
I Syringobulbia
J Vestibular neuronitis
K Wernicke's encephalopathy

For each scenario below, choose the SINGLE most likely cause from the above list of options. Each option may be used once, more than once, or not at all.

1. A 45-year-old man presents with confusion, ataxia and nystagmus. There is impairment of adduction, with nystagmus particularly affecting the abducting eye. He is otherwise normally active and works as a barman. He admits to having drunk alcohol.

2. A 25-year-old woman complains of a headache and is incidentally found to have a pendular movement of the eyes. There is no diplopia or blurring of vision. Her medication consists of Ventolin and beclometasone (beclomethasone) inhalers, and the oral contraceptive pill.

3. A 56-year-old woman complains of worsening hearing, tinnitus and unsteadiness. Examination reveals nystagmus, a sensorineural deafness, absent corneal reflex, diplopia on lateral gaze and facial weakness.

4. A 49-year-old man develops troublesome vertigo soon after recovering from a flu-like illness. It is precipitated by head movement and is worse in the lying position. There is evidence of nystagmus that diminishes with repeated testing.

5. A 62-year-old man, with a history of hypertension and ischaemic heart disease, presents with a sudden onset of unsteadiness and a tendency to fall to the left. There is evidence of nystagmus (fast component to the left) on left lateral gaze and left-sided dysdiadochokinesis with past pointing. Romberg's test is negative.

Answers to 1.42

1. **K Wernicke's encephalopathy**

    Wernicke's encephalopathy is due to thiamine deficiency causing
    haemorrhages and severe neuronal loss in the mamillary bodies. It is
    characterized by the triad of confusion, ophthalmoplegia (nystagmus,
    impaired adduction) and ataxia. If untreated, it can lead to Korsakoff's
    syndrome which consists of severe amnesia with confabulation and
    poor insight. Internuclear ophthalmoplegia (lesion in the medial
    longitudinal fasciculus) is characteristic of multiple sclerosis, but it can
    be rarely caused by a brain stem glioma, vascular lesion or Wernicke's
    encephalopathy.

2. **E Congenital**

    Congenital nystagmus is often dramatic with continuous side-to-side
    pendular movements while gazing straight ahead. It is worse on looking
    in either lateral direction.

3. **A Acoustic neuroma**

    The majority of cerebellopontine angle tumours are benign. Acoustic
    neuromas are the commonest tumours which can cause Vth (facial
    numbness, loss of corneal reflex), VIth, VIIth and VIIIth cranial nerve
    impairments and cerebellar dysfunction. Nystagmus is vestibular or
    cerebellar in origin. A magnetic resonance imaging (MRI) scan with
    gadolinium enhancement is the investigation of choice. Surgical excision
    is the only curative treatment.

4. **J Vestibular neuronitis**

    Vestibular neuronitis is a self-limiting syndrome of paroxysmal vertigo
    which may be associated with viral infections. It causes peripheral
    vestibular failure, the features of which include horizontal/rotatory
    conjugate and fatiguable nystagmus. The lesion may be associated with
    debris from damage to the utricle, collecting on the cupula of the
    posterior semicircular canal. Treatment includes vestibular sedatives and
    head exercises. Central lesions affecting the vestibular nuclei
    (cerebrovascular accident, multiple sclerosis, encephalitis, syringobulbia)
    produce both horizontal and vertical nystagmus, and multidirectional,
    dysconjugate nystagmus, often without vertigo.

5. **D Cerebellar infarction**

    This patient has a left cerebellar syndrome. Unilateral cerebellar lesions
    cause falls to the affected side, together with ipsilateral limb ataxia
    (dysdiadochokinesis, dysmetria). There is also nystagmus and dysarthria.
    In this patient with arteriopathy, the most likely cause is a cerebellar
    infarction.

Causes of cerebrospinal fluid (CSF) abnormalities

A   Bacterial meningitis
B   Benign intracranial hypertension
C   Cysticercosis
D   Encephalitis
E   Guillain–Barré syndrome
F   Multiple sclerosis
G   Subarachnoid haemorrhage
H   Tuberculous meningitis
I   Tumour
J   Vasculitis
K   Viral meningitis

For each presentation below, choose the SINGLE most likely cause from the above list of options. Each option may be used once, more than once, or not at all.

1. A 45-year-old man presents with increasing weakness of his arms and legs together with breathlessness. He is areflexic. His cerebrospinal fluid cell count is normal but the protein is raised at 1.5 g/L.

2. A 35-year-old woman presents with a 3-month history of intermittent diplopia, blurring of vision and paraesthesia in the legs. Cerebrospinal fluid reveals the presence of oligoclonal bands.

3. A 28-year-old woman is admitted with a severe headache and blurring of vision. She is overweight and is on the oral contraceptive pill. Fundoscopy reveals papilloedema. Computerized tomography (CT) of the brain is normal. Lumbar puncture is normal apart from the opening CSF pressure of 350 mm.

4. A 57-year-old man had a sudden, severe occipital headache 12 hours ago. His computerized tomography (CT) of the brain is normal. There is evidence of xanthochromia in his cerebrospinal fluid.

5. A 38-year-old woman presents with a chronic headache and lethargy and a 12-day history of diplopia and photophobia. The CSF contains 200 cells/mm^3 half of which are neutrophils and the other half lymphocytes. The protein is elevated at 1.5 g/L, and glucose reduced at 1.6 mmol/L. There are no organisms identified on Gram-staining.

Answers to **1.43**

1. **E**   Guillain–Barré syndrome

Guillain–Barré syndrome is characterized by a demyelinating polyneuropathy which may be preceded by an infection with an enterovirus, Epstein–Barr virus, Mycoplasma, HIV or *Campylobacter jejuni*. There may be the features of an ascending paralysis, distal paraesthesia and autonomic disturbance. The CSF protein is often elevated to between 1–3 g/L. Spirometry is essential to monitor the involvement of respiratory musculature. Plasma exchange or high-dose intravenous immunoglobulin may be used in those severely affected to improve the rate of recovery.

2. **F**   Multiple sclerosis

Multiple sclerosis is characterized by areas of demyelination disseminated in time and place within the brain and spinal cord. Oligoclonal bands in the CSF, a finding that indicates a production of immunoglobulin to unknown antigens in the central nervous system, occur in more than 90% of cases. MRI scanning of the brain is the first-line investigation for detecting demyelinating plaques especially in the periventricular region and brain stem.

3. **B**   Benign intracranial hypertension

Benign intracranial hypertension is the syndrome of raised intracranial pressure in the absence of mass effect or increase in ventricular size. It mainly affects obese, young women. Headache is the most common symptom with papilloedema present in virtually all cases. Permanent visual loss occurs in up to 50% of cases due to optic nerve damage. The CSF is normal but the opening pressure is greater than 200 mm CSF.

4. **G**   Subarachnoid haemorrhage

The history is suggestive of a subarachnoid haemorrhage. Xanthochromia (from oxyhaemoglobin and bilirubin) with CSF protein <1.5 g/L usually indicates a subarachnoid or intracerebral haemorrhage. Angiography is needed to determine the site of haemorrhage.

5. **H**   Tuberculous meningitis

Tuberculous meningitis is likely in view of the elevated CSF protein, mixed cellular response and a chronic illness with a recent neurological deficit. The differential diagnosis would have to include a partially treated bacterial meningitis. Viral meningitis usually develops more rapidly and the CSF glucose is usually normal except in some cases of mumps or herpes simplex/zoster meningoencephalitis.

Causes of gout

A	Chronic myeloid leukaemia
B	Chronic renal failure
C	Diuretics
D	Ethambutol
E	Hyperparathyroidism
F	Lesch–Nyhan syndrome
G	Myeloma
H	Polycythaemia rubra vera
I	Pyrazinamide
J	Sarcoidosis
K	Secondary polycythaemia

For each presentation below, choose the SINGLE most likely cause from the above list of options. Each option may be used once, more than once, or not at all.

1. A 19-year-old man presents with gouty arthritis, spasticity and choreoathetosis. He has a history of worsening behavioural problems with a recurring tendency of biting his fingers and lips that has been present for several years.

2. A 66-year-old man complains of a painful right knee, tiredness, abdominal discomfort and weight loss. On examination, he is pale and has an enlarged spleen reaching below the umbilicus. His uric acid level is elevated.

3. A normally fit 56-year-old man develops gout after several weeks of antituberculous treatment. His night sweats have resolved and his dry cough has eased considerably.

4. A 76-year-old woman presents with severe pain in her right ankle and the first metatarsophalangeal joint. She also complains of pruritus and headaches. The haematocrit, red cell mass, white blood cells, platelets and neutrophil alkaline phosphatase score are all increased.

5. A 75-year-old man with controlled hypertension on antihypertensive therapy presents with an inflamed, painful right knee joint. He has hyperuricaemia and the aspirate from the joint shows negatively birefringent needle-shaped urate crystals under light microscopy.

Answers to **1.44**

1. F   Lesch–Nyhan syndrome

Lesch–Nyhan syndrome is due to a deficiency of HPRT (hypoxanthine-guanine phosphoribosyl transferase), which is associated with purine overproduction, hyperuricaemia and gout. There are also neurological features including choreoathetosis, spasticity, mental deficiency and behavioural disturbance (particularly self-mutilation). It is an X-linked recessive disorder. Gouty arthritis usually occurs after puberty and before the age of 20 years.

2. A   Chronic myeloid leukaemia

Chronic myeloid leukaemia, like many myeloid and lymphoid proliferative disorders, is associated with an increased cell and nucleic acid turnover resulting in an increased urate production. The symptoms of the associated anaemia and splenomegaly (abdominal discomfort) are insidious. Acute gouty attacks are usually precipitated during treatment due to the increased white cell destruction.

3. I   Pyrazinamide

Tuberculosis (TB) is treated in two phases. At least three drugs (isoniazid, pyrazinamide and rifampicin) should be used during the initial phase which lasts 2 months with respiratory TB. Ethambutol is omitted if there is a low risk of resistance to isoniazid, i.e. those not previously treated for TB and patients who are not immunocompromised. Pyrazinamide causes hyperuricaemia and secondary gouty arthritis. The continuation phase lasts a further 4 months with isoniazid and rifampicin.

4. H   Polycythaemia rubra vera

This patient is likely to have primary (polycythaemia rubra vera) rather than secondary polycythaemia because of the raised white blood cells, platelets and neutrophil alkaline phosphatase score. Clinical features of polycythaemia include a plethoric appearance, headaches, pruritus, bleeding, hypertension, gout and peptic ulcers. Polycythaemia is confirmed by finding a raised red cell mass.

5. C   Diuretics

This patient is probably on a thiazide diuretic for hypertension. This causes hyperuricaemia and acute gout by reducing renal uric acid excretion. Furosemide (frusemide) also causes hyperuricaemia but its mechanism is through dehydration and not by directly inhibiting urate excretion.

Diagnosis of lung tumours

A   Adenocarcinoma
B   Carcinoid tumour
C   Hamartoma
D   Kaposi's sarcoma
E   Leiomyoma
F   Mesothelioma
G   Metastases
H   Pancoast's tumour
I   Small-cell carcinoma
J   Squamous-cell carcinoma
K   Teratoma

For each presentation below, choose the SINGLE most likely type of tumour from the above list of options. Each option may be used once, more than once, or not at all.

1. A 74-year-old retired worker in a shipbuilding yard, who has been a life-long non-smoker, presents with a cough and loss of 3 kg in weight during the past 3 months. An X-ray of the chest shows a subpleural mass in the right upper zone.

2. A 45-year-old teacher who smokes 20 cigarettes a day presents with haemoptysis and weight loss. He has clubbing of the fingers and a mass in the right mid-zone on the chest X-ray. His corrected serum calcium is elevated at 2.97 mmol/L.

3. A 71-year-old retired dockworker complains of dull, right-sided chest pain and breathlessness. The chest X-ray shows some right-sided irregular pleural thickening and a small pleural effusion.

4. A 54-year-old housewife presents with weight loss and malaise. She has severe hyponatraemia with a serum sodium level of 115 mmol/L. There is radiological evidence of mediastinal lymphadenopathy.

5. A 56-year-old machinist is referred with an abnormal chest X-ray that shows numerous rounded shadows of varying sizes in both lung fields.

Answers to **1.45**

1.   A   Adenocarcinoma

Adenocarcinomas arise in the periphery of the lungs from the mucous glands of small bronchi. They may be seen as a subpleural mass. They account for about 10% of all bronchial carcinomas. They are commoner in women and non-smokers, particularly those who have been exposed to asbestos (as this patient has who previously worked in shipbuilding) and who do not have clinically identifiable asbestosis.

2.   J   Squamous-cell carcinoma

Finger clubbing occurs in up to 30% of lung cancers (mainly with squamous-cell carcinomas and occasionally adenocarcinomas). Hypercalcaemia is usually due to bone metastases. There is non-metastatic hypercalcaemia due to the production of parathyroid hormone-related peptides in about 6% of patients with squamous-cell carcinoma.

3.   F   Mesothelioma

Mesothelioma (due to previous asbestos exposure) is most frequently diagnosed between 50–70 years of age. It commonly presents with dull chest pain, breathlessness, weight loss and cough. As the tumour progresses there is irregular lobulated pleural thickening better seen on computerized tomography (CT) of the chest. The average latent period between first exposure to asbestos and death from mesothelioma is between 20–40 years.

4.   I   Small-cell carcinoma

Paraneoplastic syndromes including the syndrome of inappropriate secretion of ADH (SIADH) occur in up to 10% of patients with small-cell lung carcinomas. This patient's low serum sodium level together with the radiological picture suggests that she has SIADH associated with a small-cell carcinoma of the lung. Small cell carcinomas metastasize early via the lymphatics and blood stream.

5.   G   Metastases

Tumours from the gastrointestinal tract, prostate, breast, kidney and bladder often metastasize to the lung. Typically these lesions are multiple, vary in size, are rounded and well-defined. As with primary lung tumours, metastatic lesions need to be at least 1 cm to be visible on the chest X-ray.

Diagnosis of lymphadenopathy

A   Brucellosis
B   Chronic lymphatic leukaemia
C   Cytomegalovirus (CMV)
D   Hodgkin's lymphoma
E   Human immunodeficiency virus (HIV) infection
F   Infectious mononucleosis
G   Metastases
H   Non-Hodgkin's lymphoma
I   Sarcoidosis
J   Toxoplasmosis
K   Tuberculosis

For each presentation below, choose the SINGLE most likely cause from the above list of options. Each option may be used once, more than once, or not at all.

1. A 27-year-old woman presents with fever, rigors, pneumonitis and lymphadenopathy. She is neutropenic following recent chemotherapy for acute myeloid leukaemia. Fundoscopy shows retinitis with a 'scrambled egg and tomato sauce' appearance.

2. A 56-year-old man presents with weight loss and haemoptysis. Examination reveals supraclavicular lymphadenopathy, finger clubbing and a right pleural effusion.

3. A promiscuous 20-year-old man returns from holiday in the Far East and presents with malaise, fever, sore throat, myalgia and generalized lymphadenopathy. There is lymphocytosis but the Paul–Bunnell test is negative.

4. A 75-year-old man complains of tiredness and lethargy. Examination reveals lymphadenopathy and hepatosplenomegaly. Numerous small lymphocytes and smear cells are present in the blood film.

5. A 35-year-old woman presents with fever and painful lesions on her shins. Her chest X-ray shows bilateral hilar lymphadenopathy.

Answers to **1.46**

1.   C   Cytomegalovirus (CMV)

CMV infection is usually asymptomatic in healthy individuals but may cause an infectious mononucleosis-like illness with fever, hepatitis and lymphocytosis. A high proportion of immunodeficient patients with renal/bone marrow transplants or AIDS (particularly when the CD4+ level <50/μL) develop active CMV infection and this can cause encephalitis, retinitis with a characteristic appearance as in this patient, pneumonitis and gastrointestinal complications.

2.   G   Metastases

This patient has bronchogenic carcinoma with metastases to the cervical lymph nodes. Finger clubbing is mainly associated with squamous-cell carcinomas occurring in up to 30% of cases.

3.   E   Human immunodeficiency virus (HIV) infection

This patient could have cytomegalovirus infection, but the history of sexual promiscuity suggests human immunodeficiency virus (HIV) infection. The risk of contracting HIV from one unprotected sexual act is 1 in 1000 for penile–vaginal sex, and may be 30 times higher for receptive penile–anal sex. The majority of HIV seroconversions are asymptomatic, but some may be accompanied by a non-specific illness. Chronic infection then follows with one-third of patients developing persistent generalized lymphadenopathy.

4.   B   Chronic lymphatic leukaemia

Chronic lymphatic leukaemia (CLL) occurs mainly in older people and is due to an uncontrolled proliferation and accumulation of mature B lymphocytes (rarely T cells). Lymphocytosis is defined as white blood cells $>15 \times 10^9$/L of which 40% are lymphocytes. It may lead to painless lymphadenopathy, hepatosplenomegaly, anaemia (autoimmune haemolysis/bone marrow failure), thrombocytopenia and infections (neutropenia with or without reduced immunoglobulins). A blood film normally shows lymphocytes and smear cells.

5.   I   Sarcoidosis

Sarcoidosis is a multisystem, non-caseating, granulomatous disease most commonly affecting young adults between the ages of 20 and 35 years. The presence of erythema nodosum and bilateral hilar lymphadenopathy are almost diagnostic of acute sarcoidosis (Lofgren's syndrome), which is associated with a good prognosis.

Diagnosis of arthropathy

A   Ankylosing spondylitis
B   Behçet's syndrome
C   Enteropathic synovitis
D   Juvenile chronic arthritis
E   Lyme disease
F   Osteoarthrosis
G   Psoriasis
H   Reiter's syndrome
I   Rheumatoid arthritis
J   Systemic lupus erythematosus
K   Whipple's disease

For each presentation below, choose the SINGLE most likely cause from the above list of options. Each option may be used once, more than once, or not at all.

1. A 45-year-old man presents with a 2-year history of recurrent, fleeting arthritis and a peripheral neuropathy. There is evidence of a symmetrical, erosive polyarthritis. He distinctly recalls being unwell at the onset with malaise, myalgia, lymphadenopathy and a painful rash over his thigh.

2. A 30-year-old man complains of a 2-week period of pain in his knees and right ankle. He has also noticed mild dysuria and a urethral discharge. Examination reveals mild conjunctivitis and a circinate balanitis.

3. A 60-year-old woman presents with arthritis particularly affecting her hands, lower back and knees. Her fingers show Heberden's and Bouchard's nodes.

4. A 55-year-old man has a stooped posture with a protruberant abdomen and back pain. His chest expansion is reduced and there is clinical evidence of apical lung fibrosis and aortic regurgitation.

5. A 45-year-old man presents with recurrent, painful oral and genital ulcers, arthritis, recurrent thrombophlebitis of the lower limb veins and relapsing uveitis.

Answers to **1.47**

1.   E   Lyme disease

Lyme disease is a tick-borne spirochaetal infection caused by *Borrelia burgdorferi*, transmitted primarily by Ixodes ticks. It is a multisystemic disease affecting skin, joints (can mimic rheumatoid arthritis), central nervous system (meningoencephalitis, peripheral neuropathy and lymphocytic meningoradiculitis) and heart (atrioventricular block, pericarditis, myocarditis and heart failure). Early disease is characterized by an expanding painful rash (erythema chronicum migrans) accompanied by lymphadenopathy, malaise, fever and myalgia.

2.   H   Reiter's syndrome

Reiter's syndrome is a triad of arthritis (HLA-B27 present in 60% cases), non-specific urethritis and conjunctivitis which may follow a gastrointestinal infection or venereal disease. Circinate balanitis is rare (a superficial penile lesion with a pale centre surrounded by erythema). Acute anterior uveitis and keratoderma blenorrhagica (affecting the soles of the feet and sometimes the palms and resembling pustular psoriasis) is present in 10% cases.

3.   F   Osteoarthrosis

Osteoarthrosis (OA) is a disease of the cartilage. There is radiological evidence of narrowing of the joint space, osteophyte formation, sclerosis and cyst formation of the underlying bone. There are often bony swellings at the distal interphalangeal joints of the hands (Heberden's nodes) and also at the proximal interphalangeal joints (Bouchard's nodes).

4.   A   Ankylosing spondylitis

Ankylosing spondylitis affects young adults (male:female 5:1), presenting with an insidious onset of back pain, early morning stiffness and radiological evidence of sacroiliitis. Extra-articular manifestations include apical lung fibrosis, cardiac conduction defects, iritis, aortic regurgitation, traumatic fracture of the rigid spine and secondary amyloidosis.

5.   B   Behçet's syndrome

Behçet's syndrome is a recurrent multifocal disorder characterized by orogenital ulceration, polyarthritis, and iritis. There may also be recurrent thrombophlebitis, neurological features (multiple sclerosis-like features, strokes and meningoencephalitis), erythema nodosum and epididymo-orchitis.

Diagnosis of neurological lesions

A   Anterior horn cell disease (motor neurone disease)
B   Autonomic neuropathy
C   Brachial plexus lesion
D   Cauda equina lesion
E   Cord compression
F   Median nerve lesion
G   Multiple sclerosis (demyelination)
H   Peripheral neuropathy
I   Radial nerve lesion
J   Sciatic nerve lesion
K   Ulnar nerve lesion

For each presentation below, choose the SINGLE most likely cause from the above list of options. Each option may be used once, more than once, or not at all.

1. A 38-year-old pregnant woman complains of a tingling sensation in her hands that is worse at night. There is no loss of muscle bulk in the hands but the Tinel and Phalen signs are positive.

2. A 72-year-old woman presents with a bilateral foot drop and a spastic weakness with fasciculation in the muscles of her legs. Recently, she has had recurrent chest infections. Her tongue is wasted with fasciculations.

3. A 55-year-old man complains of left shoulder pain and weight loss. There is evidence of meiosis and a partial ptosis of his left eye.

4. A 70-year-old diabetic man complains of impotence and intermittent vomiting, with abdominal distension after eating. He also has evidence of postural hypotension.

5. A 75-year-old man complains of bilateral lower limb weakness, numbness and urinary incontinence. His knee and ankle reflexes are absent. There is loss of sensation in the saddle area.

Answers to **1.48**

1. **F** Median nerve lesion

This patient has bilateral carpal tunnel syndrome. Tinel's sign is tingling in the distribution of the median nerve on percussion over the nerve at the wrist, and Phalen's sign is exacerbation of paraesthesiae on flexion of the wrists for 60 seconds and which is relieved when the wrists are straightened. Causes include pregnancy, the oral contraceptive pill, myxoedema, acromegaly, rheumatoid arthritis, amyloidosis and idiopathic (particularly in middle-aged women).

2. **A** Anterior horn cell disease (motor neurone disease)

Motor neurone disease is associated with degeneration of the motor neurones and somatic motor nuclei of the cranial nerves and within the cortex. There are three patterns – progressive muscular atrophy, amyotrophic lateral sclerosis and progressive bulbar palsy. The diagnosis is usually made on clinical grounds (diffuse muscular wasting with fasciculation). Denervation can be confirmed on electromyography.

3. **C** Brachial plexus lesion

This patient has a left Horner's syndrome from a Pancoast's tumour which compresses the sympathetic fibres (from T1 and T2) as they travel upwards to the superior cervical ganglion and then to the dilator pupillae as the long ciliary nerve. Carcinomas at the apex of the lung can erode the ribs and the lower part of the brachial plexus (C8, T1, T2) causing pain in the shoulder and the medial surface of the arm.

4. **B** Autonomic neuropathy

This diabetic man has impotence, postural hypotension and gastroparesis from autonomic neuropathy secondary to the diabetes mellitus. Other features include diarrhoea/steatorrhoea (due to bacterial overgrowth) and an atonic, distended bladder.

5. **D** Cauda equina lesion

Compression of the cauda equina causes bilateral leg weakness, loss of sphincter control (compression of sacral fibres) and impotence. There is loss of sensation over the sacral dermatomes (saddle area of buttocks and perineum) and loss of the ankle and anal reflexes. Causes include central lumbar disc protrusion, tumour and spondylolisthesis. Urgent surgery is required to ensure neurological recovery and to prevent permanent damage.

Diagnosis of skin lesions

A   Dermatitis herpetiformis
B   Eczema
C   Erythema multiforme
D   Erythema nodosum
E   Lichen planus
F   Pemphigoid
G   Pemphigus
H   Pityriasis versicolor
I   Pretibial myxoedema
J   Psoriasis
K   Pyoderma gangrenosum

For each patient below, choose the SINGLE most likely diagnosis from the
above list of options. Each option may be used once, more than once, or
not at all.

1. A 72-year-old woman complains of a 6-month history of tense blisters
    forming over the trunk and lower limbs. There are no lesions in the
    mouth.

2. A 45-year-old man presents with a 1-year history of pruritus.
    Examination reveals widespread excoriations with groups of vesicles,
    most of which are ruptured. He is on a gluten-free diet.

3. A 23-year-old woman has a severe sore throat and also painful, raised
    red lesions on the front of her shins.

4. A 30-year-old woman has a long history of plaque-like lesions with
    silvery scales on the extensor aspects of her elbows and also has diffuse
    pitting of her nails.

5. A 40-year-old woman has noticed elevated skin lesions with a peau
    d'orange appearance over her lower legs. She has a history of a
    thyroidectomy and examination reveals that she is euthyroid with
    exophthalmos.

Answers to **1.49**

1. F Pemphigoid

The site of the blister is at the basement membrane *between* the epidermis and the dermis (unlike pemphigus where the site is *in* the epidermis); therefore the blisters are less likely to rupture. Mucosal lesions are uncommon in pemphigoid, which affects mostly elderly patients (60–80 years). Biopsy shows IgG and complement in the basement membrane zone. Treatment is with systemic steroids and azathioprine for its steroid-sparing effect.

2. A Dermatitis herpetiformis

Dermatitis herpetiformis occurs mainly between 20 and 50 years of age and is almost always associated with coeliac disease. The vesicles occur in groups and are intensely pruritic with a burning sensation. Direct immunofluorescence showing IgA deposits in unaffected skin is diagnostic. Treatment is with a gluten-free diet and dapsone.

3. D Erythema nodosum

Erythema nodosum is an acute panniculitis that produces painful nodules on the shins. A streptococcal throat infection is the cause in this case. Other important causes include sarcoidosis, inflammatory bowel disease, rheumatic fever, tuberculosis, pregnancy, leprosy and drugs (sulphonamides, oral contraceptives).

4. J Psoriasis

There is a ten-fold increase in the speed of epidermal cell proliferation in psoriasis. The commonest type is plaque psoriasis. Others include guttate psoriasis, palmar and plantar psoriasis, flexural psoriasis and pustular psoriasis. Pitting of the nails and onycholysis are characteristic findings.

5. I Pretibial myxoedema

Pretibial myxoedema occurs in about 5% of patients with Graves' disease. In many cases, it appears several months after a patient has been rendered euthyroid with surgery or radioiodine. The superficial layer of the skin is infiltrated with hyaluronic acid (mucopolysaccharide). Classically, it is associated with acropachy and exophthalmos. Intralesional steroids may be used to treat it.

Causes of sexually transmitted diseases

A   *Chlamydia trachomatis*
B   *Gardnerella vaginalis*
C   *Haemophilus ducreyi*
D   Hepatitis A and B
E   Herpes simplex
F   Human papillomavirus
G   Molloscum contagiosum
H   *Neisseria gonorrhoea*
I   *Treponema pallidum*
J   *Trichomonas vaginalis*
K   *Ureaplasma urealyticum*

For each presentation below, choose the SINGLE most likely cause from the above list of options. Each option may be used once, more than once, or not at all.

1. A 45-year-old man presents with a flu-like illness, dysuria and severe pain around his penis. He is married and denies having any extramarital affairs. On examination, there are multiple painful penile vesicles and shallow ulceration with tender inguinal lymphadenopathy.

2. A 35-year-old woman complains of an excessive, offensive vaginal discharge. Examination reveals a frothy yellow-green discharge and erythematous vaginal walls. The cervix has multiple small haemorrhages.

3. A 45-year-old man presents with a painless, firm ulcer on his glans penis that has developed rapidly from a papule. He also has painless inguinal lymphadenopathy. He has a partner but admits to having sexual contact with prostitutes.

4. A 26-year-old woman has noticed warts developing on her vulva and perianal region. She is otherwise asymptomatic and remains well.

5. A 40-year-old man presents with a painless penile ulcer and painful inguinal lymphadenopathy. He has recently returned from a holiday in the Far East. Examination reveals tender, fluctuant lymph nodes some of which have ruptured.

Answers to 1.50

1. E   Herpes simplex

Genital herpes is most frequently caused by herpes simplex virus type 2.
Primary infection is associated with flu-like symptoms, anorexia, fever
and bilateral inguinal lymphadenopathy. In men, initial infection is
often associated with painful vesiculation and ulceration on the glans
penis and the prepuce of the penile shaft. The incubation period varies
between 2–14 days after exposure and attacks can last 20 days.
Recurrent attacks tend to be shorter and less severe.

2. J   Trichomonas vaginalis

Trichomonas vaginalis is a flagellated protozoon which causes excessive
vaginal discharge and local irritation in up to half of infected women.
Infection in males is usually asymptomatic. A strawberry cervix is
the most specific sign for trichomoniasis. Treatment is with
metronidazole.

3. I   Treponema pallidum

Syphilis is caused by *T. pallidum*, a motile spirochaete, which has an
incubation period of 3 weeks. The early stages of acquired syphilis
include a painless chancre with painless regional lymphadenopathy. The
secondary phase (4–10 weeks later) includes fever, sore throat,
arthralgia, generalized lymphadenopathy, skin rash, condylomata lata
(highly infectious plaque-like lesions found in warm, moist areas) and
snail-track ulcers in the mouth and on the genitalia. The late stages of
infection (tertiary phase, after latent period of many years) is
characterized by gumma formation (chronic granulomatous lesions)
which affect bone, viscera, central nervous system and the aorta.

4. F   Human papillomavirus

Anogenital warts are caused mainly by human papillomavirus types 6
and 11 and are the most commonly acquired sexual infection. Half of
women with vulval warts have human papillomavirus infection of the
cervix which is associated with cervical intraepithelial neoplasia.
Cryotherapy, electrocautery or laser therapy may be needed.

5. A   Chlamydia trachomatis

Chlamydia trachomatis types 1, 2 and 3 cause lymphogranuloma
venereum which is endemic in Southeast Asia. It produces a painless
ulcerating papule, painful swelling of the inguinal, femoral and iliac
lymph nodes, and an anorectal syndrome with ulcerative proctitis and
perirectal abscesses. Complications include rectal stricture, genital
elephantiasis and acute meningoencephalitis.

Diagnosis of genetic disorders

A   Fanconi syndrome
B   Friedreich's ataxia
C   Haemochromatosis
D   Haemophilia A
E   Huntington's chorea
F   Myotonic dystrophy
G   Lesch–Nyhan syndrome
H   Osler–Weber–Rendu syndrome
I   Peutz–Jeghers syndrome
J   Tuberous sclerosis
K   Von Recklinghausen's disease

For each scenario below, choose the SINGLE most likely cause from the above list of options. Each option may be used once, more than once, or not at all.

1. A 17-year-old boy presents with compulsive behavioural problems and intermittent episodes of self-mutilation. The mother recalls a normal child at birth but he was late in his development, and she is concerned that he is now mentally retarded. There is evidence of choreoathetosis and spasticity.

2. A 45-year-old man has bilateral ptosis and frontal balding. He complains of generalized weakness particularly of his hands. There is wasting and weakness of his limbs and slow relaxation of his handgrip. His past medical history includes ischaemic heart disease, diabetes and hypertension.

3. A 65-year-old man presents with recurrent severe epistaxes, which are hard to control even with nasal packing. He has telangiectasia on his face, lips, tongue and the buccal and nasal mucosa. He has a chronic iron deficiency anaemia, requiring regular blood transfusion.

4. A 45-year-old man presents with colicky abdominal pain. His wife is concerned that he may be depressed because of the recurrent nature of his pain. He has brownish-black macules on his lips, buccal pigmentation and also a laparotomy scar from a previous bowel operation.

5. A 60-year-old man has a long history of epilepsy. There are papules in the nasolabial fold, sub-ungual fibromas and plaque-like lesions on his lower back. His seizures are well controlled with phenytoin.

Answers to 1.51

1. G   Lesch–Nyhan syndrome

Lesch–Nyhan syndrome is an X-linked recessive disorder with mental retardation and behavioural problems characterized by self-mutilation. There is also pyramidal and extrapyramidal involvement producing spasticity and choreoathetosis, which is unique to this disorder.

2. F   Myotonic dystrophy

This is an autosomal dominantly inherited disorder characterized by myotonia (delayed voluntary relaxation of muscles), wasting of the masseters, temporal muscles and distal musculature with other features including frontal baldness, cataracts, cardiomyopathy, diabetes, testicular atrophy and varying degrees of mental impairment. The condition is clinically overt between the ages of 20–50 years. The signs and symptoms may get worse with successive generations.

3. H   Osler–Weber–Rendu syndrome

Osler–Weber–Rendu syndrome or familial haemorrhagic telangiectasia is inherited as an autosomal dominant disorder, and is the most common genetic cause of vascular bleeding. It is characterized by bleeding from telangiectasia (collections of non-contractile capillaries) and presents with epistaxis, gastrointestinal haemorrhage, haemoptysis or iron deficiency anaemia. Pulmonary arteriovenous malformations may occur.

4. I   Peutz–Jeghers syndrome

Peutz-Jeghers syndrome consists of mucocutaneous pigmentation and gastrointestinal polyposis (single or multiple hamartomatous polyps in the small and large bowel). It is inherited as an autosomal dominant disorder. Complications include recurrent abdominal pain, intestinal obstruction or intussusception, iron deficiency anaemia and malignant transformation of a polyp.

5. J   Tuberous sclerosis

Tuberous sclerosis is characterized by epilepsy, mental retardation (in about two-thirds of cases) facial angiofibromas and the presence of hamartomata (excessive growth of normal cells) of the skin, kidneys, retina, heart, lungs, bone and the central nervous system. It is inherited as an autosomal dominant disorder with features including shagreen patches, hypopigmented macules (ash leaf spots) and subungual fibromata.

Diagnosis of vitamin and mineral deficiencies

A	Copper
B	Niacin
C	Riboflavin
D	Selenium
E	Thiamine (Vitamin B$_1$)
F	Vitamin A
G	Vitamin B$_{12}$
H	Vitamin C
I	Vitamin D
J	Vitamin K
K	Zinc

For each presentation below, choose the SINGLE most likely cause from the above list of options. Each option may be used once, more than once, or not at all.

1. A 38-year-old vagrant presents with poor night vision and dryness of the eyes. He has had recurrent conjunctivitis and corneal ulceration.

2. A 45-year-old alcoholic is admitted with confusion, ataxia and ophthalmoplegia. He is thin and wasted.

3. A 70-year-old widower presents with confusion, diarrhoea and dermatitis. He lives alone and has little social contact.

4. A 40-year-old alcoholic presents with breathlessness for the last 4 months with orthopnoea and leg oedema. He also complains of pains and tenderness in his feet and calves. Chest X-ray shows cardiomegaly and small bilateral pleural effusions.

5. An 80-year-old nursing home resident is admitted with bony and muscular pain and a proximal myopathy. An X-ray of her pelvis reveals Looser's zones.

Answers to **1.52**

1. **F   Vitamin A**

    The clinical features of vitamin A deficiency are impaired night vision, dryness of the cornea (xerophthalmia), and corneal ulceration with frequent infections. Untreated deficiency causes blindness from corneal destruction (keratomalacia) and retinal dysfunction. There may also be thickening and dryness of the skin (follicular hyperkeratosis). A good response to replacement therapy would confirm the diagnosis.

2. **E   Thiamine (Vitamin B₁)**

    This patient has Wernicke's encephalopathy (acute confusion, nystagmus, ataxia, variable ophthalmoplegia) from thiamine deficiency. If untreated, it will lead to irreversible neurological damage.

3. **B   Niacin**

    This man has the classical triad (3Ds – dementia, diarrhoea and dermatitis) of pellagra (niacin deficiency). This is rare except in socially deprived individuals and has also been described in patients whose diet is virtually based on maize (niacin in the form of niacytin that is not bioavailable). It can also occur with isoniazid treatment, malabsorption, starvation, carcinoid syndrome and phaeochromocytoma.

4. **E   Thiamine (Vitamin B₁)**

    Thiamine deficiency can produce wet beri-beri (cardiomyopathy) with peripheral oedema, pleural effusion and ascites. There is impaired glucose metabolism with accumulation of lactate and pyruvate resulting in vasodilatation and oedema. Cardiac muscle is also affected resulting in congestive heart failure. There may be co-existing dry beri-beri (distal motor-sensory neuropathy) with aching in the extremities, cutaneous hyperaesthesia, tenderness of the soles of the feet and eventually a peripheral neuropathy. Thiamine deficiency is confirmed by a reduced erythrocyte transketolase activity which needs thiamine as a co-factor.

5. **I   Vitamin D**

    Osteomalacia is caused by a defect in vitamin D metabolism or its availability resulting in an inadequate mineralization of the osteoid. Hence the bones are soft and prone to subclinical fractures. There is often a proximal myopathy with a characteristic waddling gait. In this case, there may be inadequate sunlight exposure due to poor mobility, i.e. from being confined indoors. X-rays show defective bone mineralization – loss of bone density, thinning of the trabeculae and cortex and Looser's zones (pseudofractures consisting of short, lucent bands running through the cortex at right angles).

Infection by opportunistic organisms

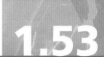

1.53

A Candida
B Cryptococcus
C Cryptosporidiosis
D Cytomegalovirus
E Herpes simplex
F Histoplasmosis
G *Pneumocystis carinii*
H Polyoma virus
I Toxoplasmosis
J Tuberculosis
K Varicella zoster

For each presentation, choose the SINGLE most likely causative organism from the above list of options. Each option may be used once, more than once, or not at all.

1. A 23-year-old patient with AIDS presents with general malaise, fever and seizures. Computerized tomography (CT) of the head shows several ring-enhancing lesions with surrounding oedema.

2. A 45-year-old man with AIDS complains of blurring of vision and 'floaters'. Fundoscopy shows retinitis with irregular white patches in the retina with haemorrhages.

3. A 35-year-old intravenous drug abuser is admitted with a dry cough, fever and breathlessness. His chest X-ray shows bilateral perihilar haze and silver-staining of bronchial lavage confirmed the diagnosis.

4. A 42-year-old woman with AIDS has had chronic, intermittent diarrhoea. She now presents with right upper abdominal discomfort and fever.

5. A 35-year-old patient with AIDS develops a sore mouth and painful dysphagia which is unresponsive to proton pump inhibitors. A barium meal shows diffuse ulceration with a cobblestone appearance of the oesophageal mucosa.

Answers to **1.53**

1. **I   Toxoplasmosis**

   Cerebral toxoplasmosis is the most common CNS infection in AIDS, usually due to reactivation of toxoplasma cysts in the brain resulting in abscess formation. Treat empirically for toxoplasmosis (using pyrimethamine and sulfadiazine (sulphadiazine)) and consider a brain biopsy if there is no improvement within 7–10 days. Differential diagnoses include cerebral lymphoma, progressive multifocal leucoencephalopathy and cryptococcoma.

2. **D   Cytomegalovirus (CMV)**

   CMV retinitis is the most common cause of loss of vision, occurring at a late stage of AIDS (CD4 count <50/mm^3). It starts peripherally and progresses towards the macula to cause blindness. Initial lesions are unilateral but it spreads to the other eye in 60%. Diagnosis is clinical, based on the appearance (bushfire, scrambled egg and ketchup) and by the response to treatment, e.g. ganciclovir or foscarnet.

3. **G   *Pneumocystis carinii***

   Pneumocystis carinii is the most common opportunistic infection in AIDS. It is now thought to be a fungus although antifungal therapy is ineffective. The clinical features of *Pneumocystis carinii* pneumonia may be subtle and there is often a prodrome for up to 7 weeks before diagnosis. Classically, there is bilateral perihilar shadowing on the chest X-ray which may be normal in up to 15% of cases. The parasites found in the lungs are small cysts which divide by binary fission. They may be identified with silver stain or immunofluorescence.

4. **C   Cryptosporidiosis**

   Chronic, intermittent diarrhoea is common in HIV disease and has no obvious cause in more than half of the cases. Cryptosporidiosis is a protozoal infection spread by contaminated food or water. In healthy subjects, it causes a self-limiting gastroenteritis but in AIDS patients it causes intractable diarrhoea or cholangitis/cholecystitis.

5. **A   Candida**

   Oesophageal candidiasis causes painful dysphagia in late HIV disease. There is often an associated oral thrush and a characteristic cobblestone appearance of the oesophageal mucosa after a barium meal. Differential diagnoses includes CMV oesophagitis (associated with large, shallow ulcers) or herpes simplex oesophagitis (multiple, deep ulcers).

Ocular features of systemic disease

A Diabetes mellitus
B Graves' disease
C Hyperlipidaemia
D Hypertension
E Infective endocarditis
F Lawrence–Moon–Bardet–Biedl syndrome
G Rheumatoid arthritis
H Sarcoidosis
I Subarachnoid haemorrhage
J Systemic lupus erythematosus
K Wilson's disease

For each ocular feature below, choose the SINGLE most likely cause from the above list of options. Each option may be used once, more than once, or not at all.

1. A 35-year-old blind man has a short stature, polydactyly and obesity. Fundoscopy reveals evidence of cataracts and black pigmentation resembling bone corpuscles.

2. A 45-year-old man is admitted with a several-day history of worsening breathlessness secondary to left ventricular failure. On fundoscopy, there is evidence of arteriovenous (AV) nipping, flame-shaped haemorrhages and papilloedema.

3. A 38-year-old woman presents with a 10-hour history of severe headache of sudden onset, drowsiness and neck stiffness. She is normally fit and well. Her only medication consists of the oral contraceptive pill. Fundoscopy shows a large, well-demarcated haemorrhage in the right eye.

4. A 67-year-old woman presents with tiredness and lethargy. She has a low-grade pyrexia, sweating and breathlessness that has been present for several weeks. Amongst other clinical signs, she is found to have small retinal haemorrhages with pale centres.

5. A 40-year-old man with a tremor, dysarthria and bradykinesia has a brownish ring in the limbus of the cornea visible on slit-lamp examination. He is also jaundiced and has gynaecomastia. He is married and drinks up to 35 units of alcohol/week.

Answers to **1.54**

1. **F Lawrence–Moon–Bardet–Biedl syndrome**

    This patient has retinitis pigmentosa (RP), which is associated with cataracts, optic atrophy and tunnel vision. It may occur with the Lawrence–Moon–Bardet–Biedl syndrome, which is an autosomal recessive condition. Other features include hypogonadism, dwarfism, mental retardation, obesity and polydactyly. RP may also occur in Refsum's disease and the hereditary ataxias.

2. **D Hypertension**

    This patient has grade 4 hypertensive retinopathy (both grades 3 and 4 indicate accelerated hypertension and the need for urgent treatment). Arteriovenous (AV) nipping, or concealment of a part of the vein where it crosses an artery, occurs due to a combination of hypertension, ageing and atherosclerosis. Flame-shaped haemorrhages indicate leakage of blood from the capillary branches supplying the nerve layer, and papilloedema may be associated with cerebral oedema. Emergency treatment with intravenous labetolol or nitroprusside is indicated in the presence of left ventricular failure, hypertensive encephalopathy or aortic dissection.

3. **I Subarachnoid haemorrhage**

    Subhyaloid (preretinal where there is a large potential space) haemorrhages have a distinct margin and are pathognomonic of subarachnoid or intracerebral haemorrhage. A computerized tomography (CT) scan of the head is needed to confirm the diagnosis.

4. **E Infective endocarditis**

    Roth spots (white-centred haemorrhages) are associated with infective endocarditis, leukaemia, severe anaemia and hyperviscosity. In infective endocarditis, they are probably a result of an immune-mediated vasculitis. Histologically, they are groups of lymphocytes in the nerve layer of the retina with surrounding oedema and haemorrhage.

5. **K Wilson's disease**

    Wilson's disease usually presents between the ages of 14 to 40 years and is inherited (autosomal recessive) with the primary defect being the failure of biliary excretion of copper. Kayser–Fleischer rings are pathognomonic of Wilson's disease and are due to the deposition of copper. They are best viewed with a slit-lamp though in advanced cases can be visible to the naked eye. Other features include cirrhosis, psychosis, parkinsonism (degeneration of the basal ganglia) and chorea. Treatment is with penicillamine (a chelating agent). Liver transplantation is reserved for young patients with severe neurological and hepatic damage.

Muscle function of the upper limb

A   Abductor pollicis brevis
B   Adductor pollicis
C   Brachioradialis
D   Deltoid
E   Dorsal interossei
F   Infraspinatus
G   Latissimus dorsi
H   Lumbricals
I   Palmar interossei
J   Subscapularis
K   Supraspinatus

For each muscle action(s) below, choose the SINGLE most likely muscle involved in producing the movement from the above list of options. Each option may be used once, more than once, or not at all.

1.   Abduction of the first 30° of the shoulder.

2.   Adduction of the fingers.

3.   Flexion of the extended fingers at the metacarpophalangeal joints.

4.   Internal rotation of the shoulder.

5.   Elbow flexion when half supinated.

Answers to **1.55**

1. **K   Supraspinatus**

    Supraspinatus, supplied by the suprascapular nerve, is involved in the abduction of the first 30° of the shoulder before the deltoid muscle (supplied by axillary nerve) takes over the full abduction. The single root value for shoulder abduction is C5.

2. **I   Palmar interossei**

    The palmar interossei adduct the fingers whilst the dorsal interossei abduct. They are supplied by the ulnar nerve and have the root value of T1.

3. **H   Lumbricals**

    The medial two lumbricals are supplied by the ulnar nerve and the lateral two are supplied by the median nerve. Their combined action with the interossei is to flex the extended fingers at the metacarpophalangeal joints.

4. **J   Subscapularis**

    Subscapularis and teres minor are involved in the internal rotation of the shoulder. They are supplied by the subscapular nerve with the root value of C5. External rotation is performed by infraspinatus which is supplied by the suprascapular nerve.

5. **C   Brachioradialis**

    Brachioradialis is supplied by the radial nerve (root value C6) and it flexes at the elbow when the forearm is in the semiprone, semisupine position. Flexion with the elbow fully supinated is performed by the biceps which is supplied by the musculocutaneous nerve (root value C5).

Muscle function of the lower limb

A   Extensor digitorum brevis
B   Gastrocnemii
C   Gluteus maximus
D   Gluteus medius and minimus
E   Hamstring muscles
F   Iliacus
G   Peroneus longus and brevis
H   Peroneus tertius
I   Quadriceps
J   Tibialis anterior
K   Tibialis anterior and posterior

For each joint movement presented below, choose the SINGLE most likely muscles involved in producing the movement from the above list of options. Each option may be used once, more than once, or not at all.

1.   Knee extension.

2.   Inversion of the foot.

3.   Abduction of the hip.

4.   Plantarflexion.

5.   Hip flexion.

Answers to **1.56**

1. **I   Quadriceps**

   The knee is extended by the quadriceps muscles which are supplied by the femoral nerve (root value L2, 3, 4). The hamstrings flex the knee and are supplied by the sciatic nerve (root value L4, 5; S1, 2, 3).

2. **K   Tibialis anterior and posterior**

   Both tibialis anterior and posterior, supplied by the tibial and peroneal nerves (root value L4), produce inversion of the foot. Eversion of the foot is performed by peroneus longus and brevis, and also extensor digitorum brevis, which are supplied by the peroneal nerve (root value S1).

3. **D   Gluteus medius and minimus**

   Abduction of the hip is performed by gluteus medius and minimus which are supplied by the superior gluteal nerve (root values L4, 5). The quadriceps (supplied by the femoral nerve) are involved in adduction of the hip.

4. **B   Gastrocnemii**

   Gastrocnemii and tibialis posterior are involved in plantarflexion. They are supplied by the tibial nerve with root values S1, 2. Dorsiflexion is performed by tibialis anterior, the long extensors, peroneus tertius and extensor digitorum brevis. They are supplied by the peroneal nerve with root values L4, 5.

5. **F   Iliacus**

   Iliacus and psoas muscles flex the hip. They are supplied by the femoral nerve and psoas nerves respectively (root values L2, 3). Hip extension is performed by gluteus maximus which is supplied by the inferior gluteal nerve (root value L4, 5).

Causes of poisoning

A   Amphetamines
B   Carbon monoxide
C   Chlorpromazine
D   Chlorpropamide
E   Ethanol
F   Ferrous sulphate
G   Opiates
H   Organophosphates
I   Paracetamol
J   Salbutamol
K   Salicylates

For each presentation below, choose the SINGLE most likely drug or toxin as the poisoning agent from the above list of options. Each option may be used once, more than once, or not at all.

1. A 45-year-old accountant is admitted with agitation, paranoid delusions and hallucinations. His temperature and blood pressure are elevated and his pupils are dilated but reactive to light and accommodation.

2. A 37-year-old housewife is brought to the A&E department drowsy and incoherent. She is icteric and has spider naevi and bilateral Dupuytren's contractures. There is no flapping tremor but her breath smells of ketones.

3. A 67-year-old retired teacher is admitted with headaches, sore throat, nausea and vomiting. He has long standing chronic obstructive pulmonary disease and hypertension. His wife complains of tiredness and lethargy for the last week, ever since they arrived at their holiday caravan.

4. A 22-year-old student is found comatose in the local park. His Glasgow Coma Scale is 5/15. His pupils are pinpoint and his respiratory rate is slow (6/min).

5. A 56-year-old farmer presents with anxiety, headache, hypersalivation, sweats, abdominal colic and diarrhoea. He has hypotension and bradycardia.

Answers to **1.57**

1. **A   Amphetamines**

    Amphetamines cause excitability, euphoria, paranoia, dilated pupils (also caused by cocaine, quinine and tricyclics), hypertension and hyperthermia (also caused by theophylline, anticholinergics and monoamine oxidase inhibitors). Convulsions, rhabdomyolysis and cardiac arrhythmias may occur in severe cases. Chlorpromazine can be used for sedation, together with beta blockers to block peripheral sympathomimetic activity. Tepid sponging may be needed.

2. **E   Ethanol**

    This patient has clinical evidence of chronic liver disease. Severe ethanol intoxication may cause stupor, hypothermia, hypoglycaemia and convulsions. It can also cause coma and death from aspiration of vomitus, respiratory or circulatory failure. Ketoacidosis may occur in alcoholics who are binge drinkers due to a combination of hypoglycaemia, dehydration, increased lipolysis and ketogenesis.

3. **B   Carbon monoxide**

    It is likely that there was inadequate ventilation in their caravan when using gas appliances including the refrigerator. The man, with a limited respiratory reserve, is affected more than his wife. Carbon monoxide has a much greater affinity than oxygen for haemoglobin forming carboxyhaemoglobin. It causes tissue hypoxia.

4. **G   Opiates**

    The features of opioid overdose include non-cardiogenic pulmonary oedema, pinpoint pupils, depressed respiration, hypothermia, bradycardia, hypotension and coma. Heroin is the most commonly abused opioid which can be injected (main-lining) or inhaled (snorted or smoked). Rhabdomyolysis, hyperuricaemia and renal failure may occur. Treatment is with naloxone.

5. **H   Organophosphates**

    This farmer may have been exposed to organophosphorus compounds during crop spraying or sheep dipping. They are absorbed through the bronchi, intact skin and gut, and inhibit acetylcholinesterase activity. The clinical features are due to the muscarinic and nicotinic effects of acetylcholine. Weakness, paralysis, tachycardia, convulsions, coma, pulmonary oedema with excessive bronchial secretions and hyperglycaemia may occur.

Management of acute medical emergencies

A   Admit to a medical ward
B   Admit to the coronary care unit (CCU)
C   Admit to the intensive care unit (ICU)
D   Arrange computerized tomography (CT) of the head
E   Call police
F   Check serum urea and electrolytes and glucose
G   Discharge patient
H   Lumbar puncture
I   Refer to social services
J   Request psychiatric opinion
K   Toxicology screen

For each presentation below, choose the SINGLE most appropriate first line management from the above list of options. Each option may be used once, more than once, or not at all.

1. A 37-year-old woman presents with a sudden onset of occipital headache, photophobia and neck stiffness. She is apyrexial and there is no neurological deficit.

2. A 55-year-old man with ischaemic heart disease, who is on antianginal treatment, presents to the A&E department with an episode of angina that lasted for 15 minutes. He has had two episodes the previous day and one brief episode earlier that day. He is in a stable state and his ECG, compared with an earlier recording, shows no new changes.

3. A 36-year-old woman comes to the A&E department complaining of a pain in her infrascapular region. She had started a decorating job that day and, while stretching up to paint the wall, she suddenly developed the pain which is now exacerbated by movement and coughing. Examination shows no abnormalities and her chest X-ray is normal.

4. A 19-year-old man is brought in a drowsy state to the A&E department by his father. The father says that his son has had some problems with his girl friend but insists that there is no reason why he should have taken an overdose. Apart from a drowsy state and small but reactive pupils there is no neurological deficit.

5. A 60-year-old man comes to the A&E department after having vomited a cupful of blood. He admits to having passed dark stools the previous day. His pulse is 90/min and the BP is 150/85 mmHg. His Hb is 14 g/dl.

Answers to **1.58**

1. D   Arrange computerized tomography (CT) of the head

The presentation suggests a diagnosis of a subarachnoid haemorrhage.
CT imaging is the initial investigation of choice and should be arranged
as the patient is admitted to a medical ward. Lumbar puncture should
be considered if the CT scan is normal.

2. B   Admit to the coronary care unit (CCU)

A cluster of anginal episodes in a previously stable patient suggests
unstable angina, which is a medical emergency requiring urgent
treatment in the coronary care unit. He should be given aspirin and
heparin in addition to his antianginal therapy before his transfer. If
untreated, unstable angina will progress to acute myocardial infarction
in about 10% of cases. He will require early coronary angiography with a
view to a revascularization procedure.

3. G   Discharge patient

This patient's pain appears to be of musculoskeletal origin caused by
unaccustomed stretching of her arms. She should be reassured, given a
simple analgesic and discharged home.

4. K   Toxicology screen

It is not unusual for a loving father to think that his son could not have
taken an overdose. He should be reassured that a blood sample will not
do any harm and may prove his point. After taking blood samples for
baseline investigations (blood count, urea and electrolytes and blood
sugar) and for a toxicology screen, he should be admitted to a medical
ward for observations and further investigations, if needed.

5. A   Admit to a medical ward

This patient has had a haematemesis and melaena and will require
admission to a medical ward for a gastroscopy and possible
sclerotherapy if oesophageal varices are found to be the cause of the
bleeding. His pulse rate and blood pressure will need to be monitored
and his haemoglobin level should be checked again to see if a blood
transfusion is required.

Management of chest pain

A   Calcium channel antagonists
B   Inferior vena cava filter
C   Low molecular weight heparin
D   Non-steroidal anti-inflammatory drug (NSAID)
E   Proton pump inhibitor
F   Radiotherapy
G   Reassure
H   Streptokinase
I   Surgery
J   Tissue plasminogen activator (TPA)
K   Warfarin

For each presentation below, choose the SINGLE most appropriate course of action from the above list of options. Each option may be used once, more than once, or not at all.

1. A 56-year-old man is readmitted 2 weeks after his first myocardial infarction with further chest pain. He received streptokinase during his last admission. He now has acute ST elevation in the inferior leads.

2. A 66-year-old woman presents with gradually worsening sharp chest pain following a flu-like illness. The pain is aggravated by deep breathing and is relieved by sitting forward. She has a pericardial rub.

3. A 73-year-old man recovering from a haemorrhagic stroke develops sudden onset right pleuritic chest pain. His ventilation perfusion scan has revealed several areas of mismatch in both lung fields. Doppler venogram confirms an extensive deep vein thrombosis in the left leg.

4. A 51-year-old man presents with episodes of angina occurring at rest and during the night. During the pain there is evidence of regional ST-segment elevation. An exercise tolerance test and coronary angiography are both normal.

5. A 65-year-old woman has troublesome burning retrosternal chest pain which is not related to exertion. Gastroscopy shows severe oesophagitis.

Answers to **1.59**

1. J   Tissue plasminogen activator (TPA)

The chest pain and electrocardiographic findings suggest a further episode of acute myocardial infarction. Thrombolysis acts by activating plasminogen to form plasmin which degrades fibrin. It is highly allergenic thereby causing a big rise in antibodies which occurs within days and persists for years. These antibodies can neutralize further doses of streptokinase rendering it ineffective. It is preferable, therefore, to use tissue plasminogen activator for a recurrent myocardial infarction. It is more effective but is about ten times more expensive.

2. D   Non-steroidal anti-inflammatory drug (NSAID)

Pericarditis is characterized by chest pain, a pericardial rub and an abnormal electrocardiograph. The chest pain is characteristically relieved by sitting up or by leaning forwards. In the majority of cases there is symmetrical ST (concave upward) elevation in all leads except a Vr. Viral infections such as coxsackie group B, echovirus type 8, mumps, rubella, Epstein–Barr and varicella can cause acute pericarditis. Milder cases can respond to NSAIDs, but severe cases need a short course of steroids.

3. B   Inferior vena cava (IVC) filter

An IVC filter may be inserted to prevent pulmonary emboli when anticoagulation is contraindicated as in this case or when anticoagulation alone fails. There is no evidence that IVC filters are better than anticoagulation. Complications include perforation of the vessel wall, filter moving out of position and device failure with emboli passing through or around it.

4. A   Calcium channel antagonists

Intense vasoconstriction or vasospasm can cause focal or near occlusion of a major coronary vessel leading to transient myocardial ischaemia. It may occur in apparently normal coronary arteries or, more commonly, in atherosclerotic vessels. The mechanism of the spasm is unclear. Nitrates and calcium channel antagonists are useful when used prophylactically or for the treatment of the variant Prinzmetal's angina.

5. E   Proton pump inhibitor

Proton pump inhibitors inhibit gastric acid by blocking the proton pump of the parietal cells. They are effective in gastro-oesophageal reflux, gastric and duodenal ulceration, eradication of *Helicobacter pylori* in combination with antibacterials, and in the treatment of the Zollinger–Ellison syndrome.

Treatment of heart failure

A   Angiotensin-converting enzyme (ACE) inhibitors
B   Beta blockers
C   Biventricular pacing
D   Digoxin
E   Dobutamine
F   Exercise
G   Heart transplantation
H   Intra-aortic balloon pump
I   Intravenous furosemide (frusemide)
J   Left ventricular assisted device
K   Nitrates

For each patient below, choose the SINGLE most appropriate treatment from the above list of options. Each option may be used once, more than once, or not at all.

1. A 44-year-old male develops cardiogenic shock following an anterior myocardial infarction. He has a loud pansystolic murmur loudest at the left lower sternal edge.

2. A 28-year-old previously fit male presents with increasing shortness of breath for the last fortnight following an upper respiratory tract infection. His echocardiogram shows a cardiac ejection fraction of 15%. He feels no better on diuretics.

3. A 50-year-old female with a dilated cardiomyopathy has gradually deteriorated despite medical therapy. She is now breathless at rest and grossly oedematous.

4. An elderly male presents with sudden onset of breathlessness. His pulse is regular at 125 beats per minute and his blood pressure is 95/60 mmHg. There are bilateral basal crackles in his chest. Pulse oximetry reveals an oxygen saturation of 86%.

5. A 46-year-old male who is awaiting cardiac transplantation becomes progressively more short of breath and has had to give up some of his usual activities (NYHA Class III). He is currently on diuretics, ACE inhibitors and digoxin.

Answers to **1.60**

1. **H   Intra-aortic balloon pump**

Cardiogenic shock is due to primary left ventricular damage, and is associated with a systolic blood pressure of less than 90 mmHg, poor urine output, peripheral cyanosis, sweating and an altered sensorium. The outlook is extremely poor with a mortality of 70% following an acute myocardial infarction (MI). In this situation, mechanical support with intra-aortic balloon pumping may help by improving coronary perfusion, decreasing afterload and hence reducing myocardial oxygen consumption. It is usually reserved for those with post-MI cardiogenic shock associated with mechanical defects such as a ventricular septal rupture (as in this patient) or papillary muscle rupture, which are both amenable to surgical correction.

2. **A   Angiotensin-converting enzyme (ACE) inhibitors**

This patient most likely has a viral myocarditis with heart failure. Most of these conditions tend to improve over time but in the meanwhile will require aggressive medical therapy with diuretics and ACE inhibitors. Digoxin and beta blockers can be added if necessary. Some patients will get worse and may require referral for cardiac transplantation.

3. **G   Heart transplantation**

The mean age for referring patients for cardiac transplantation at most centres in the UK is below 60 years. In the majority of cases the indications for transplantation include ischaemic cardiomyopathy or idiopathic dilated cardiomyopathy. Transplantation is only indicated if conventional medical or surgical treatment has failed. Most centres report a 5-year survival of 75%.

4. **I   Intravenous furosemide (frusemide)**

The history is typical of acute left ventricular failure. Intravenous furosemide (frusemide) will decrease the preload by increasing the vascular capacitance and by promoting diuresis. Apart from intravenous diuretics one should also consider diamorphine, intravenous nitrates and inotropes during the acute phase.

5. **B   Beta blockers**

Beta blockers such as metoprolol, bisoprolol and carvedilol have the proven benefit of reducing morbidity, mortality and hospitalization rates in patients with clinically stable heart failure. They can also be used to buy time for those waiting for a suitable donor. They are not to be used in those with severe heart failure (NYHA class IV) or cardiogenic shock.

Management of myocardial infarction

A   Angiotensin-converting enzyme (ACE) inhibitors
B   Bisoprolol
C   Clopidogrel
D   Diamorphine
E   Digoxin
F   Dipyridamole
G   Low molecular weight heparin
H   Nitrates
I   Refer to tertiary centre for rescue angioplasty
J   Statin therapy
K   Thrombolysis

For each patient below, choose the SINGLE most appropriate treatment from the above list of options. Each option may be used once, more than once, or not at all.

1. A 46-year-old man presents with a sudden onset of chest pain that has lasted more than an hour following a game of badminton. He looks pale and unwell. His electrocardiogram shows ST segment elevation of more than 1 mm in the inferior leads.

2. A 60-year-old female is recovering well from a myocardial infarction. Her initial biochemical results have come back showing that her serum cholesterol on the day of admission to hospital was 5.7 mmol/L.

3. A 50-year-old male complains of persistent chest pain 4 hours after thrombolysis for an acute anterior myocardial infarction.

4. A 55-year-old male complains of breathlessness following a recent myocardial infarction. He has clinical evidence of mild left ventricular systolic dysfunction.

5. A 60-year-old lady is admitted feeling generally unwell with nausea and vomiting. Her electrocardiogram is consistent with a non-Q wave myocardial infarction.

Answers to **1.61**

1. **K** Thrombolysis

Thrombolysis with streptokinase or recombinant tissue plasminogen activator (rTPA) is the mainstay of therapy for an acute myocardial infarction. Contraindications include recent surgery, bleeding diathesis, active peptic ulcer, pregnancy, head injury, recent stroke and proliferative diabetic retinopathy (relative contraindication only). It is best to treat within 4–6 hours of the onset of chest pain.

2. **J** Statin therapy

Recent trials (CARE, 4S, LIPID) showed that statins (HMG CoA reductase inhibitors) should be given to patients with a total cholesterol level of more than 4.8 mmol/L for secondary prevention of vascular disease. The infarction causes an initial fall in the serum cholesterol. Hence, the cholesterol needs to be checked within 6 hours of the event or else it must be checked 12 weeks later.

3. **I** Refer to tertiary centre for rescue angioplasty

This is a case of incomplete revascularization of the infarct-related artery following thrombolysis. Ongoing chest pain with ECG changes would suggest the presence of viable myocardium. Treatment is by rescue (salvage) angioplasty with or without coronary stenting.

4. **A** Angiotensin-converting enzyme (ACE) inhibitors

ACE inhibitors are the mainstay of therapy following an acute myocardial infarction (MI) and they help in the remodeling of the ventricle. Significant benefits are observed in patients with post-MI left ventricular systolic dysfunction (SAVE, AIRE and recently HOPE studies).

5. **G** Low molecular weight heparin

A non-Q wave myocardial infarction is considered part of the acute coronary syndrome which has an impending chance of complete vessel closure. In the initial management, patients require treatment with low molecular weight heparin, aspirin and beta blockers (metoprolol or atenolol). If there is evidence of ongoing ischaemia then urgent coronary angiography may be required. Otherwise, the acute stage may be controlled with medical therapy and coronary angiography is undertaken on a semi-elective basis (preferably within 2 weeks).

Treatment of arrhythmias

A Adenosine
B Amiodarone
C Beta blockers
D Cardiac pacing
E DC cardioversion
F Disopyramide
G Flecainide
H Lidocaine (lignocaine)
I Procainamide
J Sotalol
K Verapamil

For each presentation below, choose the SINGLE most appropriate
treatment from the above list of options. Each option may be used once,
more than once, or not at all.

1. A 15-year-old girl presents to the A&E department with a sudden onset
    of narrow-complex tachycardia with a rate of 210 beats per minute. Her
    blood pressure is 98/64 mmHg.

2. A 65-year-old man has been having runs of 'torsade de pointes' (syncope
    due to short bursts of arrhythmia) during which he feels unwell. This is
    following an acute inferior myocardial infarction. His underlying heart
    rhythm is sinus bradycardia with a rate of 42 beats per minute.

3. An elderly man presents with sudden onset of giddiness and
    palpitations. His pulse is 140/min, irregularly irregular with a blood
    pressure of 76/48 mmHg. He has severe ischaemic heart disease with a
    previous myocardial infarction 2 years ago. His jugular venous pressure
    is elevated with prominent v waves. He has a third heart sound with
    bilateral basal crackles in the chest.

4. A 25-year-old asthmatic with known Wolff–Parkinson–White syndrome
    presents with a fast and irregular pulse. He feels unwell. The ECG shows
    atrial fibrillation.

5. A 40-year-old woman with a known mitral valve prolapse complains of
    palpitations. A 24-hour ECG tape shows frequent episodes of ventricular
    ectopics.

Answers to **1.62**

1. **A** **Adenosine**

This young girl has a supraventricular tachycardia (SVT) probably due to an AV nodal re-entrant dysrhythmia. Adenosine is the treatment of choice for SVT. It produces a transient AV nodal block. It is a safe drug because of its very short half-life. Side effects can include transient flushing, chest tightness due to bronchospasm and abdominal cramps.

2. **D** **Cardiac pacing**

His arrhythmia is due to a bradycardia producing a long QT interval. This can be corrected by temporary pacing.

3. **E** **DC cardioversion**

This patient is haemodynamically unstable with uncontrolled atrial fibrillation. He needs to have sinus rhythm restored quickly and this is best done by a synchronized direct current (DC) cardioversion (defibrillator to discharge 0.02 seconds after the peak of the R wave). Flecainide is used in chemical cardioversion but is contraindicated in those with heart failure, a previous myocardial infarction and significant valvular heart disease.

4. **G** **Flecainide**

Pre-excited atrial fibrillation in the Wolff–Parkinson–White syndrome is worrying due to the very fast ventricular rate associated with fast conduction through the accessory pathway. Digoxin and verapamil are contraindicated as they may paradoxically increase the ventricular rate. Flecainide is the drug of choice. The abnormal pathway should then be destroyed by radiofrequency ablation.

5. **C** **Beta blockers**

Beta blockers are useful in those with symptomatic ventricular ectopics associated with a mitral valve prolapse.

Treatment of breathlessness

A   Aminophylline
B   Amiodarone
C   Antibiotics
D   Beclometasone (beclomethasone)
E   Chest drain
F   Diamorphine
G   Diuretics
H   Pleural aspiration
I   Psychological support
J   Salbutamol
K   Warfarin

For each presentation below, choose the SINGLE most appropriate treatment from the above list of options. Each option may be used once, more than once, or not at all.

1. A 67-year-old woman with stable chronic obstructive pulmonary disease (COPD) presents with acute onset of breathlessness and sweating. Examination reveals a tachycardia with gallop rhythm and bilateral basal crepitations in her chest.

2. A 27-year-old man with no past medical history is admitted with left-sided chest pain and breathing difficulties. A chest X-ray shows a large, simple pneumothorax.

3. A 30-year-old woman with a past history of wheezing now presents with worsening of the wheezing and breathlessness on exertion and during the night. Her peak flow rate diary shows early morning dips.

4. A 19-year-old healthy woman complains of intermittent breathlessness during which she feels dizzy and has pins and needles in her fingers and lips.

5. A 46-year-old man with a recent history of pain in his left leg is admitted with a dry cough, right-sided pleuritic chest pain and breathlessness. A chest X-ray reveals patchy shadowing in the right base and a ventilation/perfusion scan shows a large area of mismatch in the right lung.

Answers to **1.63**

1. **G**   Diuretics

Gallop rhythm, due to the presence of a third heart sound with sinus tachycardia, is associated with heart failure. Intravenous diuretics such as furosemide (frusemide) are used to relieve the breathlessness of pulmonary oedema by inducing a diuresis, and by reducing the ventricular preload through dilatation of the venous capacitance vessels. Diamorphine is best avoided initially in a patient with a history of COPD.

2. **H**   Pleural aspiration

Simple aspiration can be effective even for a large pneumothorax. The indications for a chest drain are tension pneumothorax, failed aspiration and the presence of a significant amount of blood in the pleural space.

3. **D**   Beclometasone (beclomethasone)

This patient has asthma suggested by the diurnal variation in airflow obstruction. Airway tone is greatest in the early hours of the morning, during which asthmatic symptoms are worse. The current British Thoracic Society (BTS) recommendations for the management of chronic asthma consist of five steps.

Step 1   occasional use of relief bronchodilators (if more than once daily go to step 2)

Step 2   regular standard-dose inhaled steroids

Step 3   high-dose inhaled steroids *or* standard-dose inhaled steroids with a long-acting inhaled β_2 agonist

Step 4   high-dose inhaled steroids and regular bronchodilators

Step 5   regular steroid tablets

4. **I**   Psychological support

The hyperventilation syndrome is associated with inappropriate hyperventilation, hypocapnia, dizziness and paraesthesiae in the hands and around the mouth. She needs counselling to give her some insight into her problem and to explain how these symptoms arise from the overbreathing. The breathlessness may be controlled by rebreathing from a paper bag.

5. **K**   Warfarin

The clinical diagnosis of pulmonary embolism (PE) is likely because of the history and the X-ray findings. A PE characteristically causes a mismatch on V/Q scanning (perfusion defect with normal ventilation in the same area). Treatment is initially with heparin (not on the list) and then warfarin.

Management of tuberculosis

A   Adjuvant corticosteroid treatment
B   Administer BCG vaccination
C   Extension of standard treatment to 12 months
D   Isoniazid for 6 months
E   Monitor liver function tests
F   Monitor visual acuity
G   Standard four-drug regimen for 6 months
H   Standard three-drug regimen for 6 months
I   Start pyridoxine
J   Supervised Directly Observed Therapy (DOT)
K   Tuberculin testing

For each patient below, choose the SINGLE most appropriate course of action from the above list of options. Each option may be used once, more than once, or not at all.

1. A 75-year-old woman has sputum positive for acid-fast bacilli on direct microscopy. She lives alone and has cognitive impairment.

2. A 35-year-old man presents with a dry cough, weight loss and night sweats. He is normally fit and well. Microscopy of bronchial raps confirms tuberculosis.

3. A 45-year-old man with human immunodeficiency virus (HIV) infection is due to start quadruple antituberculous treatment but is worried about the effects of ethambutol.

4. A 13-year-old boy has been in close contact with his grandfather who has been recently found to have acid-fast bacilli on Ziehl–Nielsen staining of his sputum (sputum smear-positive tuberculosis). The child has never received BCG (Bacillus Calmette-Guérin) vaccination.

5. A 29-year-old woman presents with weight loss and night sweats. She is 10 weeks pregnant and is confirmed to have pulmonary tuberculosis.

Answers to 1.64

1. **J Supervised Directly Observed Therapy (DOT)**

    Drug compliance is essential for antituberculous therapy. Alcoholics, vagrants and patients with dementia are likely to be poorly compliant with self-medication. It is best to obtain the patient's cooperation and administer the drugs three times weekly under direct supervision at home.

2. **H Standard three-drug regimen for 6 months**

    Tuberculosis is treated in two phases, the initial phase using at least three of the main drugs (isoniazid, rifampicin, pyrazinamide and ethambutol) for 2 months and a continuation phase of two drugs (isoniazid and rifampicin) for a further 4 months. Ethambutol can be omitted if the risk of resistance to isoniazid is low as with patients who have never previously been treated for tuberculosis and those who are not immunocompromised.

3. **F Monitor visual acuity**

    The side effects of ethambutol are mainly confined to visual disturbances from retrobulbar neuritis. They include loss of visual acuity, loss of red-green discrimination and restriction of the visual fields. Patients should be told to stop ethambutol immediately if this occurs. It should not be given to those unable to understand the warnings of the visual disturbances. It is contraindicated in children under 5 years old. Recovery of eyesight follows early discontinuation of the drug. Other side effects include arthralgia and, rarely, hepatitis, rashes and peripheral neuropathy. Toxic effects are more likely with excessive doses and in the presence of renal failure, as 70% of the drug is excreted unchanged in the urine.

4. **K Tuberculin testing**

    About 10% of close contacts with patients with smear-positive tuberculosis develop the disease. Children should have a tuberculin test even if they have received BCG vaccination in the past. A chest X-ray is required in those who test positive. Those with a positive tuberculin test and a normal chest X-ray should be treated with isoniazid for 6 months (or a combination of isoniazid/rifampicin for 3 months). Those with tuberculosis seen on chest X-ray need full antituberculous treatment. If both the chest X-ray and tuberculin testing are normal, then BCG vaccination should be considered as it provides 75% protection for up to 15 years.

5. **H Standard three-drug regimen for 6 months**

    The standard three-drug regimen may be used during pregnancy and breast-feeding. Streptomycin should not be used in pregnancy because of the risk of ototoxicity. There is little or no evidence of teratogenicity from isoniazid, rifampicin or pyrazinamide.

Management of nausea and vomiting

A	Betahistine
B	Dexamethasone
C	Disodium pamidronate
D	Domperidone
E	Lorazepam
F	Metoclopramide
G	Ondansetron
H	Oral laxatives and enemas
I	Proton pump inhibitor
J	Stop drug
K	Trimethoprim

For each scenario below, choose the SINGLE most appropriate course of action from the above list of options. Each option may be used once, more than once, or not at all.

1. A 45-year-old woman complains of severe nausea and vomiting following highly emetogenic chemotherapy for acute myeloid leukaemia.

2. A 56-year-old diabetic presents with troublesome nausea and upper abdominal distension after meals. He has underlying autonomic neuropathy. A recent gastroscopy was normal.

3. A 57-year-old man with known metastatic squamous-cell lung carcinoma is admitted with nausea and vomiting. His serum calcium is raised at 3.4 mmol/L.

4. A 70-year-old man with severe Parkinson's disease has troublesome nausea following treatment with apomorphine.

5. A 78-year-old woman complains of tinnitus, deafness and vertigo which is associated with nausea.

Answers to **1.65**

1. **G   Ondansetron**

   Ondansetron is a specific serotonin ($5HT_3$) antagonist which acts at the chemoreceptor trigger zone in the floor of the fourth ventricle. It is highly effective in controlling the vomiting caused by chemotherapy and radiotherapy.

2. **F   Metoclopramide**

   Autonomic neuropathy in diabetics causes postural hypotension, impotence, diarrhoea, urinary retention, gustatory sweating, gastroparesis and cardiac dysrhythmias. Gastroparesis produces gastric stagnation which can mimic pyloric stenosis. Treat with metoclopramide, a peripheral dopamine antagonist, which can improve gastric motility. Severe gastroparesis has a poor prognosis with up to 50% mortality in 2 years.

3. **C   Disodium pamidronate**

   Metabolic causes of nausea and vomiting include diabetic ketoacidosis, uraemia, hyponatraemia, liver failure and hypercalcaemia. Patients with severe hypercalcaemia (>3 mM) need urgent rehydration. Loop diuretics (e.g. furosemide (frusemide)) increase urinary calcium excretion. Bisphosphonates should be given in addition to these measures in those with hypercalcaemia of malignant origin. They reduce the rate of bone turnover by inhibiting bone resorption. Pamidronate is only given intravenously but clodronate can be given orally as well. Corticosteroids are useful for treating hypercalcaemia associated with myeloma, lymphoma, sarcoidosis and vitamin D toxicity but are ineffective in non-haematological malignancy or primary hyperparathyroidism.

4. **D   Domperidone**

   Apomorphine is used to treat the severe 'off-periods' in Parkinson's disease which are usually resistant to conventional treatment. It is a potent stimulator of D_1 and D_2 receptors and it has to be given parenterally (subcutaneous injection or continuous subcutaneous infusion). Domperidone is a dopaminergic antagonist which does not readily cross the blood–brain barrier, hence it does not cause extrapyramidal side effects to interfere with the treatment of the Parkinson's disease. It acts at the chemoreceptor trigger zone and is effective in relieving the nausea and vomiting associated with apomorphine therapy.

5. **A   Betahistine**

   Vertigo is the most distressing symptom in Ménière's disease, which lasts less than 24 hours and can occur in clusters. Betahistine (an antihistamine) is promoted as a specific treatment for Ménière's disease that will relieve vertigo and the associated nausea.

Management of jaundice

A Alpha interferon
B Colestyramine (cholestyramine)
C Corticosteroids
D Insertion of a stent via endoscopic retrograde cholangiopancreatography (ERCP)
E Liver transplantation
F Penicillamine
G Reassure patient
H Sphincterotomy via endoscopic retrograde cholangiopancreatography (ERCP)
I Splenectomy
J Ursodeoxycholic acid
K Venesection

For each scenario below, choose the SINGLE most appropriate course of action from the above list of options. Each option may be used once, more than once, or not at all.

1. A 45-year-old man with malaise and abdominal pain is found to have a raised serum bilirubin of 60 μmol/L. All the other liver function test indices are normal. The provocation test with intravenous nicotinic acid is positive and produces a further rise in the serum bilirubin level.

2. A 65-year-old man with diabetes and heart failure presents with loss of libido. He is noted to have a slate-grey pigmentation of the skin, jaundice and hepatomegaly.

3. A 23-year-old woman presents with jaundice and signs of severe hepatic encephalopathy 24 hours after a paracetamol overdose.

4. An 80-year-old woman presents with jaundice and weight loss. Computerized tomography (CT) of the abdomen suggests the presence of a carcinoma of the head of the pancreas.

5. A 45-year-old woman presents with pruritus and jaundice. Examination reveals pigmentation and excoriation of the skin with hepatosplenomegaly. Her anti-mitochondrial antibodies are positive and the serum bilirubin is elevated at 40 μmol/L.

Answers to **1.66**

1. **G** **Reassure patient**

This patient has Gilbert's syndrome which is a familial, mild, unconjugated hyperbilirubinaemia with an excellent prognosis. It is probably an autosomal dominant condition. Investigations show a rise in unconjugated bilirubin on fasting, or after provocation with nicotinic acid. The patient should be reassured that the condition is common and benign.

2. **K** **Venesection**

Idiopathic haemochromatosis is inherited (autosomal recessive) and is associated with HLA-A3. Excessive iron deposition leads to multiple organ failure. The association of heart failure, hepatomegaly, skin pigmentation (excessive melanin), diabetes mellitus, arthritis and hypogonadism is suggestive of haemochromatosis. Venesection prolongs survival and is the treatment of choice. Desferrioxamine may be used if venesection cannot be tolerated (heart disease, anaemia or hypoproteinaemia).

3. **E** **Liver transplantation**

Paracetamol overdose accounts for 50% of cases of acute liver failure with viral hepatitis as a cause in a further 40%. Major complications include cerebral oedema with raised intracranial pressure, renal failure, infection, coagulopathy, hypoglycaemia and hypotension. The patient will need intensive care in a specialized liver unit with the facilities for liver transplantation. N-acetylcysteine (not on the list) is worth trying during the 24-hour period after paracetamol ingestion.

4. **D** **Insertion of a stent via ERCP**

Surgical resection is possible, in the absence of metastases, if the tumour is <3 cm in diameter, and does not involve adjacent structures. Those not fit, or unsuitable for surgery, require a stent placed endoscopically to relieve the jaundice.

5. **J** **Ursodeoxycholic acid**

Primary biliary cirrhosis is a chronic, cholestatic liver disease mainly affecting middle-aged women. Progression is slow and will eventually lead to cirrhosis. Ursodeoxycholic acid improves liver biochemistry, reduces pruritus and the referral rate for liver transplant, but an overall increase in survival has yet to be demonstrated. Liver transplantation is indicated for end-stage disease with a bilirubin >100 μM, and in those with intractable itching or bleeding.

Management of portal hypertension

A Beta blockers
B Blood culture
C Diagnostic paracentesis
D Endoscopic sclerotherapy
E Insertion of a Sengstaken–Blakemore tube
F Octreotide
G Porto-systemic shunt
H Spironolactone
I Total paracentesis
J Transfer to an intensive care unit
K Ultrasound scan of the abdomen

For each scenario below, choose the SINGLE most appropriate course of action from the above list of options. Each option may be used once, more than once, or not at all.

1. A 56-year-old man presents with a rapid onset of general malaise and abdominal pain. Examination reveals the stigmata of chronic liver disease including ascites. He is apyrexial. What is the next step?

2. A 45-year-old woman, with known severe liver disease, is admitted with a history of rapid deterioration over the last few days. She is in stage 4 encephalopathy.

3. A 50-year-old man is admitted with significant blood loss from bleeding oesophageal varices. He is receiving a blood transfusion but has a further episode of haematemesis. He is otherwise well perfused. The endoscopist is on his way to the hospital.

4. A 65-year-old man with recently diagnosed oesophageal varices would like to reduce his risk of bleeding from them. He is not on any medication at present.

5. A 67-year-old man is admitted with tense ascites causing considerable discomfort.

Answers to **1.67**

1.   C   Diagnostic paracentesis

Spontaneous bacterial infection of the ascitic fluid needs to be excluded (occurs in up to 15% of patients with ascites, sometimes with bacteraemia). The clinical presentation is often subtle but there may be pyrexia, abdominal pain and tenderness, malaise and confusion. Ascitic Gram stains are often negative and treatment should be started with third generation cephalosporins in the presence of a raised ascitic neutrophil count (>250/mm^3).

2.   J   Transfer to an intensive care unit

Intensive care should be arranged for patients with stage 3 (very drowsy and only able to follow simple commands, or incoherent and agitated) or stage 4 (unresponsive) encephalopathy, and preferably to a unit which can perform a liver transplant, if necessary. One-third of these patients die within 2 days. Cause of death can include acute gastrointestinal haemorrhage, sepsis, renal failure and cerebral oedema. Treatment of cerebral oedema includes mannitol with careful monitoring of intracranial pressure.

3.   F   Octreotide

Octreotide is a somatostatin (growth hormone release inhibitory hormone) analogue used to relieve the symptoms associated with neuroendocrine tumours, e.g. carcinoid and acromegaly, and in variceal bleeding. Other vasoactive drugs used in variceal bleeding include vasopressin (antidiuretic hormone), desmopressin or terlipressin which vasoconstricts the splanchnic arterioles hence decreasing the portal circulation to the bleeding area. Octreotide should be given while endoscopic sclerotherapy is being arranged.

4.   A   Beta blockers

Beta blockers reduce the variceal flow by reducing cardiac output and allowing vasoconstriction of the splanchnic vessels. It can be used in primary and secondary prevention of variceal bleeding reducing the risk by up to a half.

5.   I   Total paracentesis

Total paracentesis is used for tense ascites, refractory ascites and in cases where the use of diuretics is restricted by hyponatraemia or hypovolaemia. Albumin (6–8 g), or colloid equivalent, should be infused for every litre of ascitic fluid removed, although this is not necessary in malignant ascites.

Management of diarrhoea

A Carbimazole
B Ciprofloxacin
C Corticosteroids
D Gluten-free diet
E Low fat diet
F Metronidazole
G Octreotide
H Pancreatic enzyme supplements
I Paromomycin
J Reassurance
K Surgical resection

For each patient below, choose the SINGLE most appropriate course of action from the above list of options. Each option may be used once, more than once, or not at all.

1. A 56-year-old man with a history of alcohol abuse presents with intermittent abdominal pain, diarrhoea and steatorrhoea. An abdominal X-ray shows extensive pancreatic calcification.

2. A 36-year-old woman complains of intermittent attacks of tachycardia, flushing and diarrhoea, which are precipitated by stress and exertion. She has widespread facial telangiectasia.

3. A 36-year-old woman is admitted with a 4-month history of abdominal pain and troublesome, bloody diarrhoea with mucus. She has never been abroad. Examination reveals a mass in the right iliac fossa.

4. A 67-year-old woman develops abdominal cramps and severe, watery diarrhoea several days after completing a course of antibiotics for a chest infection. A stool test for *Clostridium difficile* toxins (CDT) is positive.

5. A university student develops anorexia, weight loss and watery diarrhoea following his holiday in the tropics. Both Giardia cysts and trophozoites are found in the stools.

Answers to **1.68**

1. **H   Pancreatic enzyme supplements**

    Pancreatic enzyme supplements are useful in relieving both the pain and steatorrhoea of chronic pancreatitis, especially in those with small-duct disease and minimal to moderate exocrine dysfunction. A lateral pancreaticojejunostomy may be needed in large-duct disease (marked exocrine impairment and marked ERCP abnormalities) unresponsive to medical therapy. Alcohol should be avoided and the diet should be moderate in fat, high in protein and low in carbohydrate.

2. **G   Octreotide**

    The carcinoid syndrome occurs in 10% of patients with carcinoid tumours in association with liver metastases. The commonest sites for the primary tumours are the appendix and rectum. The syndrome consists of the carcinoid flush usually affecting the head and upper body, tachycardia and hypotension. Patients may develop a chronically reddened face with facial telangiectasia and there may be abdominal pain and diarrhoea. Octreotide (a somatostatin analogue) inhibits the release of serotonin (5-HT) and antagonizes its effects. Hence it is useful even in a carcinoid crisis.

3. **C   Corticosteroids**

    The features here are suggestive of Crohn's disease with an inflammatory mass involving the caecum. Ileocaecal tuberculosis is an important differential diagnosis particularly amongst the Asian population. If there is any doubt, corticosteroid treatment must be covered with antituberculous therapy. Surgery should be avoided if possible but may be needed if medical therapy fails, or with complications such as toxic dilatation of the colon, strictures, fistulae, perforation and abscesses.

4. **F   Metronidazole**

    Pseudomembranous colitis may follow the use of any antibiotic even up to a month after discontinuing the antibiotic. It is caused by the A and B toxins of *Clostridium difficile* which can be identified in stool specimens. Treatment involves stopping the antibiotics and starting either oral vancomycin or metronidazole for 7 to 10 days.

5. **F   Metronidazole**

    Giardia lamblia causes small intestinal disease (damaging the villous microarchitecture) and malabsorption. It is an important cause of travellers' diarrhoea with a high prevalence in the tropics. Most of those secreting Giardia cysts are asymptomatic but others will develop diarrhoea, nausea, abdominal discomfort and weight loss. Treatment is with metronidazole.

Management of the nephrotic syndrome

A   Angiotensin-converting enzyme (ACE) inhibitors
B   Aspirin
C   Calcium supplements
D   Cyclophosphamide
E   Ciclosporin (cyclosporin)
F   Dietary salt restriction
G   Furosemide (frusemide)
H   High-dose corticosteroids
I   HMG CoA reductase inhibitor
J   Vitamin D replacement
K   Warfarin

For each scenario below, choose the SINGLE most appropriate course of action from the above list of options. Each option may be used once, more than once, or not at all.

1. A 45-year-old man with a 3-year history of the nephrotic syndrome is found to have an elevated fasting cholesterol level of 7.8 mmol/L, and a triglyceride level of 3 mmol/L. He is otherwise fairly fit and well.

2. A 16-year-old boy presents with severe hypoalbuminaemia and generalized oedema. The proteinuria is highly selective for albumin and transferrin. He is haemodynamically stable.

3. A 56-year-old woman presents with left loin pain, haematuria and a sudden worsening of renal function. She has a history of the nephrotic syndrome.

4. A 60-year-old man with the nephrotic syndrome and chronic renal failure is found to have osteomalacia and secondary hyperparathyroidism.

5. A 62-year-old woman with the nephrotic syndrome complains of severe oedema of her legs which is uncomfortable and prevents her from wearing her shoes. She has tried bendroflumethiazide (bendrofluazide) with little effect.

Answers to **1.69**

1.   I   HMG CoA reductase inhibitor

Hyperlipidaemia in the nephrotic syndrome is a risk factor for accelerated vascular disease. Reduction in lipid levels may reduce vascular disease. HMG CoA reductase inhibitors (statins) inhibit the enzyme involved in cholesterol synthesis especially in the liver. They markedly reduce cholesterol and some of them, to a lesser extent, also reduce triglycerides.

2.   H   High-dose corticosteroids

Selective proteinuria (smaller molecules such as albumin and transferrin, as opposed to larger proteins like IgG or α_2-macroglobulin), suggests minimal change glomerulonephritis, whilst an unselected protein leak is more typical of proliferative glomerulonephritis. Minimal change glomerulonephritis is responsible for 80% of nephrotic syndrome in children. About 90% of children with minimal change glomerulonephritis will respond to corticosteroids within 8 weeks.

3.   K   Warfarin

Thrombosis in the venous/arterial circulation is common in the nephrotic syndrome. Abnormalities of coagulation may be due to haemoconcentration from hypovolaemia, and also proteins in the coagulation cascade are altered in concentration. Renal vein thrombosis may present with loin pain, haematuria, renal enlargement and deteriorating renal function. The diagnosis is established by selective renal venography. Up to one-third of patients with a renal vein thrombosis have pulmonary emboli. Those with symptomatic thromboses should be anticoagulated initially with heparin (not on the list) and then warfarin for 3–6 months.

4.   J   Vitamin D replacement

Vitamin D-binding protein and vitamin D are lost in the nephrotic urine. Hypocalcaemia, particularly in the presence of renal failure, can lead to osteomalacia (inadequate osteoid mineralization causing softening of the bones), and secondary hyperparathyroidism leading to severe decalcification of the skeleton. Early treatment with vitamin D is recommended.

5.   G   Furosemide (frusemide)

Diuretics are the mainstay of the treatment of oedema, but modest salt restriction (<60 mmol/24 h) and water restriction should also be instituted. The use of diuretics may be limited by postural hypotension from hypovolaemia. If large doses of oral diuretics (furosemide (frusemide) up to 500 mg twice a day) are ineffective then intravenous salt-poor albumin (has only a transient effect) and intravenous furosemide (frusemide) may be needed.

Treatment of thyrotoxicosis

A   Antithyroid treatment
B   Aspirin
C   Corticosteroids
D   DC cardioversion
E   Digoxin
F   Orbital decompression
G   Partial thyroidectomy
H   Propranolol
I   Psychological support
J   Radioiodine
K   Stop drug

For each patient below, choose the SINGLE most appropriate treatment from the above list of options. Each option may be used once, more than once, or not at all.

1. A 56-year-old woman complains of malaise, fever and a sore throat following a recent chest infection. She has a sinus tachycardia (120/min) and tenderness of her slightly enlarged thyroid gland.

2. A 67-year-old woman presents with the clinical signs of thyrotoxicosis. She has a history of hypertension and was started 6 months ago on amiodarone for paroxysmal supraventricular tachycardia.

3. A 45-year-old man is admitted with heart failure and uncontrolled atrial fibrillation of 180 beats/min. He has a moderately enlarged goitre with a loud bruit on auscultation and his blood pressure is 140/80 mmHg. What supportive measure should be initiated?

4. A 35-year-old woman with Graves' disease complains of pain in her eyes, photophobia and diplopia. She is biochemically euthyroid but has evidence of exophthalmos. Computerized tomography (CT) of the orbits confirms enlargement of the extraocular tissues.

5. A 56-year-old woman presents with depression, weight loss and agitation. She is single and looks after her elderly parents. Her thyroid function tests show elevated total thyroid hormones but the radioactive thyroid scan shows suppressed uptake of the isotope.

Answers to **1.70**

1. **B   Aspirin**

    De Quervain's, or subacute, thyroiditis is due to a viral infection of the
    thyroid gland. There is a transient thyrotoxicosis due to the release of
    preformed thyroid hormones. A radioactive thyroid scan shows
    suppression of uptake in the acute phase. Aspirin is useful in the acute
    phase although a short course of steroids may be necessary in severe
    symptomatic cases.

2. **K   Stop drug**

    Amiodarone, a class III antiarrhythmic agent, can cause thyrotoxicosis
    especially in those with iodine depletion. Thyroid function tests show an
    elevated total thyroxine, relatively normal T_3 (due to inhibition of
    peripheral conversion of T_4 to T_3) and suppressed TSH. The
    thyrotoxicosis can be refractory and amiodarone should be stopped at
    least temporarily to achieve control, although its effect will continue for
    several weeks due to its storage in adipose tissue. Antithyroid treatment
    may be required.

3. **E   Digoxin**

    The clinical picture suggests a thyrotoxic crisis or storm. Digoxin should
    be given to control the atrial fibrillation. Beta blockers are useful but
    should be avoided in heart failure. Treating sepsis, fluid replacement,
    starting heparin for atrial fibrillation and controlling fever are other
    supportive measures. The most urgent treatment for the thyrotoxic
    storm is iodine (in addition to antithyroid treatment) to block the
    release of thyroid hormones from the thyroid.

4. **C   Corticosteroids**

    Graves' ophthalmopathy usually occurs within 12 months of the onset
    of thyrotoxicosis, but may precede or accompany the onset of the
    disease. There is a risk of blindness, if untreated, due to pressure on the
    optic nerve. High dose steroids are required, sometimes given in
    conjunction with external radiation to the orbits. Orbital decompression
    is performed in the event of disease progression despite treatment, and
    if the vision is threatened.

5. **I   Psychological support**

    Thyrotoxicosis factitia usually occurs in patients with psychiatric
    problems who have some medical knowledge and access to the drugs.
    The diagnosis is confirmed by the reduced or absent uptake of isotope in
    the thyroid scan.

Management of diabetes mellitus/hypoglycaemia

A Acarbose
B Angiotensin-converting enzyme (ACE) inhibitors
C Glucagon
D Intravenous fluids
E Intravenous glucose
F Metformin
G Psychiatric referral
H Subcutaneous insulin
I Sulphonylurea
J Surgical excision
K Thiazolidinediones

For each patient below, choose the SINGLE most appropriate course of action from the above list of options. Each option may be used once, more than once, or not at all.

1. A previously fit 45-year-old man presented with diabetic ketoacidosis which is now controlled. He is still on intravenous insulin, but is feeling much better and is eating and drinking normally. His urine is free from ketones.

2. A 60-year-old woman presents with recurrent hypoglycaemic episodes associated with confusion and weakness, which are worse in the mornings. There are inappropriately high insulin levels with measurable C-peptides in the presence of low plasma glucose levels.

3. A 65-year-old man with non-insulin dependent diabetes presents with severe pain in his thighs which is unrelieved by analgesia. There is wasting of his quadriceps and a proximal myopathy with loss of the knee reflexes. His weight is steady but his diabetic control is poor (HbA1$_c$9%) despite full oral hypoglycaemic therapy.

4. A 56-year-old obese woman is recently found to have hyperglycaemia that is not properly controlled by dietary means alone. Although she has lost 2 kg in the past 2 months, her blood sugars remain around 12 mmol/L.

5. A 51-year-old diabetic is found to have microalbuminuria on urinalysis. His diabetes is otherwise well controlled and he is normotensive.

Answers to **1.71**

1. **H** Subcutaneous insulin

Diabetic ketoacidosis arises from a deficiency of insulin, resulting in an uncontrolled catabolic state. It is characterized by dehydration, hyperventilation (Kussmaul respiration) and ketosis (from rapid lipolysis producing free fatty acids which are converted to ketone bodies in the liver). Treatment includes insulin and fluid replacement (up to 6 L in the first 24 h). This patient is now stabilized and his intravenous insulin should be changed to the subcutaneous route.

2. **J** Surgical excision

The vast majority of insulinomas (pancreatic islet-cell tumours) are benign. Classically, there is fasting hypoglycaemia (with raised insulin and C-peptide levels) associated with drowsiness on waking which is relieved by giving glucose. Other symptoms include confusion, abnormal behaviour, 'funny' turns, blackouts and seizures. Insulinomas can be localized by MRI or gamma camera. An intravenous injection of labelled octreotide may be needed to visualize small tumours. Surgical excision is the main treatment option. Medical treatment with diazoxide and somatostatin may be useful for those unfit for surgery.

3. **H** Subcutaneous insulin

Diabetic amyotrophy usually occurs in older diabetics who are not on insulin. It is often rapid in onset and causes pain in the thighs with proximal weakness at the hip and knee. There is asymmetrical wasting of the quadriceps with loss or diminished knee reflexes. It is associated with poor glycaemic control and often resolves with good diabetic management with insulin. This patient would require insulin therapy even if he had no amyotrophy.

4. **F** Metformin

Metformin decreases hepatic gluconeogenesis and increases peripheral utilization of glucose. It is the drug of choice in obese patients in whom the diabetes is uncontrolled despite dieting, since it does not promote weight gain. If metformin and strict dieting fail then consider adding a sulphonylurea.

5. **B** Angiotensin-converting enzyme (ACE) inhibitors

Microalbuminuria (less than 300 mg albumin/24 h on at least three occasions) is the earliest sign of diabetic nephropathy. Treatment with ACE inhibitors, even if the blood pressure is normal, diminishes the risk of renal deterioration by reducing the intraglomerular filtration pressure.

Management of multiple sclerosis

A   Anticholinergic drugs
B   Antihistamine
C   Baclofen
D   Beta-blockers
E   Beta-interferon
F   Carbamazepine
G   Methylprednisolone
H   Papaverine
I   Phenytoin
J   Selective serotonin reuptake inhibitor (SSRI)
K   Self-catheterization

For each patient below, choose the SINGLE most appropriate course of action from the above list of options. Each option may be used once, more than once, or not at all.

1.   A 38-year-old woman with relapsing multiple sclerosis would like treatment to reduce the number of relapses. She remains fit and is still able to work full time as a teacher.

2.   A 45-year-old man with impotence related to neurological dysfunction in multiple sclerosis is keen to resume a normal sexual relationship with his wife.

3.   A 35-year-old woman is admitted with a severe, acute relapse of her multiple sclerosis. She is distressed, ataxic and has a spastic paraparesis.

4.   A 52-year-old woman with multiple sclerosis complains of intermittent, severe, sharp, right-sided facial pain lasting seconds. The pain is sometimes provoked by touching a part of her cheek.

5.   A 35-year-old man has lost interest in most things and has had early morning wakening for the last 6 months ever since the diagnosis of multiple sclerosis was made.

Answers to **1.72**

1. E   Beta-interferon

Beta-interferon is indicated in patients with relapsing, remitting multiple sclerosis (at least two attacks over 2 years, with complete or incomplete recovery) and who are still able to walk unaided. It reduces the frequency and severity of the relapses but it does not affect disability or the course of the disease. It is also licensed in secondary, progressive multiple sclerosis. Patients who fulfil the criteria should be referred to a neurologist who will make the ultimate decision.

2. H   Papaverine

Erection is under the control of the sacral erection centre via the parasympathetic nerves in S2–4. Sexual function is affected by spinal demyelination. Intracavernosal injection of papaverine (smooth muscle relaxant) or alprostadil (prostaglandin E1) is effective even in severe, organic impairment. Priapism may occur and this needs urgent urological attention should it last longer than 4 hours.

3. G   Methylprednisolone

High-dose intravenous methylprednisolone shortens the duration of a relapse by reducing oedema in the areas of acute inflammation. It also reduces macrophage activity and alters the permeability of the blood–brain barrier. It is better tolerated than steroids given orally or intramuscularly.

4. F   Carbamazepine

Trigeminal neuralgia may be associated with multiple sclerosis. The pain is characteristically unilateral, brief, severe and sharp and may be provoked by cold air on the face or by touching trigger spots on the face. Carbamazepine is the treatment of choice, although phenytoin given alone or in combination with carbamazepine may work.
Thermocoagulation of the ganglion or microsurgery to section the sensory root of the fifth cranial nerve by a posterior fossa approach, may be considered in resistant cases. A modern surgical approach is to separate a pulsating artery from the sensory nerve root, and this results in complete relief from the pain.

5. J   Selective serotonin reuptake inhibitor (SSRI)

This patient has reactive depression and will require counselling, psychotherapy and probably an antidepressant. Concentrations of noradrenaline (norepinephrine) and serotonin (5-HT) in the brain are reduced in depressive illness. SSRIs selectively inhibit the reuptake of serotonin and are less sedating and have less antimuscarinic (dry mouth, urinary retention) and cardiotoxic effects than tricyclic antidepressants.

Management of epilepsy

A Computerized tomography (CT) scan of the head
B Dexamethasone
C Diazepam
D Electroencephalogram (EEG)
E Folic acid
F Lamotrigine
G Magnetic resonance imaging (MRI)
H Phenytoin
I Sodium valproate
J Stop driving for 1 year
K Stop driving for 3 years

For each scenario below, choose the SINGLE most appropriate initial course of action from the above list of options. Each option may be used once, more than once, or not at all.

1. A 16-year-old girl presents with a 'funny turn' at home. Whilst waiting for medical attention in the A&E department she develops status epilepticus. You are the first doctor arriving on the scene.

2. A 65-year-old woman presents with her first grand mal seizure. She had a left mastectomy 10 years ago for breast carcinoma. Examination reveals no neurological signs.

3. A 20-year-old student presents with possible seizures. She has bizarre, jerky, synchronous movements of her limbs. There is no neurological deficit.

4. A recently married 28-year-old woman gives a history of three 'funny turns' which started with shaking of the right hand and then the arm before losing consciousness. Her family report that she subsequently developed a tonic–clonic fit each time. What initial treatment is appropriate for her?

5. A 35-year-old salesman has a definite single tonic–clonic fit and would like to know when he can start driving again.

Answers to **1.73**

1. C Diazepam

Status epilepticus is defined as generalized tonic–clonic fits lasting for more than 30 minutes or repeated fits without regaining consciousness between the fits. It is a medical emergency with a mortality of 10–15% from cardiorespiratory failure. It should be treated initially with intravenous diazepam or lorazepam. If the seizures fail to respond then phenytoin, clomethiazole or phenobarbital may be used. If all fails, the patient needs anaesthesia with thiopental or propofol with full intensive care support.

2. A Computerized tomography (CT) scan of the head

Anticonvulsants are indicated for recurrent seizures. It is not common practice to start treatment with the first attack. However, this patient needs a CT scan of the head to exclude cerebral metastases. Dexamethasone may be needed to reduce cerebral oedema if a space-occupying lesion is demonstrated on the CT scan.

3. D Electroencephalogram (EEG)

EEG telemetry with video recordings during an attack is useful, as a normal EEG between attacks does not exclude epilepsy. Pseudoseizures can be difficult to diagnose. Serum prolactin checked within about 20 min after a true seizure is raised to 4–5 times the normal level, but not in pseudoseizures.

4. F Lamotrigine

This woman has partial seizures evolving to secondarily generalized seizures and carbamazepine is the drug of choice but it is not available on the list. Of the options available, lamotrigine would be the best. There is an increased risk of teratogenicity associated with the use of antiepileptic drugs particularly valproate, phenytoin and carbamazepine. It is important to discuss the possible consequences of these drugs in pregnancy when dealing with women of childbearing age. Lamotrigine is probably the safest of the four drugs. Folic acid is recommended for women before and during pregnancy to reduce the risk of neural tube defects.

5. J Stop driving for 1 year

Those with one definite epileptic seizure may drive a car provided that they have been free from seizures for 1 year, or have seizures during sleep without any daytime seizures for the past 3 years. Public Service Vehicle and Heavy Goods Vehicle licences (PSV and HGV) are barred from those who have had any epileptic attack after the age of 3 years. It is advisable to record this advice in the notes and inform the patient that you have done so.

Treatment of movement disorders

A   Amantadine
B   Apomorphine
C   Baclofen
D   Beta blockers
E   Botulinum toxin
F   Levodopa
G   Penicillamine
H   Physiotherapy
I   Procyclidine
J   Tetrabenazine
K   Withdraw drug

For each patient below, choose the SINGLE most appropriate treatment from the above list of options. Each option may be used once, more than once, or not at all.

1.   A 30-year-old asthmatic patient has been admitted with an exacerbation of her asthma. She has made a good recovery with nebulized bronchodilators and oral steroids. However, she has noticed a fine tremor affecting her hands since admission.

2.   A 25-year-old man presents with dysarthria, tremor, involuntary movements and chronic liver disease. A slit-lamp examination of his eyes reveals the presence of Kayser–Fleischer rings.

3.   A 45-year-old man with Huntington's disease is distressed by his choreiform movements. He has not received any medication yet.

4.   A 19-year-old student was recently started on metoclopramide for nausea following an episode of gastroenteritis. Soon after taking her first tablet she had a severe reaction. Her eyes were forced upwards and she lost all voluntary ocular movements.

5.   A 67-year-old man presents with a 1-year history of spontaneous nodding of his head and worsening tremor when he tries to eat. Both his muscle tone and walking are normal. He finds the tremor embarrassing.

Answers to **1.74**

1. **K** Withdraw drug

Salbutamol (a beta-2 agonist) causes a fine tremor of the hands. Other side effects include tachycardia, palpitations, headaches, hypokalaemia when given in very high doses, and hypersensitivity reactions. Sometimes the tremor is disabling and the drug may have to be withdrawn.

2. **G** Penicillamine

This patient has Wilson's disease (hepatolenticular degeneration). It is inherited as an autosomal recessive gene and results in the deposition of copper in various organs, particularly the liver and the brain, causing cirrhosis and Parkinsonism. The Kayser–Fleischer ring is due to copper deposition in the Desçemet's membrane in the cornea and is best seen on slit-lamp examination. Long term treatment with penicillamine is required.

3. **J** Tetrabenazine

Tetrabenazine is used to control the movement disorders (hemiballismus and senile chorea) of Huntington's disease by depleting the nerve endings of dopamine. Side effects include depression, parkinsonism and hypotension.

4. **I** Procyclidine

Oculogyric crises can occur due to the extrapyramidal side effects of metoclopramide, which can affect children and young adults in particular. It can also occur in encephalitis or in post-encephalitic parkinsonism. The use of metoclopramide should be restricted to those over 20 years. Treatment is with anticholinergics, e.g. procyclidine.

5. **D** Beta blockers

Benign essential tremor is inherited as an autosomal dominant trait and occurs most frequently in the elderly. It affects mainly the hands when holding a cup or spoon, head (titubation) and trunk. This is slowly progressive but seldom very disabling. Treatment is often unnecessary but small doses of alcohol, beta-blockers or primidone (not on the list) may be helpful.

Management of rheumatological disorders

A   Allopurinol
B   Arthroscopy
C   Bisphosphonate
D   Colchicine
E   Cyclophosphamide
F   Exercise training programme
G   Intramuscular steroid injection
H   Local steroid injection
I   Methotrexate
J   Non-steroidal anti-inflammatory drugs (NSAIDs)
K   Splinting

For each presentation below, choose the SINGLE most appropriate management from the above list of options. Each option may be used once, more than once, or not at all.

1. A 37-year-old woman presents at 34 weeks' gestation in her second pregnancy with paraesthesiae over the lateral half of her right palm and fingers. Tinel's sign is positive.

2. A 70-year-old man with a long history of severe osteoarthrosis complains of worsening pain in his left knee. He also describes troublesome knee-locking. His only medication is regular co-codamol.

3. A 54-year-old man presents with severe pain affecting his right first metatarsophalangeal joint which has occurred several times over the last twelve months. He has a history of hypertension.

4. A 27-year-old woman is admitted with a 2-week history of symmetrical arthropathy of the small joints of the hands.

5. A 46-year-old man presents with worsening back pain and immobility. He has a past history of ankylosing spondylitis and a bleeding duodenal ulcer.

Answers to **1.75**

1. K   Splinting

This lady has the symptoms of carpal tunnel syndrome probably associated with fluid retention in pregnancy. Tinel's sign (reproduction of the tingling sensation or pain on percussion of the median nerve) confirms the diagnosis. The treatment of choice for this condition, which is often self-limiting during pregnancy, is splinting in order to reduce movement during the day. In other instances, either splinting or local steroid injection to the wrist offers temporary relief. Decompression is necessary if muscle weakness, wasting, or a sensory deficit is present or if conservative measures fail.

2. B   Arthroscopy

Arthroscopy is useful in severe osteoarthrosis of the knee and hip. It allows for therapeutic lavage to remove debris and debridement of the meniscal cartilage to relieve knee-locking. It has an important role in assessing a monoarthritis of unknown aetiology by allowing visual inspection and biopsies from within the joint.

3. J   Non-steroidal anti-inflammatory drugs (NSAIDs)

The presentation is typical of gout which may have been precipitated by thiazide diuretics used in the treatment of the hypertension. Acute gout is treated with non-steroidal anti-inflammatory drugs (NSAIDs) such as indometacin (indomethacin). Colchicine may be used in those intolerant of NSAIDs but diarrhoea may be a troublesome side effect. Allopurinol (a xanthine oxidase inhibitor) prevents further attacks of gout but should not be used within 4 weeks of the last episode.

4. J   Non-steroidal anti-inflammatory drugs

It may be difficult to differentiate the early stages of rheumatoid arthritis from other self-limiting inflammatory arthropathies especially in the absence of obvious rheumatoid changes. Analgesics, including NSAIDs, are useful for pain control. This patient may have rheumatoid arthritis which can present with an insidious onset of pain and stiffness affecting the peripheral small joints with increasing joint involvement. Disease-modifying drugs which slow the progression of erosive joint damage are used in those patients with early development of erosions and a failure to respond to NSAIDs.

5. F   Exercise training programme

As NSAIDs are contraindicated in this patient, an exercise training programme (regular daily exercises involving walking, posture and chest expansion exercises) is useful for controlling the pain from ankylosing spondylitis. Local intra-articular steroid injections may occasionally be used for peripheral synovitis.

Management of terminal care

A Antidepressants
B Bisphosphonate
C Dexamethasone
D Diamorphine pump
E Fentanyl patches
F Haloperidol
G Hyoscine
H Non-steroidal anti-inflammatory drugs (NSAIDs)
I Oral morphine
J Psychological support
K Radiotherapy

For each patient below, choose the SINGLE most appropriate course of action from the above list of options. Each option may be used once, more than once, or not at all.

1. A 67-year-old man with metastatic bronchogenic carcinoma presents with a dry, intractable cough.

2. A 50-year-old woman with breast carcinoma develops severe headaches, nausea and vomiting. A computerized tomography (CT) scan of the brain reveals several metastatic lesions.

3. A 50-year-old woman with recently diagnosed metastatic bowel carcinoma has expressed her fear of dying which is making her both anxious and depressed.

4. A 76-year-old man with prostatic carcinoma presents with nausea and vomiting. His corrected serum calcium is elevated at 3.4 mmol/L.

5. A 56-year-old woman with inoperable non-small-cell lung carcinoma presents with troublesome haemoptysis. She has a large mass in the left mid-zone of her chest X-ray.

Answers to **1.76**

1.   I   Oral morphine

Opioids can be used to suppress the cough reflex centrally. Morphine (initially 5 mg every 4 h) is often required for a severe intractable cough associated with lung carcinoma. Nebulized lidocaine (lignocaine) may be useful although it is often poorly tolerated.

2.   C   Dexamethasone

The symptoms of raised intracranial pressure are drowsiness, headache and vomiting. Deteriorating vision and level of consciousness are sinister features. Characteristically, the headaches occur in the early hours of the morning partly due to retention of carbon dioxide during sleep that causes cerebrovascular dilatation and a further rise in intracranial pressure. The headaches are worse with bending or coughing. Dexamethasone is the treatment of choice. Brain metastases do not respond well to radiotherapy.

3.   J   Psychological support

It is important to explore the patient's natural and understandable fear of death and allow open communication to address any issues of concern. Pain control, dependence, incontinence, worry about family left behind and financial problems are commonly expressed fears. A lot of the worry can be alleviated by explanation, reassurance and by offering practical advice and palliative care support. Anxiolytics or antidepressants are sometimes needed in addition to psychological support.

4.   B   Bisphosphonate

Severe hypercalcaemia (calcium >3 mmol/L) is a medical emergency that requires treatment with rehydration and bisphosphonates (inhibits osteoclastic activity), of which disodium pamidronate is the most effective. Specific treatment of the underlying cause is also needed to prevent a recurrence of the hypercalcaemia, which in this case may involve orchidectomy or gonadorelin analogues.

5.   K   Radiotherapy

Radiotherapy is useful for the palliation of distressing symptoms particularly haemoptysis and cough. It can also be used for relieving breathlessness caused by bronchial obstruction, spinal cord compression, pain from bony metastases and dysphagia and superior vena cava obstruction from lymph node compression.

Prophylactic treatment

A Chloroquine and proguanil
B Clindamycin
C Co-trimoxazole
D Isoniazid
E Mefloquine
F Nebulized pentamidine
G Penicillin
H Rifampicin
I Tetracycline
J Trimethoprim
K Zidovudine

For each patient below, choose the SINGLE most appropriate treatment from the above list of options. Each option may be used once, more than once, or not at all.

1. A 54-year-old lady with known mitral valve disease is due to have some dental work done by her own local dentist under a local anaesthetic. She is allergic to penicillin.

2. A 20-year-old student plans to travel to sub-Saharan Africa for at least 1 month. She is worried about malaria and would like the best protection available.

3. There has been an outbreak of meningococcal meningitis at the local university hall of residence. A 19-year-old student is worried as she shared a room with a fellow student who is now critically ill with meningitis.

4. A 12-year-old boy has been sharing a flat with his grandfather who has now recently been diagnosed as having tuberculosis. The boy has shown a positive reaction to tuberculin testing but his chest X-ray is normal.

5. A 35-year-old HIV-positive, pregnant woman would like to minimize the risk of transmission of the HIV to her baby.

Answers to **1.77**

1. **B Clindamycin**

   Clindamycin 600 mg should be given 1 h before the local anaesthetic for the dental procedure. Patients who can tolerate penicillin should receive amoxicillin (amoxycillin) 3 g 1 h before the procedure.

2. **E Mefloquine**

   Mefloquine is preferable to chloroquine and proguanil in this part of the world where there is a very high risk of chloroquine-resistant falciparum malaria. It is contraindicated in pregnancy. Important side effects include neuropsychiatric reactions (hallucinations, psychosis). Mefloquine should be started 2 to 3 weeks (as opposed to 1 week with chloroquine/proguanil) before the journey to determine tolerance.

3. **H Rifampicin**

   Rifampicin 600 mg twice a day for 2 days should be given to all close adult contacts. Medical and nursing staff need not be given chemoprophylaxis unless they have given mouth-to-mouth resuscitation.

4. **D Isoniazid**

   Isoniazid 300 mg once a day for 6 months (for a child 5–10 mg/kg daily; max 300 mg/day) may be used for preventive therapy when there has been contact with a patient with tuberculosis. A combination of isoniazid and rifampicin can be used for 3 months but rifampicin is not used alone.

5. **K Zidovudine**

   Zidovudine (nucleoside reverse transcriptase inhibitor) given in the last two trimesters of pregnancy, during delivery and to the neonate for 6 weeks reduces transmission of the HIV from mother to child.

Prevention of HIV infection

A   Avoid breastfeeding
B   Combination therapy – zidovudine (AZT), lamivudine and indinavir
C   Course of penicillin
D   Measure specific HIV antibodies
E   Methadone maintenance programme
F   Needle exchange programme
G   Polymerase chain reaction (PCR) screening
H   Promote caesarian section
I   Promote safe sex
J   Suck blood from wound
K   Zidovudine monotherapy

For each patient below, choose the SINGLE most appropriate course of action from the above list of options. Each option may be used once, more than once, or not at all.

1.   A sexually active 22-year-old woman presents to the clinic for sexually transmitted diseases (STD) with a chlamydial infection.

2.   A 24-year-old heroin addict is worried about catching HIV from sharing equipment with his friends. He is also aware that the habit is destroying him.

3.   A newly diagnosed HIV-infected woman has just given birth to a baby girl.

4.   A nurse in the local medical centre presents with a needle stick injury which occurred trying to resheath the needle after venesecting a known AIDS patient.

5.   There has been a shortage of blood in the UK but there is a good response to advertisements to donate blood. However, there is now a worry about HIV transmission via donated blood and blood products.

Answers to **1.78**

1. **I   Promote safe sex**

    Chlamydia trachomatis is an obligate intracellular bacterial parasite and often associated with other pathogens, e.g. gonorrhoea. It is a sexually transmitted disease; in men, it causes urethritis, epididymitis and proctitis and, in women, acute salpingitis and subfertility. Promotion of safe sex (use of condoms for any penetrative sex) is vital.

2. **E   Methadone maintenance programme**

    This addict may be helped to give up intravenous heroin and to use methadone instead which has no risk of HIV infection. Methadone is also addictive but is titrated according to the degree of dependence before gradual reduction. Addicts should be persuaded to change needles and syringes. Even cleaning the needle with bleach for those having to share needles can reduce the risk of HIV transmission.

3. **A   Avoid breastfeeding**

    Breastfeeding should be avoided as it increases the HIV transmission risk by 14% (30% if maternal infection occurs after delivery). Most babies are infected during the third trimester or during delivery, but HIV transmission can be reduced to <5% by zidovudine monotherapy (given in the 2nd and 3rd trimesters in women with CD4 counts <200/mm^3 and i.v. infusion during labour, and treatment of the infant for the first 6 weeks of life) and by caesarian section (the baby avoids ingestion of maternal blood and secretions during labour).

4. **B   Combination therapy**

    The risk of HIV transmission with a single percutaneous exposure is 1 in 300, and following a single mucocutaneous exposure is 1 in 3000. Exposure is significant if the patient is HIV positive as in this case. Irrigate with running water and offer prophylactic treatment with three-drugs (AZT, lamivudine and indinavir). AZT and lamivudine can be given if the source is not known to be HIV positive.

5. **D   Measure specific HIV antibodies**

    In the UK, where the HIV prevalence is low, screening by measuring specific HIV antibodies in the serum has reduced HIV transmission to very low levels (7 cases in 34 000 since screening started). However, there is a 3-month window period between infection and a detectable level of antibodies during which the HIV test will be negative. Potential donors are asked not to give blood if there is a chance that they may have contracted HIV in the last 3 months.

Antidotes for poisons

A   Acetylcysteine
B   Atropine
C   Desferrioxamine
D   Dicobalt edetate
E   Dimercaprol
F   Ethanol
G   Flumazenil
H   Fresh frozen plasma
I   Fuller's earth
J   Glucagon
K   Naloxone

Choose the SINGLE most appropriate antidote for the following poisons from the above list of options. Each option may be used once, more than once, or not at all.

1.   Arsenic

2.   Warfarin

3.   Methanol

4.   Iron

5.   Benzodiazepines

Answers to **1.79**

1. **E** **Dimercaprol**

Dimercaprol is the traditional treatment for arsenic poisoning. Both dimercaprol and penicillamine can also be used in mercury and lead poisoning.

2. **H** **Fresh frozen plasma**

Fresh frozen plasma is used in the event of a major haemorrhage. For less severe cases, a small dose of parenteral vitamin K (5 mg) can be used to reduce the haemorrhagic tendency without cancelling the anticoagulation. Reversing the anticoagulant state completely with larger doses of vitamin K will render the patient refractory for about 2 weeks, and it will take longer to re-establish good anticoagulant control.

3. **F** **Ethanol**

Gastric lavage should be performed in those who present less than 1 h after ingestion. When presenting later, ethanol can be given, as it inhibits methanol oxidation but it is of no use (it can even exacerbate metabolic acidosis) once the methanol is already metabolized. The infusion should continue until the methanol levels are undetectable. Ethanol can also be used in diethylene glycol poisoning.

4. **C** **Desferrioxamine**

Iron has a direct corrosive effect on the gastrointestinal tract causing haematemesis, abdominal pain and diarrhoea. Once absorbed in large quantities, it can also cause renal failure, liver failure, metabolic acidosis, coma and death. At cellular level, iron tends to concentrate around the mitochondrial cristae where it interferes with metabolism. Desferrioxamine is given parenterally to act as a chelating agent.

5. **G** **Flumazenil**

Supportive measures are often adequate. In severe cases, the use of flumazenil (a specific benzodiazepine antagonist) is indicated. Repeated doses may be necessary since the effects of benzodiazepines may persist for 24 h.

Adverse drug reactions

A   Co-codamol
B   Ethambutol
C   Gentamicin
D   Haloperidol
E   Indometacin
F   Levodopa
G   Lithium
H   Metformin
I   Prednisolone
J   Ramipril
K   Spironolactone

For each adverse drug reaction below, choose the SINGLE most likely causal drug from the above list of options. Each option may be used once, more than once, or not at all.

1.   High-pitched tinnitus

2.   Diabetes insipidus

3.   Gynaecomastia

4.   Lactic acidosis

5.   Tardive dyskinesia

Answers to **1.80**

1. C Gentamicin

All aminoglycosides may cause reversible and irreversible vestibular, cochlear and renal toxicity. This occurs more commonly in the elderly and in patients with renal failure. A high-pitched tinnitus is often the first symptom of cochlear toxicity and, if the drug is not discontinued, auditory impairment may develop within a few days. Tinnitus may persist for up to 2 weeks after the drug is stopped. Features of vestibular toxicity include nausea, vomiting, vertigo and ataxia. Monitoring of the serum concentration is essential to avoid both excessive and subtherapeutic concentrations.

2. G Lithium

Acquired diabetes insipidus may occur with lithium therapy. This is reversible with termination of the therapy. The renal tubules become insensitive to vasopressin causing polydipsia and polyuria. Other side effects include hypothyroidism, confusion, hyper-reflexia, cardiac arrhythmias, psychoses, coma and occasionally death.

3. K Spironolactone

Spironolactone may cause gynaecomastia, impotence and menstrual irregularities. The most serious side effect is hyperkalaemia as it is a potassium-sparing diuretic. It is used in treating oedema associated with cirrhosis of the liver, Conn's syndrome and severe heart failure. Other drugs known to cause gynaecomastia are oestrogens, antiandrogens, digoxin, griseofulvin, alkylating agents, phenothiazines, tricyclics, isoniazid, diazepam and heroin.

4. H Metformin

Lactic acidosis may occur with metformin in the presence of renal impairment (even in mild cases), dehydration, shock, infection, myocardial infarction, pregnancy and hepatic impairment. However, it is generally safer than phenformin which was withdrawn because of the high incidence of lactic acidosis. Metformin is a biguanide that decreases gluconeogenesis and increases peripheral utilization of glucose. It is the drug of choice in obese patients with non-insulin dependent diabetes.

5. D Haloperidol

A drug-induced extrapyramidal syndrome may be caused by neuroleptics due to the inhibition of dopamine function. There may be orofacial dyskinesia (lip-smacking, grimacing and pouting) and choreoathetosis (involuntary quasi-purposeful movements) of the limbs and trunk. It usually happens at least 3 months after the start of withdrawal of long term treatment with neuroleptics. So, it is termed tardive (late) dyskinesia as opposed to parkinsonism or acute dystonias which occur early.

SECTION 2

Surgery

Symptoms and signs in urological disease

A Anuria
B Dysuria
C Frequency
D Haematuria
E Incontinence
F Nocturia
G Oliguria
H Pneumaturia
I Polyuria
J Pyuria
K Retention

For each presentation below choose the SINGLE most appropriate symptom/sign from the above list of options. Each option may be used once, more than once, or not at all.

1. A 60-year-old man is known to have severe, sigmoid diverticular disease. He now has recurrent urinary tract infections and is also passing gas bubbles in the urine. Investigations reveal a colovesical fistula.

2. A 70-year-old man, who developed nocturia 6 months ago, is now having to make increasingly frequent visits to the toilet. His rectal examination reveals a smooth, enlarged prostate.

3. A 65-year-old man is intermittently passing dark-coloured urine. Cystoscopy reveals a frond-like growth in the bladder and histology suggests a transitional-cell carcinoma.

4. A 25-year-old healthy, pregnant (20 weeks' gestation) woman cannot go more than an hour without having to empty her bladder.

5. A 30-year-old woman who had a forceps delivery 1 month ago is having difficulty holding her water. Urine is leaking through the vagina. Investigations show that she has a small vesicovaginal fistula.

Answers to **2.1**

1. **H Pneumaturia**

   With a colovesical fistula, gas from the bowel is often passed out during micturition. In diverticulitis, the inflamed sigmoid flops onto the urinary bladder and becomes adherent to it. It can then erode through the bladder, giving rise to a fistula. The patient passes repetitive gas and faeculent material while urinating. This communication gives an increased risk of recurrent urinary tract infections.

2. **C Frequency**

   Frequency of micturition is one of the first symptoms of an enlarged prostate. At first, it is nocturnal with the patient needing to get up twice or more during the night to micturate and it later becomes diurnal. Frequent micturition at this stage is probably due to vesical introversion of the sensitive prostatic mucous membrane by the intravesical enlargement of the prostate.

3. **D Haematuria**

   Haematuria is the usual presentation for a tumour of the urinary bladder. Painless haematuria is by far the most common symptom and should be regarded as indicative of a bladder carcinoma until proven otherwise. Haematuria may occur on a single or on several occasions with the urine subsequently clearing. Many months may elapse before it recurs and causes concern. The bleeding, if severe, may give rise to clot formation in the bladder and subsequent clot retention.

4. **C Frequency**

   A gravid uterus pressing on the urinary bladder causes irritation to the bladder trigone giving rise to an increased frequency of micturition.

5. **E Incontinence**

   A difficult labour, especially if instrumentation is used, can result in a vesicovaginal fistula causing constant dribbling of urine via the vagina which the patient has no control of. This is quite distressing to the patient and initial management is to insert a urinary catheter. Most small vesicovaginal fistulae heal with this treatment. If this fails, then surgical intervention should be considered.

Physical signs in surgery

A Berry's sign
B Courvoisier's law
C Cullen's sign
D Joffroy's sign
E Kehr's sign
F Kenawy's sign
G Murphy's sign
H Signe de Dance
I Slipping sign
J Succussion splash
K Trousseau's sign

For each presentation below choose the SINGLE most appropriate sign from the above list of options. Each option can be used once, more than once, or not at all.

1. A 45-year-old man presents with a large swelling of the left lobe of the thyroid gland. On examination, the carotid arterial pulsations appear to be pushed outwards and backwards.

2. A 60-year-old woman presents with obstructive jaundice. The patient has lost weight but does not complain of any abdominal pain. On palpation, there is a tense, cystic mass in the right upper quadrant of the abdomen and an ultrasound scan reveals a distended gallbladder.

3. A 4-year-old boy presents with a 12-hour history of severe, colicky abdominal pain. In between attacks the boy seems to be comfortable. He gives a history of passing 'red currant jelly' stools, and abdominal examination shows emptiness in the right iliac fossa. A diagnosis of intussusception is made.

4. A 40-year-old man is involved in a road traffic accident and sustains a blunt injury to the abdomen. He then complains of pain in the left shoulder. In the A&E department, he has a blood pressure of 70/40 mmHg and a pulse rate of 130 beats per minute. An ultrasound scan of the abdomen reveals a ruptured spleen with free blood in the peritoneal cavity.

5. A 45-year-old man presents to the A&E department with severe upper abdominal pain after an alcoholic binge. His serum amylase level is elevated and he is treated for acute pancreatitis. A week later a bluish discoloration is seen in the periumbilical region which supports the diagnosis.

Answers to **2.2**

1.   **A**   Berry's sign

A large thyroid swelling can displace the carotid artery outwards and backwards. This is called Berry's sign and usually occurs with a benign thyroid swelling. In general, malignant tumours of the thyroid do not show this sign because they tend to envelop the carotid artery rather than displace it.

2.   **B**   Courvoisier's law

In a patient with painless jaundice which is obstructive in nature, and when the gallbladder is palpable, Courvoisier suggested that the obstruction is not due to a stone but implies a more sinister cause such as a carcinoma of the head of the pancreas. The tumour, by virtue of its relationship with the common bile duct, can obstruct it extrinsically. If gallstones were to be the cause of the jaundice then the gallbladder would not be distended because of the fibrosis from chronic infection.

3.   **H**   Signe de Dance

This is the feeling of emptiness in the right iliac fossa that suggests an intussusception. It is not a very reliable sign but it has been well described. The diagnostic feature on palpation is the finding of a curved, sausage-shaped lump in the line of the colon with a concavity directed towards the umbilicus.

4.   **E**   Kehr's sign

This is a sign generally associated with splenic rupture with the presence of free intraperitoneal blood. This blood irritates the left side of the diaphragm, which is supplied by the phrenic nerve (C4) and which also supplies the shoulder tip. This common supply causes referred pain to the tip of the left shoulder.

5.   **C**   Cullen's sign

This is a bluish discoloration of the periumbilical region. This physical sign occurs in less than 3% of patients with pancreatitis and results from blood-stained, retroperitoneal fluid tracking through the tissue plains along the falciform ligament to the umbilical area. This is a late sign and indicates the presence of a severe episode of acute haemorrhagic pancreatitis, which has an overall mortality rate of about 30%. A similar, large ecchymosis in the flank is referred to as Grey Turner's sign.

Premalignant conditions

A   Achalasia of the cardia
B   Barrett's epithelium
C   Bowen's disease
D   Familial polyposis coli
E   Gardner's syndrome
F   Leukoplakia
G   Lymphogranuloma venereum infection
H   Paterson–Brown–Kelly syndrome
I   Senile keratosis
J   Tylosis
K   Ulcerative colitis

For each of the following presentations choose the SINGLE most likely
premalignant condition from the above list of options. You may use each
option once, more than once, or not at all.

1.   A 75-year-old man presents with a white patch on the tongue, which
     cannot be removed by scraping. He has been a heavy smoker.

2.   A 56-year-old woman presents with a 6-month history of dysphagia and
     is known to have an iron deficiency anaemia. Investigations reveal that
     she has a post-cricoid web.

3.   A 35-year-old woman complains of abdominal pain and diarrhoea.
     Investigations reveal the presence of multiple colonic polyps and an
     osteoma of the mandible. Her father had a colonic carcinoma.

4.   A 60-year-old man presents with dyspepsia. Gastroscopy shows the
     lower end of the oesophagus to be pink in colour. A biopsy of this area
     shows columnar epithelium.

5.   A 45-year-old woman has a proven invasive adenocarcinoma of the
     sigmoid colon. She has a 10-year history of intermittent diarrhoea with
     blood and mucus, which had to be controlled with steroids.

Answers to **2.3**

1. **F Leucoplakia**

    Leucoplakia consists of sharply defined white patches or streaks on the
    oral mucosa which cannot be removed by scraping. In about 5% of
    cases leucoplakia undergoes malignant transformation into a squamous
    cell carcinoma, but epithelial atypia associated with hard, irregular
    plaques has a higher risk (30%). Smokers' keratosis and frictional
    keratosis are associated with a very good prognosis.

2. **H Patterson–Brown–Kelly syndrome**

    Patterson–Brown–Kelly syndrome is the triad of iron deficiency
    anaemia, dysphagia and atrophic glossitis. It predominantly affects
    women in the northern hemisphere. The dysphagia is associated with a
    post-cricoid web (circumferential mucosal folds), which causes
    narrowing of the lumen. The syndrome is associated with a high
    incidence of malignancy in the upper part of the gastrointestinal tract.

3. **E Gardner's syndrome**

    Gardner's syndrome is a variant of familial adenomatous polyposis,
    which is inherited as an autosomal dominant trait. It consists of
    gastrointestinal adenomas and mesodermal tumours (osteomas of the
    skull, mandible and long bones and soft tissue lesions such as
    fibromas, lipomas and desmoid tumours mostly on the face and limbs).
    The colon is usually involved with multiple polyps. The potential for
    malignant change is identical to that of familial adenomatous polyposis
    and carcinoma of the colon develops at a mean age of 36 years.
    Screening of family members is essential from the age of 12 years.

4. **B Barrett's epithelium**

    Barrett's oesophagus is caused by chronic gastro-oesophageal reflux and
    develops at the lower end of the oesophagus. Ulceration of the
    oesophagus is followed by regeneration of pluripotential basal cells
    which form pink, columnar epithelium in the lower oesophagus. This
    premalignant change increases the risk of adenocarcinoma by up to 40
    times.

5. **K Ulcerative colitis**

    This patient has the features of a long history of ulcerative colitis. The
    risk of developing an adenocarcinoma of the colon with ulcerative
    colitis increases with early onset and with extensive disease. About 10%
    of patients who have had the disease for 10 years develop carcinoma and
    this increases to 20% after 20 years. Screening, with annual colonoscopy,
    is essential.

Rectal bleeding

A   Amoebiasis
B   Bacillary dysentery
C   Colorectal polyps
D   Crohn's disease
E   Diverticular disease
F   Fissure-in-ano
G   Haemorrhoids
H   Intussusception
I   Ischaemic colitis
J   Neoplastic growth
K   Ulcerative colitis

For each of the clinical pictures below, choose the SINGLE most appropriate cause from the above list of options. You may use each option once, more than once, or not at all.

1.   A 45-year-old man presents with dark rectal bleeding and with no other constitutional symptoms. Flexible sigmoidoscopy shows a smooth lump on a pedicle at about 35 cm from the anal verge.

2.   A 75-year-old man has bleeding per rectum, which is associated with a sudden and severe, colicky, left lower abdominal pain. An abdominal X-ray is normal but a barium enema shows `thumb printing' of the colon at the splenic flexure.

3.   A 25-year-old woman, known to have constipation, has fresh bleeding per rectum associated with painful defecation.

4.   A 70-year-old man complains of a 6-month history of passing dark-coloured blood rectally. He also has diarrhoea, loss of weight and a feeling of incomplete evacuation. His blood tests show that he is anaemic.

5.   A 20-year-old woman presents with a 3-day history of passing bloody diarrhoea with mucus up to 15 times a day, associated with lower abdominal pain. Examination of the abdomen shows mild tenderness in the lower abdomen. This is the third similar episode in 6 months.

Answers to **2.4**

1. **C Colorectal polyps**

    These can be premalignant especially if they reach more than 3 cm in size. They may be sessile or pedunculated, and they commonly present with rectal bleeding or with iron deficiency anaemia from occult blood loss. Flexible sigmoidoscopy and colonoscopy are useful both to obtain a biopsy of the polyp and for polypectomy. Histology is essential to exclude malignancy and to establish completeness of removal.

2. **I Ischaemic colitis**

    Ischaemic colitis is characterized by intermittent bouts of abdominal pain and bloody diarrhoea. In contrast to acute mesenteric ischaemia, colonic ischaemia is not associated with a major vascular occlusion. Bleeding is not vigorous. Radiological features of ischaemic colitis are particularly characteristic, the most important being thumb-printing on barium enema, which is due to the submucosal bleeding producing a series of crescentic irregularities along the margin of the bowel.

3. **F Fissure-in-ano**

    A fissure-in-ano is a tear of the lower anal canal which may be primary (of unknown cause) or caused by the passage of hard stools or secondary to inflammatory bowel disease. It causes rectal bleeding with painful defecation. The treatment is usually conservative with laxatives, local anaesthetic cream and more recently with glycerine trinitrate creams. Most anal fissures heal spontaneously, but a few refractory cases may have to be dealt with surgically by a lateral anal sphincterotomy.

4. **J Neoplastic growth**

    Colorectal cancer is the second commonest cause of cancer death after lung cancer. Most arise from malignant transformation of adenomatous polyps over a period of 10–35 years. Two-thirds of large bowel cancers occur in the sigmoid colon and rectum. The feeling of incomplete evacuation after defecation (tenesmus) is common with rectal involvement, together with urgency for defecation and rectal bleeding with mucus discharge. The tumour may be palpable on rectal examination.

5. **K Ulcerative colitis**

    Frequent bloody diarrhoea in a young person and the two attacks preceding this suggest that she has inflammatory bowel disease. This can be either Crohn's disease or ulcerative colitis (more likely). A colonoscopy and biopsies from various parts of the colon and rectum can differentiate between these two conditions.

Constipation

A   Carcinoma of the sigmoid colon
B   Colonic stricture
C   Dietary/habitual
D   Drugs
E   Fissure-in-ano
F   Hypercalcaemia
G   Hypothyroidism
H   Inflammatory mass
I   Neoplasm of the small bowel
J   Slow colonic transit
K   Volvulus

For each of the following clinical situations choose the SINGLE most likely cause from the above list of options. You may use each option once, more than once, or not at all.

1.   A 45-year-old woman has been referred with steadily worsening constipation over the last 2 months. She has also developed menorrhagia. Her voice has become hoarse and her weight has increased. On examination, she appears listless and her skin is dry.

2.   A 75-year-old man has noticed a change in his bowel habit with marked constipation. This is associated with dark bleeding per rectum. His daughter thinks that he has lost up to 1 stone in weight over the last 6 months. On examination, he is pale and has a 5 × 7 cm painless, firm lump in his left iliac fossa.

3.   A 75-year-old woman presents with a 1-week history of constipation. She initially developed an intermittent colicky abdominal pain that later became constant. On examination, she is pyrexial (38°C) with abdominal distension and sparse bowel sounds. There is rebound tenderness with guarding in the left iliac fossa where there is also a palpable mass.

4.   A 75-year-old woman with senile dementia, normally resident in a nursing home, presents with absolute constipation of 3 days' duration and with massive distension of her abdomen. A plain X-ray of the abdomen shows gross distension of the sigmoid loop with no gas in the rectum.

5.   A 40-year-old woman seeks medical advice for long-standing constipation. She last opened her bowels 3 weeks ago. On examination, she looks fit and healthy and her recent barium enema is normal. Radio-opaque pellets are swallowed and a series of plain abdominal X-rays taken. More than 30% of the pellets are in the transverse colon after a week.

Answers to **2.5**

1.   G   Hypothyroidism

The clinical features suggest that this patient has hypothyroidism.
Unexplained and troublesome constipation, in a patient with few
obvious features of myxoedema, is the only symptom of
hypothyroidism that may take a patient to a surgeon rather than a
physician.

2.   A   Carcinoma of the sigmoid colon

This is most likely to be a colonic carcinoma. It has a high prevalence in
the western world. The presentation of a change in bowel habit (usually
towards diarrhoea but can be alternating constipation and diarrhoea)
suggests that the patient has a sinister pathology. The risk of intestinal
obstruction increases as the tumour grows in size.

3.   H   Inflammatory mass

Diverticular disease can sometimes present as complete bowel
obstruction due to inflammation and fibrous strictures. However,
incomplete obstruction is more common and this presents as severe
constipation. Other presentations include chronic abdominal pain,
rectal bleeding, acute diverticulitis, pericolic abscess, diverticular
perforation and fistula formation.

4.   K   Volvulus

Volvulus of the sigmoid colon has a curious geographical distribution; it
is uncommon in Western Europe and very common in Eastern Europe
and the East, probably due to dietary differences. In the UK it is usually
encountered in elderly institutionalized patients. They present with
constipation with a massive distension of the abdomen. The diagnostic
feature radiologically is a grossly distended sigmoid colon, the apex of
which often reaches the right upper quadrant and is referred to as the
'bent inner tube sign', in which the gas shadow is seen bent over itself
with two fluid levels, one lying in each limb of the obstructed loop.

5.   J   Slow colonic transit

Slow colonic transit probably develops secondary to a lifestyle habit of a
low fibre diet, poor fluid intake, inactivity and persistent failure to
respond to the urge to defecate. This can lead to chronic constipation
with abdominal discomfort in the absence of mechanical obstruction.
A barium enema will exclude any other pathology and if this is normal
the definitive test is the colonic transit study. This involves serial
radiographs of radio-opaque pellets taken orally and observing their
transit through the bowel. The study is positive if a high proportion of
the pellets are still seen after a week.

Diarrhoea

A Dietary indiscretion
B Drugs
C Faecal impaction
D Food poisoning
E Gut resection
F Infective diarrhoea
G Inflammatory bowel disease
H Malabsorption
I Neoplasm
J Thyrotoxicosis
K Vipoma

For each of the following clinical presentations choose the SINGLE most likely cause from the above list of options. You may use each option once, more than once, or not at all.

1. A 72-year-old lady presents with a 3-week history of diarrhoea with blood and loss of 1 stone in weight.

2. A 25-year-old woman presents with a 1-year history of intermittent bloody diarrhoea. She has had abdominal pain and weight loss of half a stone over the last few months. Examination is unremarkable. An abdominal X-ray shows faeces in the proximal transverse colon but the distal colon is dilated with mucosal islands.

3. A 60-year-old man complains of a 3-month history of profuse watery diarrhoea. He is found to have a marked metabolic hypokalaemic acidosis. He is mildly confused and has some abdominal distension. Both he and his wife have never been abroad on a holiday.

4. A 40-year-old man develops severe abdominal pain with bloody diarrhoea following his recent trip to the Indian subcontinent.

5. An 80-year-old man from a nursing home presents with diarrhoea but only passes small amounts at a time. He has also become more confused lately. His abdomen is generally distended but the bowel sounds are present.

Answers to **2.6**

1.   I   Neoplasm

The most likely cause in this patient with weight loss and rectal bleeding
is a neoplasm of the descending colon. This often presents initially with
diarrhoea. Many factors are considered to be responsible for the
diarrhoea, which include mucous discharge from the neoplasm and
colonic irritation. With a rectal lesion, because of the space occupying
effect, the patient can have the symptom of incomplete evacuation
which makes them pass frequent small amounts of mucoid diarrhoea.

2.   G   Inflammatory bowel disease

Inflammation of the large intestinal mucosa causes diarrhoea which may
often be associated with the passage of mucus and blood.
Malabsorption can occur with weight loss and hypoproteinaemia. The
inflamed colon does not contain faeces. A plain abdominal X-ray may in
showing right-sided sparing and left-sided inflammation, with
thickening of the bowel wall and mucosal islands. The colonic haustral
pattern can be lost due to mucosal oedema and thickening.

3.   K   Vipoma

Vipomas are rare pancreatic tumours that produce vasoactive intestinal
peptide (VIP) which is a neurotransmitter that stimulates adenylcyclase to
produce intestinal secretions. Half of all vipomas have metastasized to the
lymph nodes and liver by the time of diagnosis. They are characterized by
profuse watery diarrhoea (at least 3 L/day), hypokalaemic achlorhydria/
hypochlorhydria and acidosis (due to the loss of potassium and
bicarbonate in the stools), a group of symptoms which is referred to as
the WDHA syndrome (Watery Diarrhoea, Hypokalaemia,
Hypochlorhydria, Acidosis). The serum VIP is markedly raised (>200
pg/mL). Treatment is by resection in non-metastatic disease, or with
palliative chemotherapy and octreotide in metastatic disease.

4.   F   Infective diarrhoea

Organisms such as Salmonella, Shigella, Yersinia and Campylobacter
may cause infective diarrhoea with blood. These infections are more
common in tropical countries. Management is mainly supportive with
adequate fluid and electrolyte replacement.

5.   C   Faecal impaction

Severe constipation is most often seen in children and the elderly, and
also often associated with drugs (codeine, iron and opiates),
hypothyroidism and hypo/hypercalcaemia. Faecal fluid can
intermittently bypass the impacted faecal mass causing a spurious or
overflow diarrhoea.

Dysphagia

A   Benign oesophageal stricture
B   Dysmotility of the oesophagus
C   Foreign body
D   Hiatus hernia
E   Hodgkin's lymphoma
F   Neurogenic
G   Oesophageal carcinoma
H   Oesophageal ring
I   Pharyngeal pouch
J   Plummer–Vinson syndrome
K   Scleroderma

For each of the following presentations choose the SINGLE most likely
cause from the above list of options. You may use each option once, more
than once, or not at all.

1. A 70-year-old man presents with dysphagia and shortness of breath. A
    chest X-ray shows an air–fluid level in the chest.

2. A 45-year-old man develops weight loss and a slowly progressive
    painless dysphagia initially for solids and then for liquids. A barium
    meal shows an irregular narrowing in the lower oesophagus.

3. A 40-year-old woman complains of dysphagia. On examination, she is
    anaemic with a smooth, pale tongue and spoon-shaped thumbnails.

4. A 50-year-old woman with a long-standing history of heartburn
    develops progressive dysphagia. Otherwise she is in reasonably good
    health.

5. A 32-year-old man was suddenly interrupted at a business lunch when a
    bolus of steak got stuck in his gullet. He had several sips of water and
    the steak eventually passed down and he completed his lunch. He
    recalls that he has had similar episodes in the past, particularly when he
    had a hurried meal or was excited or distracted.

Answers to **2.7**

1.   D   Hiatus hernia

This patient has a para-oesophageal hiatus hernia. Reflux symptoms are uncommon but the presence of the stomach in the chest can cause obstructive symptoms and shortness of breath. A chest X-ray is useful in diagnosing this condition as the air–fluid level of the stomach can be seen in the chest.

2.   G   Oesophageal carcinoma

Most oesophageal malignancies are squamous-cell carcinomas and usually affect the middle third of the oesophagus. Adenocarcinomas, which probably arise from metaplastic gastric mucosa (Barrett's oesophagus), usually affect the lower third of the oesophagus. They usually present with progressive dysphagia and weight loss. A barium swallow usually shows an irregular filling defect or stricture. There is no proximal oesophageal dilatation as in achalasia. Carcinoma of the upper third is normally treated with radiotherapy, the lower third by surgical resection and the middle third by either method.

3.   J   Plummer–Vinson syndrome

The Plummer–Vinson syndrome (also known as the Patterson–Brown–Kelly syndrome) is characterized by the triad of dysphagia, iron deficiency anaemia and atrophic glossitis. The patient is typically a middle-aged woman who complains of dysphagia (due to a fibrous web in the upper oesophagus) and may have spoon-shaped, brittle nails (koilonychia). Treatment is with oral iron supplements and dilatation of the stricture may be necessary.

4.   A   Benign oesophageal stricture

Chronic gastro-oesophageal reflux may lead to severe persistent inflammation, fibrotic scarring and a benign oesophageal stricture. Dilatation of the stricture with oesophageal dilators may be needed if significant dysphagia is present. Barrett's oesophagus (replacement of the squamous epithelium by metaplastic gastric columnar epithelium) is a premalignant condition and is the result of chronic damage by acid reflux.

5.   H   Oesophageal ring

A low oesophageal ring is a common cause of intermittent dysphagia. It is seen in about 10% of barium meal examinations but only one third of the rings cause symptoms, more often in men between the ages of 20 and 30 years. The diagnosis can be confirmed radiologically, but only if the oesophagus is widely dilated by barium beyond the ring, with the patient lying flat. The ring may be missed if the radiologist does not examine the oesophagus with the patient recumbent.

A lump in the groin

A   Femoral aneurysm
B   Femoral hernia
C   Inguinal hernia
D   Lipoma
E   Lymphoma
F   Obturator hernia
G   Psoas abscess
H   Psoas bursa
I   Retractile testis
J   Saphena varix
K   Undescended testis

For each of the following clinical situations choose the SINGLE most likely cause from the above list of options. You may use each option once, more than once, or not at all.

1. A 28-year-old man presents with swellings in both groins and axillae. These are firm, rubbery and discrete. He complains of weight loss, fever, night sweats and pain in the swellings especially after drinking alcohol.

2. A 35-year-old woman recently noticed a painful lump in her left groin which is not reducible. The lump is located one inch below and lateral to the pubic tubercle and there is no palpable cough impulse.

3. A 35-year-old woman presents with a soft, painless lump in the groin which reduces in size on lying flat and on applying minimal pressure. There is a cough impulse. She also has varicose veins.

4. A 25-year-old man presents with a painless lump in the groin. It appears on standing and disappears on lying down. On examination in the standing position, there is a lump above the inguinal ligament which can be reduced and there is a cough impulse.

5. A 15-year-old boy presents with a lump in the right inguinal region. This cannot be reduced and there is no cough impulse. The lump feels firm and is about 3 cm in diameter. The right side of the scrotum appears underdeveloped.

Answers to **2.8**

1. **E   Lymphoma**

   Lymphoma may present with palpable lymph nodes in the groins, axillae and cervical region. This patient also has the constitutional symptoms which consist of fever, drenching night sweats and weight loss of >10% body weight. Other symptoms include fatigue and alcohol-induced pain in the enlarged lymph nodes.

2. **B   Femoral hernia**

   A femoral hernia consists of herniation of the peritoneum (which may contain omentum or small bowel) through the narrow femoral canal. Patients often seek medical advice early because of the pain and discomfort. It typically appears below and lateral to the pubic tubercle. This differentiates it from an inguinal hernia, which passes above and medial to the tubercle.

3. **J   Saphena varix**

   A saphena varix is a dilatation of the saphenous vein superficial to the deep fascia and is due to valvular incompetence at its junction with the femoral vein. It is characterized by it emptying either with lying down or the application of minimal pressure and by it refilling on release of the pressure or on standing up. A cough impulse is invariably present. Varicose veins may be present in the legs and percussion of these varicosities may transmit an impulse up towards the saphena varix (Schwartz's test).

4. **C   Inguinal hernia**

   Inguinal herniae account for 85% of herniae in the groin and occur mainly in males. They may be direct or indirect depending on whether they pass through the deep inguinal ring or not. The indirect hernia enters the deep inguinal ring and passes through the inguinal canal, but the direct hernia protrudes through the transversalis fascia and enters the inguinal canal through the posterior wall. Long standing inguinal herniae, especially the indirect ones, may become irreducible and are then at risk of obstruction and strangulation.

5. **K   Undescended testis**

   The testis develops from the genital fold during intrauterine life. Normally, the testis descends from the posterior abdominal wall into the scrotum by the time the child is born but its descent may be arrested, most commonly in the inguinal canal. Maldescended testes are often structurally abnormal and are associated with an increased risk of malignancy especially if they are retained in the abdomen. Orchidopexy (positioning of the testis into the scrotum) should be performed before the age of 2–4 years, otherwise the testis should be removed.

Haematemesis

A Carcinoma of the stomach
B Duodenal ulcer
C Gastric ulcer
D Haemophilia
E Mallory–Weiss syndrome
F Multiple gastric erosions
G Oesophageal varices
H Oesophagitis
I Osler–Weber–Rendu syndrome
J Thrombocytopenia
K Von Willebrand disease

For each of the following presentations choose the SINGLE most likely cause from the above list of options. You may use each option once, more than once, or not at all.

1. A 50-year-old office worker develops nausea and vomiting after a party during which he drank 10 pints of beer. Initially he brought up gastric contents but later he noticed a considerable amount of blood in the vomitus.

2. A 60-year-old vagrant presents with a large haematemesis but is haemodynamically stable. He has palmar erythema, spider naevi, splenomegaly and ascites.

3. A 70-year-old retired man is admitted with a history of weight loss, poor appetite and upper abdominal pain. He has had a few episodes of haematemesis although the amount of blood loss is minimal.

4. A 45-year-old sales executive presents with an episode of haematemesis amounting to about 500 mL in volume. He has a recent history of a gnawing pain in the upper abdomen which radiates to the back and is relieved by eating. His weight is stable.

5. A 75-year-old housewife with long standing osteoarthrosis presents with a haematemesis. She is otherwise fit and well apart from occasional dyspepsia.

Answers to 2.9

1. **E   Mallory–Weiss syndrome**

    The Mallory–Weiss syndrome is caused by a sudden increase in intra-
    abdominal pressure usually from a bout of coughing or retching which
    results in a superficial, longitudinal tear of the mucosa at the
    oesophagogastric junction. It may cause a severe haematemesis. This
    condition is classically associated with an alcohol binge. Most cases
    settle spontaneously although, rarely, surgery to oversew the tear may be
    required.

2. **G   Oesophageal varices**

    This patient has the peripheral stigmata of chronic liver disease (palmar
    erythema, spider naevi) and evidence of portal venous hypertension
    (ascites, oesophageal varices, splenomegaly). It is likely that he is
    haemorrhaging from the oesophageal varices which are dilatations of
    the normal submucosal oesophageal veins. However, upper GI
    endoscopy should be performed to exclude a peptic ulcer which may
    coexist. Cirrhosis of the liver, which is usually the end point of severe
    long standing alcohol abuse, is the commonest cause and the extent of
    the blood loss can be life-threatening. Management consists of
    controlling the initial bleeding (resuscitation, sclerotherapy via
    endoscopy, octreotide/vasopressin to restrict portal inflow by splanchnic
    vasoconstriction, and balloon tamponade) and prevention of further
    bleeding (beta blockade, long-term sclerotherapy, portosystemic shunt).

3. **A   Carcinoma of the stomach**

    This patient's symptoms are classic for a gastric malignancy. The
    anorexia leads to loss of weight and anaemia leads to tiredness, lethargy
    and pallor. Unfortunately, by the time of diagnosis most cases are too
    advanced for curative surgery.

4. **B   Duodenal ulcer**

    The pain of a duodenal ulcer occurs typically at night, several hours after
    food (hunger pain) and is relieved by eating. There is usually no loss of
    weight. When the ulcer becomes chronic it can erode into the
    gastroduodenal artery giving rise to massive haematemesis. In contrast,
    the pain of a gastric ulcer is exacerbated by food and patients may lose
    weight as a result of low dietary intake.

5. **F   Multiple gastric erosions**

    Scattered small, round or linear submucosal haemorrhages are typically
    seen in acute erosive gastritis. About 50% of these patients give a history
    of long standing ingestion of non-steroidal anti-inflammatory drugs
    (NSAIDs). Acute alcoholism may cause similar but short-lived changes.
    Upper GI endoscopy is required to make the definitive diagnosis.

Haematuria

A   Benign prostatic hypertrophy
B   Carcinoma of the bladder
C   Cystitis
D   Hypernephroma
E   Polycystic kidney disease
F   Renal calculus
G   Schistosomiasis
H   Trauma to the kidney
I   Tuberculosis of the kidney
J   Ureteric calculus
K   Wilm's tumour

For each of the following presentations choose the SINGLE most likely cause from the above list of options. You may use each option once, more than once, or not at all.

1. A 60-year-old man presents with frank haematuria. He has lived for many years in the Middle East. Cystoscopy reveals pseudo-tubercles and sandy patches.

2. A 25-year-old woman presents with urinary frequency, dysuria and fever. Urine microscopy shows 20–50 red blood cells and 10–20 leucocytes in each field.

3. A 70-year-old man presents with severe, right-sided colicky loin pain radiating towards the inguinal region. Urine microscopy shows 50–100 red blood cells in each field.

4. A 40-year-old man presents with haematuria. On examination, both his kidneys are easily palpable and non-tender and his blood pressure is 190/110 mmHg. His father had the same symptoms and died at the age of 55 years.

5. A 65-year-old man complains of haematuria, frequency, hesitancy and nocturia. He reports that on certain occasions he finds it difficult to control the urge to pass urine. Urine microscopy confirms the presence of blood but shows no other features.

Answers to **2.10**

1.   G   Schistosomiasis

Schistosoma haematobium mainly affects the urinary tract and is found in Egypt, East Africa and the Middle East. The organism has an affinity for the vesical venous plexus and eventually some of the ova reach the lumen of the bladder. Clinical features include urticaria associated with a high evening temperature, sweating and asthma. Chronic inflammation of the bladder, ureters and urethra may cause urinary frequency with painless, terminal haematuria and eventually it can progress to chronic pyelonephritis, renal failure and contraction of the bladder. Examination of the urine may reveal the ova. Samples should be obtained midday when excretion of the eggs is maximal. Cystoscopy shows the characteristic nodules, sandy patches and sometimes ulcers and papillomas.

2.   C   Cystitis

This patient has the classic symptoms of a urinary tract infection which are urinary frequency, dysuria and pyrexia. Urine microscopy characteristically shows both red and white blood cells but the latter are in excess of their normal ratio with the former.

3.   J   Ureteric calculus

The symptom of colicky loin pain radiating to the groin with associated microscopic haematuria is a classic presentation of a ureteric calculus. The pain is due to the migration of the calculus in a confined tubular structure. In contrast, renal calculi may be asymptomatic or present with just a dull aching pain in the loin.

4.   E   Polycystic kidney disease

Abdominal pain and haematuria are the most common initial symptoms of adult polycystic kidney disease. It is an inherited autosomal dominant disease. It may be detected during infancy but symptoms usually do not develop until adult life. Both kidneys are enlarged to several times the normal size and contain numerous cysts. The clinical features can include pain in the renal angles, haematuria, uraemia and hypertension. Associated berry aneurysms of the cerebral vessels may lead to a subarachnoid haemorrhage.

5.   A   Benign prostatic hypertrophy

The prostate gland generally enlarges with age due to hyperplasia of the periurethral glandular tissue. Urinary frequency, urgency and dysuria are common and haematuria may occur. Other symptoms include urinary hesitancy, a poor stream and terminal dribbling. Rectal examination reveals a smooth and symmetrically enlarged prostate that is rubbery in consistency. The median groove between the two lateral lobes is usually retained, whereas asymmetry, or a hard consistency, is suggestive of a malignancy.

Investigation of breast disease

A Blood biochemistry
B Bone scan
C Computerized tomography (CT) scan
D Ductography (galactography)
E Fine needle aspiration
F Genetic studies
G Mammography
H Thermography
I Trucut biopsy
J Ultrasound scan of the breast
K Xeromamography

For each of the following scenarios choose the SINGLE most appropriate investigation from the above list. Each option may be used once, more than once, or not at all.

1. A 55-year-old woman who is asymptomatic with no family history of breast cancer is now worried that she may have breast cancer and requests investigations.

2. A 60-year-old woman, who has had a wide, local excision with axillary clearance and subsequent radiotherapy for a right breast cancer 2 years ago, now presents with right anterior chest pains. On palpation, she has tenderness over the third and fourth ribs on the right side.

3. A 20-year-old woman with a strong family history of breast cancer presents to the clinic seeking advice about the probability of her developing breast cancer. She requests investigations to reassure her. Her mother developed breast cancer at the age of 45 years and her two maternal aunts at 50 years.

4. A 25-year-old anxious woman with no family history of breast cancer finds two lumps in her right breast, each measuring about 1.5 cm. These were aspirated yielding a greenish brown fluid. The lumps disappeared and have not refilled after an observation period of 4 weeks. This lady remains anxious despite these interventions.

5. A 60-year-old woman who has had a previous mastectomy for breast cancer 20 years ago now develops severe thirst and polyuria.

Answers to **2.11**

1.   **G**   Mammography

In general, all women in the UK above the age of 50 years are now offered a screening mammogram. This lady should have had this investigation as a screening procedure by now, so her GP needs to ensure that she is on the call-up register and that she has her first mammogram soon.

2.   **B**   Bone scan

Cancer of the breast tends to metastasize most commonly to the bone, liver and brain. Bony metastases are often in the ribs and spine and present with pain. An isotope bone scan will show these areas as hot spots.

3.   **F**   Genetic studies

This patient is at high risk of developing breast cancer since she has one first degree and two second degree relatives who have had the disease. This lady needs to be referred for genetic studies and counselling. They will look at the degree of the risk of this patient for developing breast cancer and based on this will initiate the appropriate management.

4.   **J**   Ultrasound scan of the breast

From the history and the subsequent disappearance of the breast lumps on aspiration, these appear to be cysts. The fact that they do not refill suggests that they are benign. Also, the colour of the aspirate is that of a typical benign breast cyst. These do not need further investigation especially in a young woman, but to allay anxiety an ultrasound scan of the breast should be done.

5.   **A**   Blood biochemistry

The presence of severe thirst and polyuria in someone with a previous history of malignancy is suggestive of hypercalcaemia. This can be checked by biochemical investigations. The hypercalcaemia is most likely to be a result of bony metastases.

Investigation of abdominal pain

A   Abdominal X-ray
B   Angiography
C   Barium enema
D   Barium meal
E   Chest X-ray
F   Colonoscopy
G   Computerized tomography (CT) scan of the abdomen
H   Gastroscopy
I   Intravenous urogram
J   Serum biochemistry
K   Ultrasound scan of the abdomen

For each presentation below choose the SINGLE most appropriate investigation from the above list of options. Each option can be used once, more than once, or not at all.

1. A 35-year-old man who drinks 30 pints of beer per week develops severe, upper abdominal pain, which radiates to the back. A plain abdominal X-ray shows a sentinel loop (dilatation of a loop of bowel adjacent to the pancreas) in the left upper quadrant.

2. A 70-year-old man who has been progressively losing weight develops severe, colicky abdominal pain and has not opened his bowels for a week.

3. A 35-year-old overweight woman has a 6-month history of colicky abdominal pain, which radiates to her back. On examination, Murphy's sign is positive.

4. A 45-year-old man has a 3-month history of upper abdominal pain that wakes him at night. He reports that the pain is worsened by hunger and tends to be relieved by eating. His weight is stable.

5. A 70-year-old hypertensive man develops severe, left-sided, loin pain of 6 hours' duration. On examination, he is sweaty, his blood pressure is 90/60 mmHg and the pulse rate is 110/min. Blood investigations show that he has a haemoglobin level of 8 g/dl.

Answers to **2.12**

1.   J   Serum biochemistry

The investigation of choice is the serum amylase to confirm acute pancreatitis. One of the causes for acute pancreatitis is excessive alcohol intake. Symptoms usually start after an alcoholic binge with severe abdominal pain radiating to the back. An abdominal X-ray is important to exclude perforation of a duodenal ulcer, and it may show a slightly dilated air-containing loop of small bowel in the left upper quadrant called the sentinel loop. This is produced by a local ileus of small bowel adjacent to the pancreas. Absence of gas in the transverse colon, the so-called colon cut-off sign, may also be seen.

2.   A   Abdominal X-ray

This patient has symptoms suggestive of intestinal obstruction and in view of his age and loss of weight it is likely to be a carcinoma, most probably in the large bowel. The initial investigation should be a plain abdominal film which will show a distended large bowel proximal to the point of obstruction. Once this is diagnosed further management can be planned depending upon the patient's condition.

3.   K   Ultrasound of the abdomen

Upper abdominal pain in an obese patient, particularly if it is in the right hypochondrium, is suggestive of biliary colic. This is usually due to gall stones in which case Murphy's test is often positive. The investigation of choice is an ultrasound scan of the upper abdomen.

4.   H   Gastroscopy

This patient probably has a peptic ulcer. A duodenal ulcer causes pain that improves after a meal whereas the pain from a gastric ulcer is worsened by eating. A definitive investigation is an upper gastrointestinal endoscopy.

5.   G   Computerized tomography (CT) scan of the abdomen

This patient has the classic symptoms suggestive of a leaking abdominal aortic aneurysm. The investigation of choice is a computerized tomography scan of the abdomen which will clearly show the retroperitoneal haematoma. Being a non-invasive investigation, it is preferable to aortography.

Investigation of suspected intestinal obstruction

A   Abdominal X-ray
B   Barium enema
C   Computerized tomography (CT) scan of the abdomen
D   Electrolyte estimation
E   Flexible sigmoidoscopy
F   Gastrograffin enema
G   Intravenous urography
H   MRI scan of the abdomen
I   Rigid sigmoidoscopy
J   Small bowel enema
K   Ultrasound scan of the abdomen

For each presentation below choose the SINGLE most appropriate investigation from the above list. Each option may be used once, more than once, or not at all.

1.   A 60-year-old lady presents with increasing constipation and colicky abdominal pain. She has lost weight and examination reveals a mass in the left iliac fossa. An abdominal X-ray shows a grossly distended colon as far as the sigmoid and distally there is a paucity of gas.

2.   An 80-year-old man presents with a 2-day history of vomiting with abdominal pain and distension. Examination reveals a distended abdomen with tenderness in the right iliac fossa but the bowel sounds are normal.

3.   A 70-year-old lady presents with an acute abdomen and, at laparotomy, there is a perforated appendix with free pus in the pelvis. Seven days post-operatively she has not opened her bowels or passed flatus. Her abdomen is distended, the bowel sounds are absent and there is minimal tenderness all over her abdomen. An abdominal X-ray shows distended loops of small bowel.

4.   A 65-year-old man has a 2-month history of weight loss of 1 stone associated with three episodes of abdominal pain, distension and constipation. More recently, he has passed some dark blood per rectum with a feeling of incomplete evacuation.

5.   A 30-year-old lady has a 3-week history of abdominal pain, distension and vomiting. Before this she has had a long history of recurrent diarrhoea but a barium enema performed 3 months ago was normal. She appears pale and thin. Abdominal examination reveals tenderness in the right iliac fossa with a suggestion of a mass in this region.

Answers to **2.13**

1.   F   Gastrograffin enema

This patient has a large bowel obstruction. If she does not require immediate operation then investigations need to be done to determine the cause of the obstruction. In this case, a barium enema cannot be performed without adequately preparing the bowel so a water-soluble contrast enema is preferred.

2.   A   Abdominal X-ray

This patient has signs suggestive of intestinal obstruction. The first investigation that must be done, along with routine blood tests, is a plain abdominal X-ray. This can generally be very informative and in this case may show distended loops of small or large bowel.

3.   D   Electrolyte estimation

This lady has had major abdominal surgery and in most cases the bowel starts to work a few days after the operation. From the clinical picture given, this patient appears to have a paralytic ileus. In addition to an abdominal film, her bloods need to be checked for an electrolyte imbalance. Hypokalaemia is a common contributory factor.

4.   E   Flexible sigmoidoscopy

This patient's symptoms warrant urgent investigation. It is most likely that he has either a rectal or a colonic neoplasm. Sigmoidoscopy uncovers up to 75% of large bowel carcinomas and enables one to obtain a biopsy. It should precede a barium enema.

5.   J   Small bowel enema

The clinical picture here suggests that this patient has inflammatory bowel disease probably in the small bowel since the barium enema is normal. She now has a subacute intestinal obstruction and requires a small bowel enema in order to determine the mucosal appearance of the small intestine.

Investigation of rectal bleeding

A Angiography
B Barium enema
C Barium meal
D Coagulation screen
E Colonoscopy
F Computerized axial tomography
G Faecal occult blood
H Flexible sigmoidoscopy
I Gastroscopy
J Proctoscopy
K Technetium-labelled red cell scan

For each of the presentations below choose the SINGLE most appropriate investigation from the above list. Each option may be used once, more than once, or not at all.

1. A 30-year-old man has a long history of painless, bright red bleeding per rectum which usually stains the toilet paper. He is otherwise asymptomatic. Digital rectal examination is normal.

2. A 60-year-old woman presents with dark red bleeding per rectum with loss of weight and a change in bowel habits towards looser motions. The patient did not tolerate an attempt at endoscopic assessment.

3. A 30-year-old woman presents with a history of passing loose stools with blood and mucus about eight to ten times a day for the past 3 months. She also complains of intermittent abdominal pain and weight loss.

4. A 60-year-old woman is referred with a history of passing large amounts of dark blood per rectum with no associated abdominal pain. Her vital signs are stable and her haemoglobin has dropped from 10 g/dl to 8 g/dl over 3 days. This is the fifth episode that she has had in 2 years. During her previous admissions, she has required repeated transfusions and has been investigated with a colonoscopy and a barium enema which were both normal.

5. A 70-year-old woman has presented with a history of passing altered blood per rectum associated with vague abdominal pain. A digital rectal examination reveals black residue on the glove. The only medication that she takes regularly is indometacin for her osteoarthrosis.

Answers to **2.14**

1. J   Proctoscopy

This man has haemorrhoids. Proctoscopy is the first line of
investigation. This will show the presence and degree of the
haemorrhoids which appear as bluish masses beneath the anal mucosa
and are commonly referred to as piles. Most haemorrhoids are 'internal',
covered by mucosa and may be first degree (never prolapse through the
anal canal), second degree (prolapse during defecation but return
spontaneously) or third degree (remain outside the anal margin). First
and second degree haemorrhoids can be banded or injected with a
sclerosant. Haemorrhoidectomy is reserved for third degree piles and for
the first and second degree haemorrhoids that have not responded to
treatment.

2. B   Barium enema

This lady has the symptoms of a colonic malignancy. Flexible
sigmoidoscopy or colonoscopy allows visual inspection and biopsy of
suspicious lesions and is the investigation of choice. A barium enema is
an alternative in patients who are unable to tolerate endoscopy although
the lower rectum is not always clearly visualized. A rectal examination
and rigid sigmoidoscopy should be performed before the barium enema.

3. E   Colonoscopy

This patient has symptoms suggestive of inflammatory bowel disease.
She needs a full assessment of the colon and rectum to establish both
the diagnosis and the extent of the disease. This is achieved by taking
multiple biopsies from various parts of the colon and rectum and this
can only be done effectively by colonoscopy.

4. K   Technetium-labelled red cell scan

This patient may have angiodysplasia which are small hamartomatous
vascular lesions in the bowel wall. These lesions cannot always be
visualized by colonoscopy. Selective mesenteric arteriography may reveal
the source of bleeding but there has to be active bleeding at a high rate
for this test to be useful. Following the course of technetium-labelled red
cells is the investigation of choice in this scenario as it helps to locate
the source of relatively slow bleeding. The affected segment of the bowel
may have to be removed if the lesions cannot be treated with electric
coagulation via the colonoscope.

5. I   Gastroscopy

This patient probably has an upper gastrointestinal source of bleeding
secondary to her anti-inflammatory medication. The black stools are
highly suggestive and the investigation of choice would be a gastroscopy.

Investigation of diarrhoea

A Barium enema
B Colonoscopy
C Computerized tomography (CT) of the abdomen
D Hydrogen breath test
E Jejunal biopsy
F Lactose tolerance tests
G Pancreatic exocrine function tests
H Rectal biopsy
I Small bowel follow through
J Stool specimen for *Clostridium difficile* toxin
K Thyroid function tests

For each of the following presentations choose the SINGLE most appropriate investigation from the options above. Each option may be used once, more than once, or not at all.

1. A 25-year-old woman presents with a 3-month history of weight loss and bloody diarrhoea with mucus. She has had the diarrhoea about ten times a day with associated abdominal pain.

2. A 65-year-old woman presents with tiredness and lethargy. She also has abdominal discomfort, weight loss of half a stone and steatorrhoea. Endomysial antibodies are present in her serum.

3. A 70-year-old woman presents with fever, diarrhoea and abdominal pain. She is still recovering from a recent hospital admission for pneumonia.

4. A 25-year-old woman with anxiety passes loose stools, sometimes with mucus, this occurrs up to ten times a day but there is no history of rectal bleeding. On examination, she looks unwell and has a tender lump in the right iliac fossa. Her recent barium enema is normal and her serum albumin is 27g/L.

5. A 32-year-old man who had a past history of episodic diarrhoea has developed persistent diarrhoea and flatulence, since he was started on treatment for a duodenal ulcer in surgical outpatients. His initial symptoms of the ulcer have subsided but he now has excessive abdominal gurgling and profuse diarrhoea.

Answers to **2.15**

1. **B Colonoscopy**

This patient's symptoms are suggestive of inflammatory bowel disease. The study of any patient with bloody diarrhoea must begin with a sigmoidoscopy (not in the list), but colonoscopy is more valuable in determining the extent of involvement of the bowel in inflammatory bowel disease. It is also of diagnostic importance in determining the distinction between ulcerative colitis and Crohn's disease (the latter shows segmental disease with areas of bowel spared).

2. **E Jejunal biopsy**

Coeliac disease may present at any age with a peak incidence in adults between 30 and 40 years of age. Symptoms include diarrhoea, steatorrhoea, weight loss, mouth ulcers and angular stomatitis. There is sensitivity to gluten (present in wheat, rye, barley and oats), which causes damage to the mucosa of the proximal small bowel (subtotal villous atrophy). There may be malabsorption of folate and iron with hypoalbuminaemia in more severe cases. A jejunal biopsy is diagnostic.

3. **J Stool specimen for *Clostridium difficile* toxin**

Pseudomembranous colitis is caused by colonization of the colon by *Clostridium difficile*. This may occur up to a month following antibiotic therapy. Sigmoidoscopy reveals inflammation, ulceration and plaque formation of the rectal mucosa. The presence of the toxin in the stools is diagnostic. Treatment with vancomycin or metronidazole may be required.

4. **I Small bowel follow through**

This patient has symptoms suggestive of inflammatory bowel disease. The presence of diarrhoea without bleeding and a tender right iliac fossa mass is highly suggestive of Crohn's disease affecting the terminal ileum. The colon seems to be spared but a small bowel follow through may show Crohn's disease with ileal involvement, with deep ulceration, strictures and a cobblestone appearance.

5. **F Lactose tolerance test**

This patient with a history of episodic diarrhoea has lactose intolerance, and the increase in his diarrhoea with gas and upper digestive complaints result from drinking too much milk for his duodenal ulcer. This link is sometimes missed when the duodenal ulcer is blamed for the symptoms and treated more energetically with worsening of flatulence and diarrhoea. The hydrogen excretion breath test is appropriate but a lactose tolerance test will provide the definitive evidence.

Investigation of dysphagia

A   Barium swallow
B   Chest X-ray
C   Computerized tomography (CT) of the chest
D   Electromyography
E   Endo-oesophageal ultrasound scan
F   Gastroscopy
G   Laryngoscopy
H   Manometry
I   pH monitoring studies
J   Rigid oesophagoscopy
K   Thoracic inlet X-ray

For each of the presentations below choose the SINGLE most appropriate investigation from the above options. Each option may be used once, more than once, or not at all.

1. A 60-year-old man complains of intermittent dysphagia with regurgitation of undigested food. There is a swelling in his neck which produces a gurgling sound when he swallows.

2. A 40-year-old woman presents with gradually worsening dysphagia for both liquids and solids. She also complains of regurgitation of food, a retrosternal discomfort, foetid flatulence and recurrent chest infections.

3. A 70-year-old man presents with dysphagia, initially with solids and now also with fluids. Gastroscopy reveals a squamous-cell carcinoma of the oesophagus in the middle third of the oesophagus. He would like the tumour resected if possible.

4. A 45-year-old woman complains of intermittent chest pain associated with dysphagia which clears after a drink of water. Both symptoms are exacerbated by emotional stress. Her electrocardiogram and gastroscopy are normal.

5. A 60-year-old man has progressive dysphagia and chokes when eating. His mobility has also deteriorated over the last 12 months. On examination, he has evidence of muscle wasting, fasciculation and bilateral foot drop.

Answers to **2.16**

1. **A** Barium swallow

A pharyngeal pouch is a mucosal herniation through the lower pharyngeal muscles, probably due to lack of coordination between the contraction of the pharynx and the relaxation of the upper oesophageal sphincter. The symptoms described are classic although it is unusual to be able to palpate the swelling in the neck. To confirm the diagnosis, a barium swallow is preferable to gastroscopy as the latter can perforate the pouch.

2. **A** Barium swallow

This patient has symptoms suggestive of achalasia. In this condition, there is a high resting pressure throughout the oesophagus, loss of propulsive peristalsis and failure of the lower oesophageal sphincter to relax on swallowing. The underlying cause is usually due to degeneration of Auerbach's plexus. Dysphagia is the predominant presenting symptom but regurgitation of food is also common. Aspiration may cause an aspiration pneumonitis and pulmonary fibrosis. The investigation of choice is a barium swallow which will show a tapered narrowing of the lower segment with gross proximal dilatation of the oesophagus.

3. **C** Computerized tomography (CT) of the chest

This patient has oesophageal carcinoma and about 40% are resectable. CT scans are useful to assess resectability and to stage the disease. An endo-oesophageal ultrasound scan may be used to show the degree of oesophageal wall invasion.

4. **H** Manometry

Diffuse oesophageal spasm is a poorly understood and equally poorly treated motility disorder, in which the patient experiences chest pain and dysphagia from oesophageal hypermotility and spasm. Diagnosis is difficult because of the intermittent nature of the condition but radiography and motility studies are both used. Manometry will show simultaneous contractions and a hypertensive lower oesophageal sphincter. A barium meal may show a 'cork-screw' oesophagus in about 50% of cases. Acid perfusion may elicit the chest pain of oesophageal spasm.

5. **D** Electromyography

This patient has motor neurone disease which has caused bulbar palsy and progressive muscular atrophy. The diagnosis is made on clinical grounds. Of the options listed, electromyography would be appropriate, as it would confirm lower motor neurone degeneration and exclude other disorders of the neuromuscular junction such as myasthenia gravis.

Investigation of haematuria

A   Coagulation screen
B   Computerized tomography
C   Cystoscopy
D   Intravenous pyelography
E   Renal angiography
F   Renal biopsy
G   Renogram
H   Retrograde urography
I   Ultrasound scan
J   Urine culture and sensitivity
K   Urine cytology

For each presentation below, choose the SINGLE most discriminating investigation from the above list of options. Each option may be used once, more than once, or not at all.

1. A 65-year-old woman presents with haematuria. Clinical examination is unremarkable except for a prosthetic second heart sound.

2. A 30-year-old man has a sudden, colicky pain in the left flank which radiates to the groin. He finds it difficult to get into a comfortable position. Urine microscopy shows 20–50 RBC (red blood cells) and only an occasional WBC (white blood cell) in each high power field.

3. A 75-year-old man presents with a 12-month history of worsening nocturia. A smooth, enlarged prostate is palpable per rectum and there is evidence of microscopic haematuria.

4. A 70-year-old man has episodes of frank haematuria with clots, and intermittent dysuria. He has lost about half a stone in weight in the last 3 months. Intravenous urography is normal.

5. A 50-year-old man presents with frank haematuria and pain in the right loin. He also complains of weight loss and night sweats. On examination, there is fullness in the right loin. His ESR (erythrocyte sedimentation rate) is elevated and the full blood count is suggestive of secondary polycythaemia.

Answers to **2.17**

1. A Coagulation screen

This patient will be on warfarin because of the prosthetic aortic valve. Warfarin is a vitamin K antagonist and decreases the biological activity of vitamin K-dependent factors II, VII, IX and X. The haematuria may be due to overcoagulation and partly due to fragmentation of some red blood cells as they strike the artificial valve. It is important to check the INR (International Normalized Ratio). If it is high then the patient should be reassured and the dose of warfarin adjusted. It may be sufficient to stop the warfarin for several doses. A full reversal of anticoagulation should not be attempted, as this would render the patient refractory for 2 weeks and may lead to thrombosis on the prosthetic valve. If the haematuria is gross then a small dose of vitamin K_1 (5 mg) should be given.

2. D Intravenous pyelography

This patient has the classic symptoms of ureteric colic for which intravenous pyelography is the investigation of choice. It gives valuable information regarding renal function, the anatomical outline of the upper renal tract and the degree of obstruction. A plain abdominal X-ray can occasionally be useful though radiolucent calculi will be missed.

3. I Ultrasound scan

This man has symptoms and signs of having benign prostatic hyperplasia which affects 50% of men over the age of 60. An ultrasound scan is the investigation of choice in order to demonstrate the size of the prostate and also the effects of the bladder outflow obstruction by estimating the residual urine volume. It is quick, safe and non-invasive.

4. C Cystoscopy

Haematuria (often macroscopic) and irritative bladder symptoms, such as urgency, dysuria and frequency, are the most common presenting symptoms of bladder cancer. In the absence of infection, these symptoms should lead to an evaluation for malignancy. In this case, the normal intravenous pyelography suggests normal kidneys and ureters. Small lesions in the bladder, especially if the lesion is flat, can be easily missed on X-rays. A cystoscopy is essential to examine the bladder and urethra.

5. B Computerized tomography

Renal cell carcinomas arise from the proximal tubular epithelium and account for up to 3% of malignancies. Symptoms include haematuria, loin pain, malaise, weight loss and pyrexia. Occasionally, there may be secondary polycythaemia due to inappropriate erythropoietin secretion. Computerized tomography with contrast is useful in identifying the renal lesion and any involvement of the renal vein or the inferior vena cava and for the identification of metastases.

Investigation for vascular diseases

A   Colonoscopy
B   Computerized tomography (CT) with intravenous contrast
C   Doppler studies
D   Duplex scan
E   FBC/U&E/LFTs/lipid studies/blood glucose
F   Femoral arteriogram
G   Magnetic resonance imaging (MRI) scan
H   Selective mesenteric arteriogram
I   Ultrasound scan of the abdomen
J   Venogram
K   Ventilation–perfusion scan

For each patient below, choose the SINGLE most appropriate investigation from the above list of options. Each option may be used once, more than once, or not at all.

1. A 60-year-old man presents with a severe, tearing chest pain radiating to the back and both arms. He is hypertensive. Femoral pulses are not palpable and he complains of diminished sensation below the umbilicus. A chest X-ray suggests widening of the mediastinum.

2. A 65-year-old female has developed severe, right-sided chest pain. She had an abdominal hysterectomy 4 days ago. Her oxygen saturation is low but the ECG and chest X-ray are inconclusive.

3. A 70-year-old male smoker presents with a 3-year history of developing pain in his left leg when he walked about 100 metres, after which he had to take rest. At present, he gets pain when he walks 30 metres and on occasions he gets rest pain as well. Arterial pulses below the femoral artery are not palpable. The base-line blood studies are normal.

4. A 75-year-old male has started to have transient ischaemic attacks. Otherwise, he is fit and well and had stopped smoking about 2 years before this presentation. He has requested non-invasive investigations.

5. A 65-year-old male presents with a pulsatile mass in the abdomen which is not tender. The mass is just to the left of the midline and extends from the epigastrium to the umbilicus and measures about 7 cm in diameter.

Answers to **2.18**

1. **B** **Computerized tomography (CT) with intravenous contrast**

This patient's history suggests a dissection of the thoracic aorta. Urgent computerized tomography is required to confirm the diagnosis. The definitive management should be started before the tomography and involves stabilizing the blood pressure with hypotensive agents (intravenous labetalol and nitroprusside) to a systolic BP of <100 mmHg. As there is end-organ ischaemia with loss of pulses and diminished sensation, urgent surgical intervention is indicated to replace the affected segment with a graft.

2. **K** **Ventilation–perfusion scan**

This patient is most likely to have had a pulmonary embolus. The initial investigations are chest X-ray, ECG and blood gases which can all give clues to the diagnosis but the investigation of choice would be a ventilation–perfusion scan using radionuclides.

3. **F** **Femoral arteriogram**

This patient has peripheral vascular disease and smokers are more at risk. A femoral arteriogram is the investigation of choice as it gives a 'roadmap' of the vascular tree and highlights specific areas of occlusion, the extent of the disease, run off beyond any point of occlusion and the presence of collateral blood supply. Management can then be planned appropriately.

4. **D** **Duplex scan**

This patient probably has internal carotid artery disease and there is a need to assess its extent. The duplex technology was developed in the 1980s specifically to improve the non-invasive diagnosis of carotid artery disease. The image, which is obtained by scanning with ultrasound pulses and re-assembling the return pulses with an image on computer, is combined with the pulse Doppler to improve the accuracy.

5. **I** **Ultrasound scan of the abdomen**

This patient's symptoms and findings suggest that he has an abdominal aortic aneurysm. Ultrasound measurement of the size of the abdominal aortic aneurysm is reproducible and has a reported sensitivity and positive predictive value of 100%, as verified by subsequent surgery or computerized tomography. This mode of investigation is inexpensive, readily available and the initial investigation of choice. However, computerized tomography is superior in the delineation of the extent of the aneurysm as well as its relation to surrounding structures.

Investigation of postoperative complications

A   Abdominal X-ray
B   Chest X-ray
C   Computerized tomography (CT) with intravenous contrast
D   Duplex ultrasonography
E   Electrocardiogram
F   Gastroscopy
G   Intravenous pyelography
H   Small bowel contrast study
I   Ultrasound scan
J   Urine culture/sensitivity
K   Water-soluble contrast enema

For each scenario below choose the SINGLE most appropriate investigation from the above list. Each option may be used once, more than once, or not at all.

1. A 75-year-old man has recently had an anterior resection with end-to-end anastomosis. He was fine until the seventh postoperative day when he developed a spiking temperature and severe, lower abdominal pain. On examination, there are signs of localized peritonism.

2. A 10-year-old boy has had surgery for a perforated appendix. Postoperatively he recovered well and was discharged home on the fourth day. He was brought back to hospital on the fifth day with a high pyrexia, lower abdominal pain and diarrhoea. A rectal examination reveals a boggy swelling anteriorly.

3. A 65-year-old woman has had an uneventful hysterectomy. On the fourth postoperative day, she developed a painful swelling of the right leg. On examination, the right calf is swollen, hot and tender to touch.

4. A 75-year-old male has had an emergency Hartmann's procedure for faecal peritonitis secondary to perforated diverticular disease. The operation note describes that there was a large inflammatory mass with extensive adhesions in the left iliac fossa. Postoperatively on the second day he is discharging a urine-like fluid through the drain.

5. A 60-year-old man known to suffer from ischaemic heart disease has just had a distal gastrectomy. In the immediate postoperative period, he had 2 L of crystalloid intravenously because of a falling urine output. He has suddenly become dyspnoeic and is coughing up frothy sputum with flecks of blood. He looks cyanosed and auscultation of the chest reveals bilateral crepitations.

Answers to **2.19**

1. **K Water-soluble contrast enema**

   This patient probably has an anastomotic leak. This usually occurs a few days postoperatively. If there is doubt about the diagnosis, a water-soluble contrast enema will confirm the leak. This is preferable to using barium as it is less irritant to the peritoneal cavity should there be a leak. This patient will need active resuscitation, antibiotics and conservative management which may suffice if it is a contained leak. However, many patients need a laparotomy, peritoneal lavage and a stoma formation.

2. **I Ultrasound scan**

   This patient has the clinical features of a pelvic abscess. It is well-known to complicate surgery performed for a perforated appendix. An ultrasound scan is the investigation of choice as it is non-invasive and confirms the diagnosis with a high degree of accuracy. Sometimes the abscess can be aspirated and a drain inserted under ultrasonic guidance thus avoiding the need for a laparotomy.

3. **D Duplex ultrasonography**

   This patient has the classic symptoms of a deep vein thrombosis. The risk of this complication increases with age, obesity, cardiovascular disease, immobility and pelvic surgery. A duplex scanner uses B mode ultrasound to provide an image of the vessels based on the fact that different tissues have differing abilities to reflect the ultrasound beam. Venography (not on the list) is an alternative means of diagnostic evaluation.

4. **G Intravenous pyelography**

   This patient has a urinary leak most likely due to damage caused to the left ureter during surgery. Due to the severe inflammation in these situations, the anatomy can be distorted and great care is required to avoid damage to the ureter. Intravenous pyelography will confirm the diagnosis.

5. **B Chest X-ray**

   This patient has pulmonary oedema secondary to fluid overload on a background of a compromised cardiac status resulting in left ventricular failure. A chest X-ray is useful in confirming the diagnosis. The treatment involves immediate administration of diuretics and careful monitoring of the central venous pressure.

Investigation of swellings in the neck

A Calcitonin levels
B Calcium profile
C Carotid arteriography
D Computerized tomography (CT) scan
E Fine needle aspiration
F Isotope thyroid scan
G Magnetic resonance imaging (MRI) scan
H Sestamibi imaging
I Sialogram
J Thyroid function tests
K Ultrasound scan

For each of the presentations below choose the SINGLE most appropraite investigation from the above list. Each option may be used once, more than once, or not at all.

1. A 40-year-old man presents with a painful swelling in the right anterior triangle. This appears after a meal and then slowly disappears. On examination, the swelling is firm, about 2 cm in size and is bimanually palpable.

2. A 45-year-old woman presents with polyuria, polydypsia and dyspeptic symptoms. Serum calcium and parathyroid hormone (PTH) levels are both elevated.

3. A 50-year-old woman presents with a central swelling in the neck. This is found to be a cold nodule in the thyroid from radionucleide studies.

4. A 40-year-old woman presents with a swelling at the level of the upper border of the thyroid cartilage. It has been growing in size slowly over several years. It is now 2 cm in diameter, hard, pulsatile, lobulated and is located under the upper third of the sternomastoid muscle. The swelling can be moved laterally but not vertically. A computerized tomography scan has been inconclusive in establishing the diagnosis.

5. A 60-year-old man, who has been a heavy smoker, presents with a swelling in the right posterior triangle of the neck. The lump is 2 cm in size and is hard and non-tender. A chest X-ray shows an opacity in the apex of the right lung.

Answers to 2.20

1. I Sialogram

This patient has the typical presentation of a submandibular gland swelling and the history that the swelling appears after a meal suggests that there is a calculus causing obstruction. A submandibular sialogram will show this obstruction, if it is present.

2. D Computerized tomography (CT) scan

This patient has a suspected parathyroid adenoma. This can be localized using a number of radiological modalities. High resolution, real-time ultrasonography is useful. However, in the most recent studies, computerized tomography appeared to be as effective as the ultrasound scan but also superior in identifying ectopically-situated parathyroid glands, particularly when in the mediastinum.

3. E Fine needle aspiration

Thyroid swellings which do not take up the isotope are referred to as cold nodules and may be benign or malignant. The diagnosis can often be achieved by performing a fine needle aspiration and subjecting the sample to cytological examination. Whenever evaluating thyroid nodules, this investigation should be done in preference to any isotope scans.

4. C Carotid arteriography

This patient appears to have a carotid body tumour. The diagnosis can sometimes be achieved with computerized tomography, but carotid arteriography will provide a definitive diagnosis. In addition, arteriography also provides valuable information for planning surgical treatment such as the exact blood supply, the presence of concomitant atherosclerotic disease, etc.

5. E Fine needle aspiration

The swelling in the neck is most likely a metastatic lymph node from a bronchogenic carcinoma. A fine needle aspiration of this lump will usually provide a sufficient sample for cytological diagnosis and confirmation of the primary lesion.

Radiological features seen with an acute abdomen

A   Air in the biliary tree
B   Air under the diaphragm
C   Bent inner tube sign
D   Distended air-filled caecum
E   Distended air-filled transverse colon
F   Double bubble appearance
G   Featureless colon
H   Ground glass appearance
I   Multiple fluid levels
J   Sentinel loop
K   Step ladder sign

For each of the scenarios below choose the SINGLE most appropriate X-ray appearance from the above list. Each option may be used once, more than once, or not at all.

1.   A 45-year-old man known to suffer from dyspeptic symptoms develops sudden onset of severe upper abdominal pain, which becomes progressively worse. On examination of the abdomen, there is tenderness and guarding all over the abdomen and the liver dullness is obliterated on percussion. An erect chest X-ray is taken.

2.   A 62-year-old man with a history of chronic constipation presents with a sudden, severe, twisting pain in the right lower quadrant of his abdomen. On examination, the abdomen is distended and tender with guarding. An abdominal film is obtained.

3.   An 85-year-old man with senile dementia develops severe abdominal pain with distension. He is known to have chronic constipation. On examination, he has a grossly distended abdomen. An abdominal X-ray shows massive distension of the sigmoid colon, the apex of which appears to almost reach the right upper quadrant of the abdomen. There is paucity of gas in the rectum.

4.   A 75-year-old woman has presented with distal, small bowel obstruction. A laparotomy shows that she has a 2 cm calculus in the ileum which is the cause of the obstruction. A preoperative abdominal X-ray confirms the presence of ileal obstruction but, in addition, also gives a vital clue to the probable underlying pathology.

5.   A 40-year-old man, with ulcerative colitis, was improving with lessening of diarrhoea when he felt diffuse pain in his abdomen, aggravated by cough and movement. His temperature is hectic reaching up to 41°C. The abdomen is soft but very tender. A plain film of the abdomen is taken.

Answers to **2.21**

1. B Air under the diaphragm

This patient has a good story for a perforated peptic ulcer. Free intraperitoneal air is generally due to perforation of the stomach, small intestine or colon and can be seen, on an erect chest X-ray, as a crescent under the diaphragm, more commonly under the right than the left.

2. D Distended air-filled caecum

Caecal volvulus may occur with sudden tight twisting of the mesentery leading to early fulminating gangrene with features like any other abdominal emergency. It can be recognized on an abdominal film by the marked distension of the caecum, arising from the right lower quadrant and reaching the left upper quadrant. If operation is long delayed, the mortality rate is 30–60%.

3. C Bent inner tube sign

This patient has a sigmoid volvulus. Plain abdominal X-rays often reveal a dilated colon that forms the so-called bent inner tube or omega loop sign. Two air-fluid levels, commonly at different levels, are frequently seen within the sigmoid loop. This condition results in total large bowel obstruction and so there is no gas seen distal to the level of obstruction. This appearance on an abdominal film is striking enough to suggest the diagnosis, but in doubtful cases a barium enema should be performed. This will show a narrowing at the site of the twist, the so-called bird-beak or ace-of-spades deformity.

4. A Air in the biliary tree

This patient has a gall stone ileus. Plain abdominal X-rays will often show air in the biliary tree. Chronic cholecystitis can sometimes result in a large gall stone perforating into the duodenum through a cholecystoduodenal fistula, and the gall stone travels distally and sometimes gets impacted in the distal ileum causing intestinal obstruction. Unfortunately, this finding is frequently missed.

5. E Distended air-filled transverse colon

The combination of decreased frequency of diarrhoea, diffuse, persistent abdominal pain and tenderness should alert the surgeon to the possibility of acute toxic megacolon. A plain film of the abdomen will show massive dilatation of the bowel, often limited to the transverse colon. The very presence of air in the transverse colon, even if slightly dilated, in a patient with ulcerative colitis should suggest the possibility. Abdominal films should be examined carefully for evidence of air lying free in the peritoneal cavity and in the bowel wall where it may have leaked through an ulcer crater.

Tumour markers

A   AFP (alpha fetoprotein)
B   CA 125
C   CA 153
D   CA 199
E   CA 242
F   CEA (carcinoembryonic antigen)
G   Erb B2
H   NSE (neurone specific enolase)
I   PAP (prostatic acid phosphatase)
J   PSA (prostate specific antigen)
K   Tissue polypeptide antigen

For each presentation below choose the SINGLE most appropriate investigation from the above list of options. Each option can be used once, more than once, or not at all.

1. A 40-year-old woman notices increasing, lower abdominal distension with little or no pain. On examination of the abdomen, a lobulated cystic mass is felt which seems to be arising from the pelvis.

2. A 75-year-old man has urinary symptoms of hesitancy, frequency and nocturia. Rectal examination reveals a large, hard prostate.

3. A 25-year-old man notices a lump in his right testis and he has a heavy, dragging sensation in the right side of his scrotum. An ultrasound scan suggests that this swelling is probably malignant. Histological examination of the excised testis has shown this to be a teratoma.

4. A 65-year-old woman had an excision of a colonic tumour 3 years ago. Now she is losing weight and feels lethargic. On examination, she is pale but there are no abdominal findings.

5. A 55-year-old man develops back pain and loss of weight. A computerized tomography (CT) scan of the abdomen shows the presence of a mass in the head of the pancreas.

Answers to **2.22**

1.   B   CA 125

The symptoms and clinical findings are suggestive of an ovarian tumour. The diagnosis can usually be confirmed with radiological imaging. However, there are a few tumour markers for this condition, the most common being CA 125. This is a glycoprotein antigen and is associated with an epithelial ovarian cancer.

2.   J   PSA (prostatic specific antigen)

The history and clinical findings are suggestive of prostatic cancer. One of the first tests should be a serum PSA. This is a glycoprotein specific for prostatic tissue. This is present in all males and can be raised, both in benign prostatic hypertrophy and in prostatic cancer. Levels above 10 ng/mL are suspicious of a cancer.

3.   A   AFP (alpha fetoprotein)

Although both AFP and beta-HCG (human chorionic gonadotrophin) are important tumour markers for testicular cancers, 75% of patients with non-seminomatous testicular germ-cell tumours have increased levels of serum AFP. A few of these patients will have raised beta-HCG as well. The levels drop after orchidectomy. Monitoring these tumour markers is part of the management after surgery and a further elevation often signifies metastatic disease.

4.   F   CEA (carcinoembryonic antigen)

This is a useful investigation for colorectal cancer. Although CEA is not colorectal-tumour-specific, nevertheless high concentrations in tissue and serum are found in patients with colorectal cancer. However, its usefulness for screening purposes is compromised, as cigarette smoking, pulmonary inflammation, hepatitis, pancreatitis and inflammatory bowel disease can all raise CEA levels.

5.   D   CA 199

This is a circulating marker that has sensitivity and specificity for pancreatic cancer. It is generally not detectable in the serum of normal subjects but may be present in patients with colorectal and gastric cancer. About 82% of patients with pancreatic cancer will have an elevated CA 199 level.

Common pathogenic organisms seen in surgical practice

A   Actinomycosis
B   Bacteroides
C   *C. trachomatis*
D   *E. coli*
E   *E. histolytica*
F   Proteus
G   Pseudomonas
H   *Staphylococcus epidermidis*
I   *Streptococcus faecalis*
J   *Streptococcus pneumoniae*
K   *Streptococcus pyogenes*

For each of the following clinical situations choose the SINGLE most likely causative organism from the above list. Each option may be used once, more than once, or not at all.

1. A 35-year-old man has an incision and drainage of a perianal abscess and then develops a persistent, purulent discharge from the abscess site. Examination under anaesthesia reveals a posterior fistula-in-ano.

2. A 55-year-old man had a splenectomy following a blunt injury to his abdomen. Two months later he develops pyrexia, a cough with purulent sputum and pleuritic chest pain on the right side.

3. A 60-year-old alcoholic man presents with a tender swelling in the right hypochondrium. He has a history of recurrent diarrhoea with mucus. He is pyrexial and an ultrasound scan of the abdomen reveals the swelling to be an abscess in the liver. This is drained and the pus is described as being similar to anchovy sauce.

4. A 20-year-old obese woman develops multiple, pustular skin lesions. One of the lesions progresses into an abscess, which requires incision and drainage.

5. A 30-year-old sailor presents with bilateral, tender lumps in the groin. He gives a history of transient skin lesions on his penis. Following this he developed bilateral inguinal lymphadenitis that has progressed to bubo formation by the time of the examination.

Answers to 2.23

1. **D** *E. coli*

A large percentage of patients with a fistula-in-ano would have had a preceding anorectal abscess. Since there is a communication between the bowel and the skin it is expected that the infecting organism would be the one that is commonly found in the bowel. *E. coli* is the commonest organism grown in about 60% of cases. Other organisms implicated in this condition are Bacteroides, Streptococcus, or *B. proteus*. In many cases the infection is mixed.

2. **J** *Streptococcus pneumoniae*

The spleen helps to destroy bacteria, particularly encapsulated organisms. Splenectomized patients show reduced antibody production when challenged with particulate antigens. Hence, they are at risk of infection particularly to encapsulated bacteria such as *Streptococcus pneumoniae*. It is usual for post-splenectomy patients to be given Pneumovax II and long term penicillin prophylaxis.

3. **E** *E. histolytica*

This is the protozoa that causes amoebiasis. Five percent of patients will develop a hepatic abscess. This is usually drained radiologically and occasionally by open surgery. The characteristic pus from an amoebic liver abscess is chocolate-coloured (like anchovy sauce) and consists of broken down liver cells, leucocytes and red blood cells.

4. **H** *Staphylococcus epidermidis*

This condition is commonly known as a boil and is due to an acute staphylococcal infection of a hair follicle. There is perifolliculitis, which usually proceeds to suppuration with central necrosis. Multiple lesions can occur when the condition is described as furunculosis. Occasionally some of the lesions can turn into a full-blown abscess.

5. **C** *C. trachomatis*

Lymphogranuloma venereum is the result of sexually transmitted infection with *C. trachomatis*. The infection is characterized by a transient lesion on the skin or mucous membrane of the genitalia or rectum and it is painless. Subsequently (2–4 weeks later), the infected person develops painful, regional lymphadenitis which often progresses to bubo formation. There are usually systemic features including fever, rigors, headache and myalgia.

Assessment of a lump in the groin

A Arteriogram
B Colour flow duplex ultrasonography
C Computerized tomography (CT)
D Excision biopsy
E Fine needle aspiration
F History and examination only
G Isotope bone scan
H Laparoscopy
I Lumbosacral spine X-ray
J Magnetic resonance imaging (MRI) scan
K Ultrasound scan

For each of the presentations below choose the SINGLE most appropriate mode of assessment from the above options. Each option may be used once, more than once, or not at all.

1. A 60-year-old man presents with a pulsatile swelling below the right inguinal ligament after a recent coronary angiogram which was performed via a right femoral artery cannulation.

2. A 60-year-old woman presents with hard masses in both inguinal regions. She had radiotherapy for a squamous carcinoma of the anus 3 months previously.

3. A 6-year-old boy is noticed by his mother to have a lump in the right groin. Clinical examination confirms a 3 cm soft, mobile lump in the inguinal region and an absent right testicle in the scrotum.

4. A 40-year-old man presents with a 3-month history of a painless lump in the right inguinal region. The swelling appears when he stands upright and disappears on lying down. There is a palpable cough impulse.

5. A 45-year-old woman complains of weight loss and low-grade fever. On examination, she has firm lumps in both groins and axillae and splenomegaly.

Answers to **2.24**

1.   B   Colour flow duplex ultrasonography

This patient seems to have developed a false aneurysm. When the wall of an artery is pierced, a haematoma may form which develops into a pulsatile lump. Colour duplex ultrasonography is very useful in the assessment of false aneurysms, allowing the measurement of size, direction of flow, and delineation of the track. Small false aneurysms usually resolve with no intervention but those larger than 3 cm may expand and leak and so require surgical repair.

2.   E   Fine needle aspiration

The inguinal masses are probably metastatic lymph nodes secondary to the anal carcinoma. A fine needle aspiration of a node is the first investigation of choice in order to obtain cytological evidence of malignancy. If this fails then an excision biopsy of the lymph node can be performed.

3.   K   Ultrasound scan

Undescended testes are often present in the superficial subinguinal pouch and are usually clinically palpable. The diagnosis can be confirmed with an ultrasound scan. Laparoscopy may be useful to locate and remove an intra-abdominal testis. It is possible to perform a staged repair and relocate the testis in the scrotum (orchidopexy).

4.   F   History and examination only

From the history, the lump is most likely to be an inguinal hernia. A detailed clinical examination will suffice to make a conclusive diagnosis.

5.   D   Excision biopsy

The patient is likely to have a lymphoma. An excision biopsy of an intact lymph node is preferable to a fine needle aspiration in order to provide samples for histological examination. This can usually be performed under a local anaesthetic.

Causes of an acute abdomen

A Appendicitis
B Cholecystitis
C Colitis
D Dissecting aortic aneurysm
E Diverticulitis
F Gastritis
G Gastroenteritis
H Pancreatitis
I Pelvic inflammatory disease
J Renal colic
K Urinary tract infection

For each of the following presentations choose the SINGLE most likely cause from the above list of options. You may use each option once, more than once, or not at all.

1. A 38-year-old man presents with a 6-hour history of nausea, vomiting and a severe, boring, upper abdominal pain radiating through to his back. He is known to consume alcohol heavily. On examination, there is generalized tenderness of his abdomen. A plain X-ray of the abdomen shows a dilated loop of small bowel in the left upper quadrant.

2. A 25-year-old man presents to the A&E department with a 12-hour history of severe, right loin pain radiating to the right groin. Abdominal examination is essentially normal apart from tenderness in the right loin.

3. A 16-year-old girl has a 2-day history of lower abdominal pain. Her temperature is 37.5°C. Palpation of the abdomen shows tenderness in the right iliac fossa associated with rebound discomfort and guarding. Her full blood count shows a moderate leucocytosis.

4. A 17-year-old girl presents with a 24-hour history of lower abdominal pain and urinary frequency. She has a pyrexia of 38°C and mild suprapubic tenderness.

5. A 45-year-old woman presents to the A&E department with severe upper abdominal pain which radiates to her back and right shoulder and which followed a heavy meal. On examination, she is pyrexial and is markedly tender in the right upper quadrant of her abdomen. Her serum amylase is 460 U/L.

Answers to **2.25**

1.   **H   Pancreatitis**

The history of nausea, vomiting and severe upper abdominal pain radiating through to the back should suggest pancreatitis. The main causes of acute pancreatitis are gall stones and excessive intake of alcohol. Other causes include viral infections (mumps, coxsackie), hyperparathyroidism, hypertriglyceridaemia, hypothermia, pancreatic carcinoma and iatrogenic (ERCP, angiography). The diagnosis is usually based on clinical suspicion and a high serum amylase (often above 1000 U/L). A plain X-ray of the abdomen may show a slightly dilated loop of small bowel in the left upper quadrant of the abdomen which is called a sentinel loop.

2.   **J   Renal colic**

Renal colic is characteristically unilateral and usually due to the passage of a renal stone (calculus) through the ureter causing severe loin pain radiating to the groin and occurring in waves. During an attack, the patient is usually very restless being unable to find any position of comfort. Urine examination may reveal red blood cells. Intravenous urography is used to confirms the diagnosis, and treatment in the first instance is with analgesics.

3.   **A   Appendicitis**

Acute appendicitis is a very common acute surgical condition characterized by lower abdominal pain and right iliac fossa tenderness with guarding and rebound. The patient may have a low-grade fever with a leucocytosis. Early surgery is indicated before the onset of gangrene and perforation.

4.   **K   Urinary tract infection**

Fever, urinary frequency and dysuria indicate the possibility of a urinary tract infection (UTI). A microbiological examination and culture of a mid-stream urine specimen is needed to confirm the diagnosis.

5.   **B   Cholecystitis**

The condition is characterized by intermittent episodes of colicky pain in the right upper quadrant. When the biliary tree is inflamed, the patient may be febrile and Murphy's sign (pain on inspiration while gallbladder area is pressed) is usually positive. There may be slight elevation of the serum amylase levels. Acute cholecystitis is caused by an obstruction of the neck of the gallbladder or the cystic duct, usually by a stone. An ultrasound scan of the abdomen may show stones within a thickened gallbladder.

Causes of hepatomegaly

A Amyloidosis
B Budd–Chiari syndrome
C Cirrhosis
D Congestive cardiac failure
E Hepatitis
F Hepatoma
G Hydatid cyst
H Leukaemia
I Liver abscess
J Metastases
K Portal hypertension

For each of the following clinical scenarios choose the SINGLE most likely cause from the above list of options. You may use each option once, more than once, or not at all.

1. A 55-year-old publican is admitted with weight loss, fever and anorexia. He has an enlarged liver with an irregular edge. His blood tests reveal an elevated serum alpha-fetoprotein.

2. A 75-year-old retired teacher has had a previous laparotomy and colostomy for intestinal obstruction 2 years ago. He now presents with a palpable, irregularly enlarged liver.

3. A 50-year-old farmer presents with intermittent jaundice and upper abdominal pain. Examination reveals non-tender hepatomegaly of 7 cm below the right costal margin.

4. A 50-year-old housewife is admitted with pyrexia, a high white cell count and a tender lump in the liver. She has a recent history of bloody diarrhoea with mucus after she returned from a holiday in Mexico.

5. A 65-year-old retired secretary presents with right upper quadrant pain in the abdomen, anorexia, weight loss, haematemesis and ascites. She has a tender hepatomegaly but no jaundice or any other signs of chronic liver disease.

Answers to **2.26**

1. F Hepatoma

Hepatoma is common worldwide and carriers of hepatitis B and C viruses are at a higher risk of developing the disease. Cirrhosis, from alcohol or haemochromatosis, is present in more than 80% of cases. In non-cirrhotic patients, the hepatoma may reach a considerable size before presenting with abdominal pain or swelling. The serum alpha-fetoprotein, an α_1-globulin produced in foetal, regenerating and malignant hepatocytes, is elevated.

2. J Metastases

This patient probably had a colonic cancer previously resected and a palpable liver would now suggest metastatic disease. Large bowel carcinomas metastasize mainly via the lymphatics and the blood stream. Lymphatic spread involves the mesenteric nodes and later the para-aortic nodes. Spread via the blood stream is predominantly to the liver.

3. G Hydatid cyst

Hydatid disease is prevalent in livestock-raising areas of various countries, mainly Australia, Argentina, the Middle East and Wales. It is caused by the parasite *Echinococcus granulosus* for which canines are the definitive hosts and sheep and humans are the intermediate hosts. Infection usually occurs in childhood from direct contact with infected dogs or food contaminated by infected canine faeces. The cysts grow slowly and present as hepatomegaly (the liver is the most common organ affected by the hydatid cysts) many years later.

4. I Liver abscess

The clinical findings are suggestive of a liver abscess which may be caused by a bacterial or protozoal infection. This patient's history of bloody diarrhoea is suggestive of amoebiasis which is caused by *Entamoeba histolytica*. The disease is frequently encountered in developing countries. Complications include toxic colonic dilatation and perforation, stricture formation, liver abscess and amoebic meningoencephalitis. Medical management is with metronidazole but a liver abscess should also be drained with ultrasound-guided placement of the drain.

5. F Hepatoma

The course of a hepatoma may be brief and rapidly downhill with weight loss and ascites. Bleeding may occur in as many as 50% of the cases and this may be in the gut or the peritoneum.

Causes of intestinal obstruction

A Adhesions
B Carcinoma
C Faecal impaction
D Femoral hernia
E Gall stones
F Ileus
G Inguinal hernia
H Intussusception
I Meconium ileus
J Stricture
K Volvulus of sigmoid colon

For each of the following scenarios choose the SINGLE most likely cause from the above list of options. You may use each option once, more than once, or not at all.

1. An 85-year-old man with senile dementia is found to have gross abdominal distension. He is known to have chronic constipation. On examination, the abdomen is distended and rectal examination reveals an empty ballooned rectum. A plain X-ray of the abdomen reveals a grossly distended sigmoid colon which extends to the right hypochondrium. There is a paucity of gas in the rectum.

2. An 80-year-old woman presents with a 2-day history of vomiting with abdominal pain and abdominal distension. On examination, a tender lump is found in the right groin below and lateral to the pubic tubercle. There is radiological evidence of small bowel obstruction.

3. A 26-year-old woman develops symptoms suggestive of intestinal obstruction. She has been taking mesalazine for a number of years and her recent small bowel enema demonstrates the string sign of Kantor.

4. An 80-year-old woman presents with abdominal pain and vomiting. She has had recurrent attacks of colicky pain for some days. An abdominal X-ray shows air in the biliary tree and a distal small bowel obstruction.

5. A 32-year-old woman presents with a 2-day history of abdominal discomfort and distension. She also reports that she has not been passing much flatus. In the past, she has had a cholecystectomy and an appendicectomy.

Answers to 2.27

1. **K   Volvulus of sigmoid colon**

    Patients with chronic constipation (usually the elderly) may develop a distended and relatively atonic colon, especially the sigmoid colon, which is prone to twisting on its mesenteric attachment. This can cause a large bowel obstruction and venous infarction. Perforation of the bowel may follow. Abdominal X-rays usually show a grossly dilated sigmoid loop with an 'inverted U' of bowel gas in the upper abdomen with two fluid levels. It is often possible to deflate the sigmoid loop with a flatus tube. A limited barium enema without prior bowel preparation may untwist the bowel; otherwise an urgent laparotomy is needed.

2. **D   Femoral hernia**

    In a patient who has had no previous abdominal operations and who presents acutely with a small bowel obstruction, the most likely underlying cause is a hernia. In this case, a strangulated femoral hernia is causing the mechanical obstruction. A femoral hernia should be treated surgically because of the risk of strangulation. Inguinal herniae are medial and superior to the pubic tubercle.

3. **J   Stricture**

    This patient is on mesalazine (5-aminosalicylic acid) which is used for the maintenance of remission in inflammatory bowel disease. The string sign of Kantor (narrow, featureless intestinal tube with proximal dilatation) seen in the small bowel on a barium enema suggests that there are areas of narrowing from chronic inflammation. Surgery for small bowel strictures may involve multiple stricturoplasties. If the disease is limited, then resection of the diseased segment may be possible.

4. **E   Gall stones**

    Gall stone ileus usually occurs in the elderly. A large gall stone can become impacted in the narrow distal ileum causing small bowel obstruction. On a plain abdominal X-ray, air can be seen in the biliary tree as a result of the gall stone perforating into the duodenum. Dilated loops of small bowel and possibly a stone may be seen in the terminal ileum.

5. **A   Adhesions**

    In patients who have had previous surgery, adhesions and bands are the commonest cause of intestinal obstruction. Initial management includes a conservative approach with intravenous fluids and nasogastric decompression. Operative intervention may occasionally be required.

Causes of a mass in the right iliac fossa

A   Actinomycosis
B   Amoebic typhilitis
C   Appendicular mass
D   Caecal carcinoma
E   Crohn's disease
F   Ectopic kidney
G   Faecoliths
H   Hyperplastic ileocaecal tuberculosis
I   Lymphosarcoma
J   Tubo-ovarian mass
K   Twisted ovarian cyst

For the following presentations choose the SINGLE most likely cause from the above list of options. You may use each option once, more than once, or not at all.

1. A 20-year-old Caucasian man presents with a 3-day history of a swinging pyrexia and constant pain in the right iliac fossa. On examination of the abdomen, there is a 5 cm × 7 cm tender mass in the right iliac fossa.

2. A 25-year-old Welsh woman presents with a 12-month history of weight loss and diarrhoea occurring several times each day. In addition, there has been intermittent nausea, vomiting and colicky abdominal pain. Examination reveals a distended abdomen, hyperactive bowel sounds and a mildly tender mass in the right iliac fossa. An abdominal X-ray shows distal small bowel obstruction.

3. A 20-year-old Afro-Caribbean woman is admitted with sudden onset of pain in the right iliac fossa which is exacerbated by walking. On examination, she is apyrexial and extremely tender in the right iliac fossa where a cystic mass is palpable.

4. A 60-year-old Caucasian woman presents with tiredness and lethargy and she has noticed a lump in the right lower abdomen. On examination, she is clinically anaemic and there is a non-tender mass in the right iliac fossa measuring approximately 10 cm × 8 cm.

5. A 40-year-old Asian woman presents with a 6-month history of fever with progressive loss of weight and appetite and intermittent pain in the right lower abdomen. On examination, she is thin, pale and undernourished with a non-tender mass palpable in the right iliac fossa.

Answers to **2.28**

1. **C** Appendicular mass

The short history, with constitutional symptoms, suggests an acute inflammatory process. A tender mass is usually palpable in the right iliac fossa by the third day after the onset of acute appendicitis. The mass usually consists of greater omentum, oedematous caecal wall and small intestine and within this there may be a perforated or inflamed appendix. Between 5–10 days later, the mass may get smaller as the inflammation subsides or it may enlarge as an appendicular abscess develops.

2. **E** Crohn's disease

The long history of chronic diarrhoea with loss of weight in a young person is suggestive of inflammatory bowel disease. Crohn's disease can affect any part of the gut from the mouth to the anus but it most commonly affects the terminal ileum. Chronic inflammation of the small bowel can sometimes form a mass and intestinal obstruction may result from inflammation, adhesions or fibrosis. Other complications include fistulae, abscess formation, malabsorption and perianal sepsis.

3. **K** Twisted ovarian cyst

Torsion of an ovarian cyst may cause sudden onset of severe abdominal pain usually associated with a palpable tender mass in the lower abdomen. It may be diagnosed by bimanual pelvic examination and with an ultrasound scan. Some cysts may be malignant, so care must be taken to avoid rupture during surgery.

4. **D** Caecal carcinoma

Carcinoma of the right side of the colon often presents with vague symptoms such as tiredness and lethargy usually from anaemia due to occult blood loss. Hypochromic anaemia is a well-known consequence of a right colonic neoplasm. Sometimes, the patient presents with a mass in the right iliac fossa. Caecal carcinoma sometimes presents as an emergency with small bowel obstruction. A colonoscopy or barium enema is essential for diagnosis.

5. **H** Hyperplastic ileocaecal tuberculosis

This patient has symptoms of tuberculosis. In Asian immigrants to the UK, hyperplastic ileocaecal tuberculosis is a more common cause of a mass in the right iliac fossa than Crohn's disease.

Causes of splenomegaly

A   Bacterial endocarditis
B   Chronic lymphocytic leukaemia
C   Felty's syndrome
D   Gaucher's disease
E   Hodgkin's lymphoma
F   Idiopathic thrombocytopenic purpura
G   Infectious mononucleosis
H   Myelofibrosis
I   Polycythaemia rubra vera
J   Tropical splenomegaly syndrome
K   Typhoid

For each of the following clinical situations choose the SINGLE most likely cause from the above list of options. You may use each option once, more than once, or not at all.

1. A 28-year-old woman presents with a sore throat and bilateral cervical lymphadenopathy. She has a small, palpable spleen. A full blood count reveals pleomorphic atypical lymphocytosis.

2. A 60-year-old woman with a history of rheumatoid arthritis is found to have a palpable spleen. Her full blood count shows a haemoglobin of 11.2 g/dl, white cell count of 2.6×10^9/L and platelets of 181×10^9/L.

3. A 25-year-old man, who has recently been abroad, presents with a 4-day history of persistent pyrexia, malaise and arthralgia. Initially, he complained of constipation but later developed diarrhoea. After the end of the first week, he developed a rash on the back and abdomen. The rash consists of sparse, slightly raised, rose-red spots which fade on pressure. There is splenomegaly and evidence of leucopenia.

4. A 70-year-old man presents with weight loss, anorexia, abdominal discomfort and anaemia. Examination reveals massive splenomegaly.

5. A 20-year-old woman, who has recently come from East Africa presents with anaemia, recurrent chest infections and a dragging pain in her abdomen. She is found to have massive splenomegaly.

Answers to 2.29

1. G Infectious mononucleosis

Infectious mononucleosis (glandular fever) is caused by the Epstein–Barr virus. It is characterized by fever, sore throat, lymphadenopathy and the presence of atypical lymphocytes. A palpable spleen occurs in over half the patients and hepatomegaly in about 15%. The Paul–Bunnell and monospot tests are positive.

2. C Felty's syndrome

Felty's syndrome is the combination of rheumatoid arthritis, splenomegaly and neutropenia. It tends to occur in patients with seropositive, long-standing, advanced but inactive arthritis. Splenectomy produces a temporary increase in the neutrophil count but does not help to prevent recurrent infections so it is mainly reserved for patients with severe anaemia from hypersplenism.

3. K Typhoid

Typhoid fever (caused by *Salmonella typhi*) is characterized by a fever that is persistent and increases in severity in a step-ladder fashion. There is initially constipation which is followed by diarrhoea. During the second week, 'rose spots' appear on the chest and upper abdomen. Splenomegaly occurs in about three-quarters of patients. Blood cultures are most helpful in the first week. The Widal test, which measures serum agglutinins to the bacterial antigens, is useful. Treatment is with ciprofloxacin or cotrimoxazole.

4. H Myelofibrosis

Myelofibrosis usually presents with tiredness, weight loss and discomfort in the upper abdomen. In a quarter of cases, there is a previous history of polycythaemia rubra vera. There is evidence of anaemia (leucoerythroblasts, tear-drop cells), thrombocytopenia and fibrosis of the bone marrow. The Philadelphia chromosome (translocation of part of the long arm of chromosome 22 to chromosome 9) is absent. This is useful in distinguishing this condition from chronic myeloid leukaemia.

5. J Tropical splenomegaly syndrome

The tropical splenomegaly syndrome is found in areas where malaria is hyperendemic. Repeated malarial infection causes a marked elevation in serum IgM levels and IgM macromolecular aggregrates (cryoglobulins). These stimulate the reticuloendothelial system to cause massive hepatomegaly and splenomegaly. Anaemia (from haemolysis or hypersplenism) and immunosuppression (from neutropenia or poor activation of neutrophils) may occur. Malarial parasites are not found in the spleen or blood smears.

Causes of a scrotal swelling

A Clotted hydrocele
B Epididymal cyst
C Epididymo-orchitis
D Filarial scrotum
E Haematocele
F Hydrocele
G Inguinoscrotal hernia
H Pyocele
I Spermatocele
J Testicular tumour
K Varicocele

For each of the following scenarios choose the SINGLE most likely cause from the above list of options. You may use each option once, more than once, or not at all.

1. A 30-year-old man who is being investigated for infertility is found to have a swelling in the scrotum which is separate from the testes. It is soft on palpation, and it appears on standing and disappears on lying down. The patient admits to an aching pain in the scrotum.

2. A 20-year-old man develops a painful swelling of the right side of the scrotum after injuring himself during a tackle in a rugby match.

3. A 35-year-old man who is fit and well has developed a painless swelling of his right testis over the last few months. There is a sensation of heaviness. On examination, the body of the testis is found to be enlarged, smooth and heavy.

4. A 60-year-old man who has frequency of micturition now develops a fever and malaise and increasing pain in the scrotum. On examination, the scrotum is red and there is a tender enlargement of the left testis.

5. A 40-year-old man develops a right-sided scrotal swelling over a period of 6 months. On examination, the swelling is painless but the fluctuation and transillumination tests are both positive.

Answers to **2.30**

1. K Varicocele

One of the causes of infertility is the presence of a varicocele which increases the blood supply and raises the scrotal temperature. A primary varicocele is usually left-sided and presents at puberty. A secondary varicocele, due to invasion or compression of the intra-abdominal portion of the spermatic vein by a renal or retroperitoneal mass, affects either side at any age. Clinically, there is a swelling which is separate from the testis, is soft and has a cough impulse. On lying down, the swelling tends to disappear. Surgical treatment is indicated for symptomatic patients.

2. E Haematocele

After trauma to the testis there may be damage to the testicular tissues resulting in a collection of blood. Clinically, the affected side of the scrotum is enlarged and very tender. The diagnosis can be confirmed with an ultrasound scan. In general, it is treated conservatively.

3. J Testicular tumour

The usual age of presentation of a seminoma is 30–50 years. The patient first notices a heaviness and swelling of the testis. Initially, it is painless but later an ache may develop. On examination of the testis, it is generally found to be enlarged, firm and smooth. Testicular sensation is lost early in the disease process. There may be enlarged lymph nodes in the left supraclavicular region. An ultrasound scan helps to establish the diagnosis. Treatment is by orchidectomy followed by radiotherapy. The prognosis in seminoma without metastases is favourable.

4. C Epididymo-orchitis

The history of frequency of micturition and fever suggests that this patient has a urinary infection. Sometimes this can cause an infection of the testes and epididymis. Urine should be examined to identify the organism. Treatment is bed rest with the scrotum supported, analgesics and appropriate antibiotics.

5. F Hydrocele

The usual presentation is a painless scrotal swelling that has been present for months. The patient usually seeks medical help because of its increasing size. It is a uniformly smooth swelling and the testis cannot be felt separately. Fluctuation suggests the presence of fluid and the transillumination test is positive.

Types of fistulae

A   Arteriovenous fistula
B   Biliary fistula
C   Branchial fistula
D   Colovaginal fistula
E   Colovesical fistula
F   Enterocutaneous fistula
G   Fistula-in-ano
H   Gastrocolic fistula
I   Tracheo-oesophageal fistula
J   Urethral fistula
K   Vesicovaginal fistula

For each of the following clinical presentations choose the SINGLE most likely diagnosis from the above list. Each option may be used once, more than once, or not at all.

1. A 78-year-old man presents with faeculent fluid discharging from a midline wound 4 weeks after a right hemicolectomy. The patient is otherwise comfortable with no pain or tenderness. An ultrasound scan of the abdomen does not show any collection of fluid.

2. A 60-year-old man who is known to have diverticular disease of the sigmoid colon, complains of recurrent urinary infections and states that he sometimes passes urine which contains tea leaves.

3. A 40-year-old man had a perianal abscess drained 1 month ago. He has now developed a persistent, pustular discharge from an opening about an inch posterolaterally from the anal verge.

4. A 75-year-old man presents with weight loss and has diarrhoea after every meal associated with eructation of foul gas. Once or twice he has vomited formed faeces. He looks cachetic and a gastroscopy shows a large malignant looking growth in the greater curve of the stomach. A barium enema confirms the complication that has arisen.

5. A 20-year-old woman presents with a slightly tender area on the right side of her neck. On examination, there is an orifice at the lower third of the anterior border of the right sternomastoid muscle. On further examination, there is a mirror image orifice on the left side of the neck.

Answers to **2.31**

1. F Enterocutaneous fistula

This patient probably has an anastomotic leak from the bowel resection. It can sometimes present in this manner if the anastomosis is close to the abdominal incision. At other times it can present more dramatically if the bowel contents leak into the abdominal cavity.

2. E Colovesical fistula

This is a complication of diverticular disease. Recurrent inflammation can cause the sigmoid colon to become adherent to the urinary bladder. This can eventually erode into the bladder causing a fistula when faecal particles are passed in the urine. The condition is much commoner in men since the uterus intervenes between the sigmoid colon and the bladder in women.

3. G Fistula-in-ano

This usually results from an anorectal abscess, which originates in the crypts of the anal column and ruptures spontaneously. The fistula continues to discharge and, because of constant reinfection from the anal canal or rectum, it rarely closes permanently without surgical intervention.

4. H Gastrocolic fistula

An advanced gastric tumour can sometimes involve the adjacent transverse colon forming a fistula between these two structures. The patient has diarrhoea after almost every meal; eructates foul gas and can vomit fragments of formed faeces. Loss of weight, dehydration and anaemia also occur. Once a fistula has formed, the patient deteriorates rapidly and becomes very ill within 2 to 3 weeks. The diagnosis of the fistula is established by a barium enema.

5. C Branchial fistula

These may be unilateral or bilateral and represent a persistent second branchial cleft. Nearly always the external orifice of the fistula is situated in the lower third of the neck near the anterior border of the sternomastoid muscle. The internal orifice can be located on the anterior aspect of the posterior pillar of the fauces, just behind the tonsil, but more often the track ends blindly (branchial sinus). They can become infected.

A   Branchial cyst
B   Carotid body tumour
C   Cystic hygroma
D   Dermoid cyst
E   Ludwig's angina
F   Lymphadenopathy
G   Plunging ranula
H   Sternomastoid tumour
I   Submandibular gland
J   Thyroglossal cyst
K   Thyroid swelling

For each presentation below choose the SINGLE most appropriate cause from the above list. Each option can be used once, more than once or not at all.

1. A 48-year-old man presents with a long-standing, eccentrically situated swelling in the right lower neck. On examination, the swelling is found to be hard, ovoid and lobulated and it moves only in the lateral plane.

2. A 2-year-old girl develops a slow-growing swelling in the neck measuring about 6 cm × 4 cm. It is compressible, fluctuant and transilluminant.

3. A 28-year-old woman notices that the front of her neck has gradually swollen. She is easily irritable and has warm, sweaty palms and a resting tachycardia.

4. A 6-year-old boy presents with a painful diffuse swelling of the neck which started below the mandible and extends down to the level of the clavicle. The swelling is tender and indurated and causes him difficulty with his breathing.

5. A 16-year-old boy presents with a painless, midline swelling of the neck. The swelling moves up with protrusion of his tongue.

Answers to **2.32**

1.   B   **Carotid body tumour**

A carotid body tumour lies in the axis of the carotid artery. It is a slow growing, potentially malignant tumour. It is usually unilateral and becomes more obvious in middle age. A long-standing history, and a lump at the carotid bifurcation that moves from side to side, suggest the diagnosis. Arteriography shows the carotid fork to be splayed and there is a blush outlining the abnormal tumour vessels.

2.   C   **Cystic hygroma**

This is usually a congenital, slow growing, compressible and brilliantly translucent swelling. It manifests itself during early infancy and occasionally is present at birth. Typically, the swelling occupies the lower third of the neck. The swelling is cystic due to intercommunication between many of its compartments. It visibly increases in size when the child coughs or cries.

3.   K   **Thyroid swelling**

This lady has the typical systemic symptoms of thyrotoxicosis associated with the swelling of the thyroid gland. This patient may also have heat intolerance, diarrhoea, menstrual irregularities and eye signs in the form of exophthalmos and lid lag.

4.   E   **Ludwig's angina**

This is a serious form of cellulitis of the neck that can cause respiratory embarrassment due to oedema around the glottis. Ludwig described this clinical entity as characterized by a brawny swelling of the submandibular region combined with inflammatory oedema of the mouth. The usual cause is a streptococcal infection of the cellular tissues surrounding the submandibular gland. It can also be a complication of an advanced carcinoma of the floor of the mouth.

5.   J   **Thyroglossal cyst**

A thyroglossal cyst is usually congenital and may present in any part of the thyroglossal tract. The swelling usually occupies the midline of the neck and moves upwards on protrusion of the tongue or on swallowing because of the attachment of the tract to the foramen caecum. A history of recurrent infection is often obtained and sometimes its rupture causes a fistula. A thyroglossal cyst should be excised.

Diagnosis of ulcers

A   Aphthous ulcer
B   Bazin's ulcer
C   Diabetic ulcer
D   Marjolin's ulcer
E   Meleney's ulcer
F   Rodent ulcer
G   Syphilitic ulcer
H   Traumatic ulcer
I   Trophic ulcer
J   Tuberculous ulcer
K   Varicose ulcer

For each presentation below choose the SINGLE most likely diagnosis from the above list of options. Each option may be used once, more than once, or not at all.

1.   A 26-year-old man presents with a 2 cm painless ulcer on the penis. On examination, it is shallow, indurate and does not bleed easily. The inguinal lymph nodes are enlarged, non-tender and rubbery in consistency.

2.   A 76-year-old man presents with a 6-month history of a non-healing ulcer at the outer canthus of the right eye. On examination, it has a well-defined, hard, rolled-out edge.

3.   A 15-year-old girl presents with an ulcer on the side of the face, which is about 3 cm in diameter. She had this before coming to the UK from India 5 months ago. On examination, the ulcer is superficial and appears to be healing in the centre but is active at the periphery.

4.   A 50-year-old man presents with an ulcer on his left leg which has been present for many months. In the past 4 weeks, it has started to increase in size. He gives a history of severe burns to both lower limbs as a child.

5.   A 60-year-old lady has a chronic ulcer at the right medial malleolar region. She gives a history of dilated veins in both lower extremities for several years.

Answers to **2.33**

1. G Syphilitic ulcer

This is a primary syphilitic ulcer commonly called a chancre. It develops at the site of entry of the spirochaetes and is characteristically painless. The rubbery lymph nodes are a further clue. Diagnosis is by finding *Treponema pallidum* on smears.

2. F Rodent ulcer

This has the characteristics of a basal cell carcinoma of the skin commonly called a rodent ulcer. Its burrowing nature gives its name and it is usually seen on the face. It is a common tumour of low-grade malignancy. Though the tumours are slow growing, if ulcerated they will gradually erode deeper tissues, i.e. muscles, cartilage and bone. Metastases are extremely rare and surgical excision, controlled cryotherapy, curettage and desiccation and fractionated radiation all achieve a cure rate of >90%.

3. J Tuberculous ulcer

This is a tuberculous ulcer also known as lupus vulgaris. It is typically active in the periphery while healing starts in the centre. It normally occurs in children and young adults mainly affecting the face and arms. Lupus vulgaris is less common in those parts of the world where tuberculosis is endemic but more common in Northern and Eastern Europe. It occurs more commonly in females, children and the elderly.

4. D Marjolin's ulcer

This is a carcinoma arising in a scar. Initially, these are slow growing, painless ulcers due to the avascularity of the scar tissue. Once the ulcer invades normal tissue beyond the scar it behaves like any other squamous-cell carcinoma of the skin.

5. K Varicose ulcer

Long standing varicose veins can cause ulceration due to stasis and venous hypertension. This is usually a painless, callous ulcer typically situated over the medial side of the lower leg and never penetrates the deep fascia. There is pigmentation or eczema around it. The presence of varicose veins in the upper part of the leg or thigh clinches the diagnosis.

Diagnosis of malignant tumours

A   Adenocarcinoma
B   Choriocarcinoma
C   Fibrosarcoma
D   Lymphoma
E   Malignant melanoma
F   Nephroblastoma
G   Neurofibrosarcoma
H   Renal cell carcinoma
I   Squamous-cell carcinoma
J   Teratoma
K   Transitional-cell carcinoma

For each of the scenarios below choose the SINGLE most likely tumour from the list of options above. Each option may be used once, more than once, or not at all.

1. A 27-year-old man presents with a small, painless testicular lump and cervical lymphadenopathy. A chest X-ray shows mediastinal lymphadenopathy and several cannon-ball lesions. His alpha-fetoprotein level is elevated.

2. A 70-year-old man presents in the outpatient clinic with frank haematuria. Cystoscopy reveals a frond-like tumour in the bladder.

3. A 70-year-old man presents with a history of worsening dysphagia, initially affecting solids and then liquids. Gastroscopy shows a malignant-looking lesion in the oesophagus at about 25 cm. The gastro-oesophageal junction is at 40 cm from the incisor teeth.

4. A 62-year-old man with vague abdominal pains is found to have red blood cells but no white cells or organisms in his urine. He is pale with a Hb level of 11 g/dl. An ultrasound scan of the abdomen shows a mass in the right lumbar region.

5. A 60-year-old woman presents with a history of colicky abdominal pain, weight loss and altered bowel habits. A barium enema shows an 'apple core' lesion in the splenic flexure of the colon.

Answers to **2.34**

1. J Teratoma

Any painless testicular lump in a young man should be treated with suspicion. Seminomas and teratomas account for about 90% of all testicular tumours which occur between the ages of 20–40 years. Seminomas are derived from spermatocytes and teratomas from multipotent germ cells. They spread via the lymphatics to para-aortic nodes, supraclavicular nodes and then into the systemic circulation. Pulmonary metastases are commoner with teratomas. Serum alpha-fetoprotein and human chorionic gonadotrophin levels are elevated.

2. K Transitional-cell carcinoma

The most common tumour of the urothelial (tumours arising from the transitional-cell lining of the urinary tract) system is the transitional-cell carcinoma which mainly occurs in the bladder. Risk factors include cigarette smoking and industrial carcinogens (aromatic amines). The bladder tumour is usually frond-like in appearance and invariably presents with painless haematuria but may, occasionally, cause urinary retention (obstruction from blood clot) and hydronephrosis (obstruction of the ureteric orifice by tumour).

3. I Squamous-cell carcinoma

The majority of oesophageal malignancies are squamous-cell carcinomas which most commonly affect the upper and the middle third of the oesophagus. Adenocarcinomas occur in the lower third of the oesophagus. Squamous-cell carcinomas protrude into the lumen and cause dysphagia for solids. Patients often recall that they used to have difficulty eating a steak but unfortunately the realization comes too late. Irradiation is the treatment of choice.

4. H Renal cell carcinoma

Haematuria is the most frequent presenting symptom of renal cell carcinoma. The classic triad of haematuria, pain and abdominal mass occurs in only a small proportion of cases. Patients may also have systemic symptoms such as fever, weight loss, anaemia, polycythaemia, hypercalcaemia and non-metastatic liver dysfunction.

5. A Adenocarcinoma

The presentation and barium enema findings suggest that this is a colonic tumour. Most bowel carcinomas are adenocarcinomas which metastasize via the lymphatics and blood stream. Prognosis is dependent upon the stage at diagnosis and can vary from 90% 5-year survival for Dukes' stage A to 40% for Dukes' stage C. Patients with metastases rarely survive for 5 years.

Diagnosis of right-sided abdominal pain

A   Acute cholecystitis
B   Acute pancreatitis
C   Carcinoma of the caecum
D   Gastroenteritis
E   Meckel's diverticulitis
F   Mesenteric adenitis
G   Post-herpetic pain
H   Ruptured ectopic pregnancy
I   Salpingitis
J   Torsion of an ovarian cyst
K   Ureteric colic

For each patient below, choose the SINGLE most likely diagnosis from the above list of options. Each option may be used once, more than once, or not at all.

1. A 35-year-old woman presents with severe, right-sided abdominal pain which radiates to the right scapula. She is mildly icteric and pyrexial, and has tenderness in the right upper quadrant of the abdomen which is worsened during deep inspiration.

2. An 8-year-old girl is admitted with high-grade fever, sore throat and abdominal pain. On examination, her throat is congested and there is tenderness in the right iliac fossa.

3. A 23-year-old woman presents with a sudden onset of severe, right-sided lower abdominal pain which is exacerbated by lying on her side. On examination, she is apyrexial, and has a very tender, smooth mass in the right iliac fossa.

4. A 65-year-old woman presents with abdominal pain, tiredness and lethargy. She has lost a stone in weight in the past 3 months. On examination, she is pale and has a mildly tender mass in the right iliac fossa.

5. A 26-year-old woman presents with severe, right-sided lower abdominal pain. She is pale and hypotensive (80/40 mmHg) with a pulse rate of 120 beats/min. There is generalized tenderness with guarding and rebound in the lower abdomen. Her cervix is soft and very tender.

Answers to **2.35**

1.   A   Acute cholecystitis

Pain in the right upper quadrant of the abdomen radiating to the subscapular area, together with vomiting, tachycardia, fever and leucocytosis is typical of acute cholecystitis. Murphy's sign is usually present. There may be a palpable, inflammatory mass around the gallbladder. The development of a high pyrexia and rigors indicates empyema formation or cholangitis. These are both indications for early intervention in the form of cholecystectomy or endoscopic retrograde cholangiopancreatography.

2.   F   Mesenteric adenitis

Abdominal pain accompanied by a sore throat and/or a viral illness in children is suggestive of mesenteric adenitis, a condition that is most probably viral in origin. The symptoms and signs can mimic appendicitis, but the clue to the adenitis is either a concurrent or a recent history of an upper respiratory infection. Cervical lymphadenopathy may be present. The abdominal tenderness tends to be more diffuse than that of acute appendicitis and may shift when the patient moves.

3.   J   Torsion of an ovarian cyst

Ovarian cysts can often be asymptomatic but when torsion occurs the pain is severe, is often referred to the loin and is exacerbated by movement. Tenderness and guarding may be present and rupture of the cyst may cause peritonitis. There is usually no pyrexia but a tender, mobile mass is often palpable in the suprapubic region or on vaginal examination. Ultrasonography of the pelvis is useful to confirm the diagnosis.

4.   C   Carcinoma of the caecum

The symptoms and signs are suggestive of a caecal carcinoma. This often presents very insidiously and an iron deficiency anaemia is sometimes the only presenting feature. Occasionally, caecal neoplasms can present with acute small bowel obstruction when the ileocaecal valve is involved.

5.   H   Ruptured ectopic pregnancy

Sudden, severe abdominal pain, vaginal bleeding and circulatory collapse in a woman of childbearing age are strongly suggestive of a ruptured ectopic pregnancy (occurs at about 6 weeks' gestation). Cervical softening and tenderness points to a possible pregnancy. The fallopian tube is the most common site of an ectopic pregnancy.

Clinical diagnosis of swellings

A Cystic hygroma
B Dermoid cyst
C Fibroma
D Haemangioma
E Haematoma
F Implantation dermoid
G Lipoma
H Lymph node
I Neurofibrosarcoma
J Sebaceous cyst
K Thyroglossal cyst

For each of the presentations below choose the SINGLE most likely diagnosis from the options above. Each option may be used once, more than once, or not at all.

1. A 50-year-old male presents with a painless swelling on the shoulder which has been growing very slowly for the past 5 years. On examination, the swelling is found to be soft, non-tender and measures 3 cm in diameter. It lies in the subcutaneous plane and is semi-fluctuant with well-defined edges and slips easily under the palpating finger.

2. A 60-year-old woman presents with multiple, small nodules of varying size located all over the trunk and upper limbs. One swelling in the neck has recently increased in size and now measures 6 cm in diameter. She also has axillary freckling and patchy areas of pigmentation on the skin.

3. A 25-year-old man presents with a soft swelling on the scalp. On examination, it is approximately 1.5 cm in size, attached to the skin, is non-tender and has a punctum.

4. A 20-year-old man presents with a swelling situated at the outer angle of the right orbit. The swelling is about 2 cm in size and is painless. On palpation, it appears to be fixed to the deeper structures.

5. A 30-year-old man presents with a lump in the right cervical region. On examination, he has about four discrete lumps, which are non-tender, rubbery and each measure about 1 cm. He also has similar lumps in the axillae and groins.

Answers to **2.36**

1.   G Lipoma

This patient has the characteristic findings of a subcutaneous lipoma. This is a common, benign tumour of the subcutaneous tissue occurring particularly in the region of the shoulder, back and buttocks. The subcutaneous lipoma is painless, slow growing, lobulated and is semifluctuant with a definite edge that slips under the palpating finger.

2.   I Neurofibrosarcoma

Neurofibromatosis is characterized by the presence of multiple, small nodules which vary in size and occur along the fibrous sheath of the cutaneous nerves. An important accompaniment of this condition is patchy pigmentation of the skin. A well-recognized complication is a malignant change to a neurosarcoma in one of the neurofibroma nodules. The increase in size of one of the swellings in her neck is suggestive of this change.

3.   J Sebaceous cyst

This arises from blockage of the duct of a sebaceous gland, the point of blockage being marked as a blue spot – the punctum. These cysts are fixed to the skin and can be found in places where sebaceous glands are plentiful, e.g. the scalp, face and scrotum.

4.   B Dermoid cyst

This occurs in the line of embryonic fusion. Therefore, it can be found anywhere in the midline but is most frequently seen at the outer angle of the orbit where the adjacent bone may be deficient. Diagnosis is made by its position and its relative fixation to the deeper structures.

5.   H Lymph node

This patient has similar swellings in the typical areas where lymph nodes can easily be palpated. Also, the description of the swelling seems to be that of a lymph node. Some infections and the lymphomas present with lymphadenopathy in the neck, axillae and groins.

Diagnosis of a hernia

A Direct inguinal hernia
B Epigastric hernia
C Hiatus hernia
D Incisional hernia
E Indirect inguinal hernia
F Lumbar hernia
G Obturator hernia
H Paraumbilical hernia
I Richter's hernia
J Spigelian hernia
K Umbilical hernia

For each of the presentations below choose the SINGLE most likely hernia from the above options. Each option may be used once, more than once, or not at all.

1. A 48-year-old obese woman was referred to a surgeon for a surgical procedure to reduce her weight. Apart from obesity (weight 130 kg) examination was unremarkable. A plain film of the chest showed an air shadow behind the heart.

2. A 40-year-old man presents with a 2-cm lump situated midway between the xiphoid process and the umbilicus. It is occasionally painful. Clinical examination confirms a hernia of the abdominal wall.

3. A 60-year-old woman is operated on for a strangulated, right femoral hernia and is found to have only a portion of the circumference of the small intestine in the sac.

4. A 50-year-old woman presents with a soft, reducible mass at the lateral border of the rectus abdominis muscle and below the level of the umbilicus. This is diagnosed as a specific type of hernia.

5. A 60-year-old man presents with a swelling around the umbilicus. It is reducible with a palpable cough impulse.

Answers to **2.37**

1. **C   Hiatus hernia**

   The shadow of air behind the heart suggests that a part of the stomach
   has passed into the chest through the oesophageal hiatus. The
   symptoms of hiatus hernia are mostly those of its complications,
   especially of associated oesophagitis (reflux oesophagitis, spasm,
   dysphagia and bleeding). The symptoms may be episodic or may be
   brought on for the first time after undue stress such as heavy lifting,
   rapid gain of weight (as in this patient), pregnancy or ascites.

2. **B   Epigastric hernia**

   An epigastric hernia occurs through the linea alba anywhere between the
   xiphoid process and the umbilicus, usually midway between these
   structures. It starts as a protrusion of extraperitoneal fat through the
   linea alba, where the latter is pierced by a small blood vessel.

3. **I   Richter's hernia**

   This is a hernia in which the sac contains only a portion of the
   circumference of the intestine. It usually complicates femoral and, rarely,
   obturator hernias.

4. **J   Spigelian hernia**

   This is a type of interparietal hernia occurring commonly at the level of
   the arcuate line. The fundus of the sac, clothed by extraperitoneal fat
   may lie beneath the internal oblique muscle. It advances through that
   muscle and spreads out like a mushroom between the external and
   internal oblique muscles, giving rise to a diffuse swelling which is often
   not fully reducible. Computerized tomography is often used for
   confirmation of the diagnosis.

5. **H   Paraumbilical hernia**

   In an adult herniae around the umbilicus are called paraumbilical
   herniae. These are acquired herniae rather than the congenital umbilical
   herniae seen in young children. The protrusion of the abdominal
   contents through the abdominal wall is caused by weakness in the latter,
   usually due to a wasting disease.

Management of breast lumps

A Chemotherapy
B Lumpectomy
C Mammogram
D Mastectomy/axillary clearance
E Observation
F Radiotherapy
G Simple mastectomy
H Tamoxifen
I Trucut biopsy/fine needle aspiration (FNA)
J Ultrasound scan
K Wide local excision/axillary clearance

For each presentation below choose the SINGLE most appropriate management from the above list. Each option can be used once, more than once, or not at all.

1. A 20-year-old girl presents with a 2-month history of a 1-cm smooth lump in the inner quadrant of her left breast that moves well on palpation and is firm in consistency.

2. A 19-year-old girl presents with a 1-year history of bilateral breast lumps, which are painful before her periods. Each lump measures approximately 1 cm in diameter.

3. A 70-year-old otherwise fit woman presents with a fungating lump in the right breast, which has eroded through the skin. She also has right axillary lymphadenopathy. A fine needle aspiration shows this to be malignant.

4. A 45-year-old woman presents with a left-sided breast lump situated in the outer upper quadrant. This measures about 3 cm in size and is hard on palpation. She also has left-sided axillary lymphadenopathy. Fine needle aspiration from the lump shows malignant cells.

5. A 45-year-old woman presents with a right-sided, firm lump situated centrally about 3 cm in size.

Answers to **2.38**

1.   E   Observation

A smooth breast lump that moves easily on palpation in a young woman is a fairly common occurrence. This is most likely to be a pericanalicular fibroadenoma which is most commonly encountered between the ages of 20 and 30 years. The first line of management is observation. It is slow-growing and seldom exceeds 2 cm in length. It can be removed electively through a small radial or submammary incision.

2.   E   Observation

The most likely diagnosis here is fibroadenosis, which is a benign condition that tends to worsen during the menstrual periods and improve during pregnancy. It requires reassurance, observation and symptomatic treatment with a well-fitting brassiere and analgesics. Hormonal therapy with the synthetic androgen danazol or the prolactin inhibitor, bromocriptine, is effective in relieving pain and swelling.

3.   D   Mastectomy/axillary clearance

This is an advanced fungating carcinoma of the breast. The best option is to perform a simple mastectomy with axillary clearance. Sometimes, in a frail elderly patient who is not fit for surgery, tamoxifen therapy is the management of choice.

4.   K   Wide local excision/axillary clearance

The options available for this patient are a wide local excision or a mastectomy, both with axillary clearance. However, in a young patient, breast preservation is preferred and studies have shown that both modes of treatment have equal long term results. For a wide local excision to be an acceptable option, it is important that the lump is situated in the outer region of the breast. Most often an axillary clearance is done. Depending upon the histology and nodal involvement further treatment can be initiated.

5.   I   Trucut biopsy/fine needle aspiration (FNA)

The nature of this breast lump needs to be determined. A FNA is easily done at the first clinic appointment. Most breast clinics are now 'one-stop-clinics' at which clinical examination, FNA and mammography are all performed.

Management of fistulae

A   Anal flap advancement
B   Closure of fistula and oesophageal anastomosis
C   Colostomy
D   Continuous bladder drainage by catheterization
E   Detachment of fistula and colectomy
F   Drainage and removal of the distal obstruction
G   Endoscopic retrograde cholangiopancreatography (ERCP) and
      sphincterotomy
H   Excision of fistula
I   Intravenous urography
J   Separation of vagina and bladder with a gracilis flap or omental
      insertion
K   Seton insertion

For each scenario below choose the SINGLE most appropriate
management from the above list of options. Each option can be used once,
more than once, or not at all.

1.   A 40-year-old woman who had a vaginal hysterectomy 6 months ago
presents with a watery, vaginal discharge that has been present since the
removal of her urinary catheter. The discharge smells of urine and
investigations reveal the presence of a small vesicovaginal fistula.

2.   A 25-year-old man develops a fistula-in-ano. On examination of the
rectum under general anaesthesia, he is found to have a posterior fistula-
in-ano with the internal opening 2 cm above the dentate line.

3.   A 40-year-old man has had multiple fistulae-in-ano. Conservative
management and seton insertion were unsuccessful and he continued to
be symptomatic with an almost continuous discharge from his fistulae.

4.   A 45-year-old woman develops a biliary fistula after a routine
cholecystectomy. She is not symptomatic and an ultrasound scan of the
abdomen shows a calculus in the common bile duct with proximal
dilatation.

5.   A 65-year-old woman presents with a 6-month history of pneumaturia
and passing faeculent material in the urine. A barium enema reveals
severe sigmoid diverticular disease and a colovesical fistula.

Answers to 2.39

1. **D   Continuous bladder drainage by catheterization**

   Small vesicovaginal fistulae that occur after vaginal or pelvic surgery may close spontaneously if the urine is diverted by using a Foley's catheter. If this fails, then surgical intervention should be considered.

2. **K   Seton insertion**

   An internal opening above the dentate line means it is above the sphincter mechanism. A simple laying open of the fistula can damage this mechanism causing incontinence. In these situations a seton (a thin thread of silk, linen or nylon) is inserted. This is done by passing a nylon thread from the internal opening to the external opening of the fistula. This functions as a wick or drain. Once the fistula is dry then definitive surgical treatment can be undertaken.

3. **C   Colostomy**

   A fistula-in-ano is usually treated by laying open the fistula if it is a low type. A high fistula is treated with a seton insertion. Sometimes, despite an extended period of conservative treatment, this treatment does not succeed especially in the presence of multiple fistulae, in which case a diversion stoma can dry up the perineal region. This is usually achieved by performing a colostomy. When the fistula stops discharging and the perineum is dry then a definitive surgical procedure for the fistulae can be performed after which the colostomy can be closed.

4. **G   ERCP and sphincterotomy**

   A persistent bile leak may be the result of a divided cystic duct where the surgical tie has slipped. Generally, a drain will solve the problem. However, if there is a distal blockage, as in this case, there will be a persistent leak until the blockage is removed. This can be done easily via ERCP and sphincterotomy.

5. **E   Detachment of fistula and colectomy**

   This patient has developed a colovesical fistula secondary to her severe diverticular disease. Repeated inflammation of the colon can sometimes involve the adjacent urinary bladder and this can occasionally lead to the above condition. Surgical management involves excision of the affected colon after detaching the fistula.

Types of colorectal operations

A   Abdominoperineal resection
B   Anterior resection
C   Endoanal excision
D   Loop colostomy
E   Panproctocolectomy
F   Perineal rectosigmoidectomy
G   Reilly's sigmoid myotomy
H   Restorative proctocolectomy with ileal pouch
I   Right hemicolectomy
J   Sigmoid colectomy
K   Total colectomy

For each clinical situation below, choose the SINGLE most appropriate surgical intervention from the options above. Each option may be used once, more than once, or not at all.

1. An 85-year-old man has symptoms of large bowel obstruction. Rectal examination reveals a large circumferential rectal tumour 5 cm above the dentate line and almost occluding the lumen. The anaesthetist advises that the patient is not fit for a definitive procedure to excise the rectal tumour.

2. A 75-year-old lady who is being investigated for an iron deficiency anaemia is found to have an apple-core lesion in the caecum on barium enema.

3. A 65-year-old man presents with rectal bleeding. Rigid sigmoidoscopy shows an eccentric 2 cm lesion which is about 10 cm from the anal verge. Biopsies of the lesion confirm an invasive adenocarcinoma. Staging investigations reveal no evidence of metastases.

4. An 84-year-old woman presents with a 15-cm full-thickness prolapse of the rectum causing considerable discomfort with mucous discharge and bleeding.

5. A 27-year-old woman presents with active ulcerative colitis involving the whole colon and rectum. Prolonged medical treatment has failed and she has been referred for surgical treatment. However, she does not want a permanent stoma.

Answers to **2.40**

1.   D   Loop colostomy

This patient has a large bowel obstruction due to a rectal tumour. This needs surgical intervention and ideally he should have a resection of the rectal neoplasm. However, since he is considered to be unfit for a major surgical procedure, he needs an appropriate and quick procedure which in this case is a loop colostomy of either the sigmoid or the transverse colon.

2.   I   Right hemicolectomy

Tumours of the caecum and ascending colon will need a right hemicolectomy. This involves removal of the terminal ileum, caecum, ascending colon and proximal half of the transverse colon with an ileotransverse anastomosis.

3.   B   Anterior resection

Tumours of the upper and middle rectum can be treated surgically with excision of the rectum and sigmoid colon with a primary anastomosis between the descending colon and the lower rectum or the anal canal. This procedure is referred to as an anterior resection of the rectum.

4.   F   Perineal rectosigmoidectomy

There are many operations for rectal prolapse including an abdominal approach such as suture rectopexy, mesh rectopexy or anterior resection, and perineal approach such as perineal rectosigmoidectomy and Delorme's procedure, etc. The perineal rectosigmoidectomy procedure involves the removal of the prolapsed rectum and sigmoid colon with a coloanal anastomosis. This perineal approach, without the need for a laparotomy, is a safer option for an elderly patient.

5.   H   Restorative proctocolectomy with ileal pouch

Ulcerative colitis is a form of inflammatory bowel disease limited to the colon and rectum and should therefore be curable by surgery. In the past, surgery involved the resection of the entire colon, rectum and anal canal with the terminal ileum brought out as a permanent end-ileostomy. Advances over the past couple of decades have led to the development of the pouch procedure. This involves resection of the entire colon and rectum and fashioning the terminal ileum as a pouch. This pouch acts as a reservoir and is anastomosed to the anal canal, thus avoiding a stoma.

Management of intestinal obstruction

A Caecostomy
B Defunctioning stoma
C Division of congenital band
D Enterotomy
E Excision of growth and primary anastomosis
F Hartmann's procedure
G Intestinal bypass
H Palliative analgesia
I Release of adhesions
J Repair of hernia ± resection of bowel
K Small bowel resection with anastomosis

For each of the scenarios below choose the SINGLE most appropriate intervention from the list of options above. Each option may be used once, more than once, or not at all.

1. An 85-year-old man has an inoperable tumour in the descending colon which has caused bowel obstruction with a distended proximal bowel. His past medical history includes chronic obstructive pulmonary disease, two myocardial infarctions and senile dementia.

2. At laparotomy for a small bowel obstruction, an 80-year-old woman is found to have a large gall stone impacted in the ileum. There is no evidence of bowel necrosis.

3. A 79-year-old woman presents with peritonitis. At laparotomy, it is noted that she has faecal peritonitis from a perforation due to an obstructing but mobile tumour in the sigmoid colon. The proximal colon is loaded with faeces.

4. A 60-year-old woman presents with signs of acute intestinal obstruction. There is a 3-cm tender lump in her right groin situated below and lateral to the pubic tubercle.

5. A 40-year-old woman with Crohn's disease presents with colicky abdominal pain and vomiting. Abdominal X-rays show evidence of small bowel obstruction. A 10-cm length of strictured bowel is found at laparotomy.

Answers to **2.41**

1.   B   Defunctioning stoma

The patient is unfit for a major procedure. Although this is an inoperable tumour there is still a need to relieve the intestinal obstruction. The shortest procedure to tide over this emergency is a simple defunctioning stoma. Depending on whether the ileocaecal valve is competent or not, this procedure may take the form of either a transverse colostomy or ileostomy.

2.   D   Enterotomy

Gall stone ileus is caused by a large gall stone impacting in the narrow distal ileum. This is a complication of chronic cholecystitis when a cholecystoduodenal fistula occurs. A plain X-ray of the abdomen may show air in the biliary tree. At laparotomy, a simple enterotomy and extraction of the stone will suffice if the affected bowel is healthy.

3.   F   Hartmann's procedure

This lady has faecal peritonitis from a perforated colonic tumour. The only option is to resect this lesion. In view of the contamination in the peritoneal cavity and the faecal loading of the proximal bowel, a primary anastomosis will be at risk of dehiscence. Hence the safest option is a Hartmann's procedure, which entails resection of the affected bowel and bringing the proximal end to the surface as an end colostomy. The distal end can be stapled or sutured. It may be possible to reconnect the proximal and distal ends of the bowel at a later stage.

4.   J   Repair of hernia ± resection of bowel

This lady has an obstructed femoral hernia. Release of the hernia will usually resolve the situation but, if the bowel is gangrenous, a formal laparotomy may be needed for bowel resection.

5.   K   Small bowel resection with anastomosis

A conservative surgical approach is generally undertaken in Crohn's disease due to the recurrent nature of the disease. Multiple stricturoplasties may be required for recurring small bowel strictures. However, resection of a limited segment of the bowel with end-to-end anastomosis may be possible in limited disease.

Management of vascular diseases

A   Angioplasty
B   Anticoagulation
C   Aortobifemoral bypass graft
D   Carotid endarterectomy
E   Embolectomy
F   Femoral popliteal bypass graft
G   High ligation of the saphenofemoral junction and multiple avulsions
H   Hypotensive therapy
I   Lifestyle changes
J   Sclerotherapy
K   Stripping of the long saphenous vein

For each patient below, choose the SINGLE most appropriate intervention from the above list of options. Each option may be used once, more than once, or not at all.

1. A 60-year-old woman develops sudden, severe pain in the right hand while driving. Her right radial and brachial pulses are absent, and her right hand and forearm feel cool to touch with some numbness and limitation of finger movements. Her left radial pulse is irregularly irregular.

2. A 65-year-old man has had an abdominoperineal resection for a low rectal tumour. On the sixth postoperative day, he complains of pain and swelling in the right calf. He is otherwise well.

3. A 75-year-old man presents with a 4-year history of intermittent claudication of the left leg. He now has rest pain with ischaemic changes in the toes. He has chronic obstructive airways disease and a previous myocardial infarction. Femoral arteriography reveals a stenosis in the left femoral artery at the adductor canal.

4. A 60-year-old smoker presents with a 2-year history of intermittent claudication in both lower limbs. On examination, he has diminished femoral pulses and ischaemic changes in the toes of both feet. Arteriography shows bilateral iliac atherosclerotic disease with multiple stenoses but with reasonable distal run-off.

5. A 45-year-old woman presents with varicosities of the left leg. Her past medical history includes hypertension and ischaemic heart disease. Examination of her leg reveals distended veins on the back and medial aspects of the calf with saphenofemoral incompetence.

Answers to **2.42**

1.   E   Embolectomy

This lady presents with the classic symptoms and signs of an acute arterial occlusion. Atrial fibrillation is the likely cause. Surgical exploration and embolectomy with heparinization is needed urgently to prevent irreversible ischaemic changes in the limb. Oral anticoagulation may be required for at least 6 months, or life-long if atrial fibrillation is confirmed.

2.   B   Anticoagulation

This patient has a deep vein thrombosis following major pelvic surgery. He should be started on therapeutic low molecular weight heparin injections while awaiting confirmation of the clot with a venogram or duplex scan. He will need subsequent stabilization with warfarin therapy.

3.   A   Angioplasty

This patient has a chronic occlusion of his superficial femoral artery. Balloon angioplasty can dilate a stenosis and reopen short occlusions of major arteries thus avoiding the need for major arterial reconstructive surgery. It is less successful with distal vessel disease. Other possible percutaneous techniques can include the insertion of a stent.

4.   C   Aortobifemoral bypass graft

This patient has a significant degree of bilateral iliac artery disease. The fact that there are multiple stenoses bilaterally makes angioplasty an unsuitable option. He needs a bypass graft from the abdominal aorta to both femoral arteries.

5.   G   High ligation of saphenofemoral junction and multiple avulsions

Conservative treatment and sclerotherapy is reserved for mild varicose vein disease with incompetence of the local perforators. Surgery is required for saphenofemoral or saphenopopliteal incompetence. The saphenofemoral junction is identified and all the tributaries to the saphenous vein are ligated and divided, before the long saphenous vein itself is ligated and divided close to the femoral vein. Stripping of the long saphenous vein is less commonly performed and should be avoided in those who may require coronary artery bypass surgery in the future. Prominent varices may be removed by making multiple tiny incisions (avulsion).

Management of bleeding per rectum

A   Anterior resection of rectum
B   Colonoscopic electrocoagulation
C   Conservative treatment
D   Endoscopic polypectomy
E   Haemorrhoidectomy
F   Injection/banding of haemorrhoids
G   Laser ablation of tumour
H   Lateral anal sphincterotomy
I   Resuscitation
J   Topical steroid treatment
K   Total colectomy

For each of the scenarios below choose the SINGLE most appropriate mode of management from the list of options above. Each option may be used once, more than once, or not at all.

1. A 70-year-old man presents with bleeding per rectum. On examination, he is found to have a rectal tumour at 6 cm from the anal verge. Biopsies of this have shown an invasive adenocarcinoma.

2. A 26-year-old man presents with bleeding per rectum and severe pain on defecation which lasts for an hour after opening his bowels. Conservative treatment with laxatives, local anaesthetic and glycerine trinitrate (GTN) cream has not produced any improvement.

3. A 75-year-old woman presents as an emergency admission with a short history of profuse bleeding per rectum. On examination, her pulse is 120/min and thready. Her blood pressure is 70/50 mmHg and the haemoglobin is 6 g/dl.

4. A 30-year-old man presents with a history of recurrent fresh bleeding per rectum seen on the toilet paper after defecation. He is not constipated. Proctoscopy shows small first-degree haemorrhoids.

5. A 65-year-old woman presents with occasional darkish-red blood loss per rectum. This occurs in small quantities associated with mild left-sided abdominal pain. Clinically, she is not anaemic. A barium enema shows diverticular disease of the sigmoid colon.

Answers to **2.43**

1.   A   Anterior resection of rectum

This patient has rectal carcinoma and the best mode of treatment is surgical excision. Rectal tumours do not respond well to radiotherapy so, depending upon the distance from the anal verge, they can be treated surgically either with an anterior resection or an abdominoperineal resection.

2.   H   Lateral anal sphincterotomy

A fissure-in-ano is usually managed conservatively with laxatives and local anaesthetic, and sometimes with drugs such as glyceryl trinitrate cream that act by producing a chemical sphincterotomy. In chronic cases, this line of treatment may be ineffective and so a surgical option is needed. The most common operation is a lateral anal sphincterotomy.

3.   I   Resuscitation

This patient is in hypovolaemic shock. The first priority is to initiate active resuscitation in the form of replacing fluid, blood transfusion and monitoring the jugular venous pressure and urinary output. The second priority, once the patient is stable, would be to investigate further to find the cause.

4.   F   Injection/banding of haemorrhoids

This patient has bleeding from haemorrhoids. If the blood loss is minimal, then measures to avoid constipation including a high-fibre diet are usually enough. However, persistent bleeding from haemorrhoids can be treated either with injection or rubber band ligation. Surgery is generally reserved for third-degree haemorrhoids or for complications.

5.   C   Conservative treatment

This patient has diverticular disease and one of its presentations is bleeding from the rectum. Most cases are treated conservatively with a high-fibre diet and avoidance of constipation. Only a minority of patients with uncomplicated diverticular disease will need surgery.

Management of haematuria

A Antibiotics/fluids
B Correct excessive anticoagulation
C Cystodiathermy
D Dormia basket
E Extracorporeal shock wave lithotripsy
F Isoniazid/rifampicin
G Nephrectomy
H Niridazole/praziquantel
I Transurethral resection of bladder tumour
J Transurethral resection of the prostate
K Ultrasonic lithotripsy

For each of the scenarios below choose the SINGLE most appropriate
mode of management from the above list of options. Each option may be
used once, more than once, or not at all.

1. A 30-year-old male presents with right-sided loin to groin pain,
   associated with haematuria. Intravenous pyelography shows delayed
   excretion on the right side with a dilated right ureter extending down to
   the lower third. At this point, there is evidence of obstruction caused by
   a 4-mm calculus. This does not appear to have moved from a previous
   pyelogram performed 7 days earlier. The patient is now complaining of
   increasing pain.

2. A 60-year-old healthy man presents with nocturia up to five times a
   night. He also complains of hesitancy, haematuria and dribbling. A
   rectal examination reveals a smooth, moderate enlargement of the
   prostate.

3. A 55-year-old man presents with haematuria. Cystoscopy reveals
   nodules, tubercles and sandy patches in the urinary bladder. Of
   relevance is the history that he has recently returned to this country after
   working in Egypt for 10 years.

4. A 65-year-old woman presents with haematuria. Examination of the
   abdomen reveals a palpable, non-tender left kidney. Computerized
   tomography (CT) shows a mass in the left kidney and urine cytology
   shows malignant cells. The chest X-ray is clear.

5. A 25-year-old man presents with haematuria. Investigations reveal a
   2-cm calculus in the right renal pelvis.

Answers to **2.44**

1.   D   Dormia basket

If calculi do not move completely down the ureter they can cause an obstructive uropathy. It is imperative that this obstruction is relieved as soon as possible. Through a ureteroscope this basket can be used to extract the calculus. Sometimes, even upper-third ureteric calculi can be removed using this method.

2.   J   Transurethral resection of the prostate

This man has the signs and symptoms of an enlarged prostate, most likely to be due to benign hypertrophy. The aim of the operation is to widen the urethral channel by resecting the obstructing prostatic tissue. This could be effectively performed endoscopically via a transurethral approach.

3.   H   Niridazole/praziquantel

Bilharzia of the bladder is endemic in the greater part of Africa, Israel and Arabia and bladder infestation will present as haematuria. In the early stages of the disease, cystoscopy will show Bilharzia pseudo-tubercles, nodules and sandy patches. At this stage, treatment is with the above drugs.

4.   G   Nephrectomy

This patient has a malignant tumour of the kidney. The treatment of choice for this, if the disease is confined to the kidney, is by radical nephrectomy.

5.   K   Ultrasonic lithotripsy

This patient has a fairly large calculus in the right kidney. A piezoceramic crystal is used to generate a high-frequency sound-wave vibration, which is transmitted through an acoustic horn, thus focusing the sound-wave longitudinally down a rigid, hollow, steel rod concentrating the energy at the end of the rod. The renal calculus is broken when the end of the probe is in contact with it. This procedure is usually performed through a nephroscope which also facilitates removal of the debris.

Postoperative complications

A   Aortoduodenal fistula
B   Bile-stained drainage
C   Deep vein thrombosis
D   Dumping syndrome
E   Enterocutaneous fistula
F   Haematuria
G   Hydronephrosis
H   Malabsorption syndrome
I   Pulmonary embolism
J   Urinary incontinence
K   Wound dehiscence (burst abdomen)

For each of the scenarios below choose the SINGLE most likely
complication that has occurred from the above list. Each option may be
used once, more than once, or not at all.

1. A 75-year-old woman presents with diarrhoea and a 4-kg weight loss.
    Five months previously, she had a laparotomy for peritonitis. At surgery,
    150 cm of the small bowel had been found to be gangrenous and
    required resection and anastomosis.

2. A 40-year-old woman has recently had a hysterectomy for uterine
    fibroids. During the operation, there were dense adhesions found
    around the uterus and the operation was completed with difficulty. On
    the fourth postoperative day, she has developed pain in the left loin
    with severe tenderness in the left renal angle.

3. A 75-year-old man had an abdominoperineal resection for a large rectal
    tumour. The tumour was adherent to the prostate so it had to be shaved
    away from the gland. The patient has now developed a urinary
    complication on the sixth day after the operation when his catheter was
    removed.

4. A 65-year-old woman has had an anterior resection of the rectum for a
    rectal cancer. On the eighth postoperative day, she produces a large
    volume of a serosanguinous discharge from the abdominal incision. She
    looks unwell, is hypotensive with abdominal distension and the
    peristaltic bowel sounds are not heard.

5. A 70-year-old man had an abdominal aortic aneurysm repair 2 years
    before this presentation. He now complains of abdominal pain with
    passing altered blood in the stools. He is found to be anaemic and
    hypotensive.

Answers to **2.45**

1. **H** Malabsorption syndrome

A patient who loses a large length of small bowel can develop malabsorption due to several factors. Intestinal transit time is decreased, especially with resection of the distal small intestine and ileocaecal valve, which affects absorption of many different nutrients. There may also be vitamin B_{12} deficiency. The enterohepatic circulation of bile salts can also be affected causing steatorrhoea.

2. **G** Hydronephrosis

The ureters run very close to the uterus and in a situation where the anatomy is distorted with adhesions, the ureter can be damaged or even tied off causing an obstructive uropathy on that side.

3. **J** Urinary incontinence

In a pelvic dissection to remove the rectal tumour, the sacral nerves can easily be damaged especially if the tumour is large. Hence, this procedure can cause urinary incontinence. Another factor to consider for this patient's urinary incontinence is that the normal angulation of the urethra to the bladder is lost.

4. **K** Wound dehiscence (burst abdomen)

This is a complication after major abdominal surgery especially in patients with risk factors such as malnutrition, diabetes, jaundice and those on immunosuppressive therapy. Characteristically, a thin blood-stained discharge is noted after the first week and the treatment of choice is early repair of the wound under general anaesthesia.

5. **A** Aortoduodenal fistula

This is an uncommon, but eminently treatable, complication of abdominal aortic repair surgery. It should be suspected whenever haematemesis or melaena occurs in the months or years after the operation.

Management of dysphagia

A Cervical oesophagomyotomy
B Dietary restriction of alcohol, tobacco and fatty foods
C Dilatation of the oesophagus
D Dilatation of the oesophagus and correction of nutritional deficiency
E Heller's cardiomyotomy
F H_2 receptor blockers
G Nissen's fundoplication
H Oesophagectomy
I Oesophageal stent insertion
J Radiotherapy
K Thyroidectomy

For each of the following presentations choose the SINGLE most preferable line of management from the above list. You may choose each option once, more than once, or not at all.

1. A 45-year old man presents with complaints of progressive dysphagia and regurgitation which are worse on taking cold fluids. He has had recurrent chest infections. A barium swallow shows massive dilatation of the lower oesophagus with stricturing distal to this. Hydrostatic dilatation failed to correct this.

2. A 50-year-old woman with a 2-year history of reflux oesophagitis presents with a recent onset of minimal dysphagia to solids. All modalities of medical treatment have failed and she now opts for a surgical option.

3. A 40-year-old woman presents with increasing dysphagia. On examination, she is found to be anaemic with a pale, smooth tongue and brittle spoon-shaped fingernails.

4. A 70-year-old man presents with dysphagia and gurgling noises in the left side of the neck when he swallows. On examination, a visible swelling is seen in the neck.

5. A 70-year-old man who has significant chronic obstructive airways disease develops progressive dysphagia, initially to solids and then for liquids, associated with significant weight loss. A barium swallow shows an irregular narrowing in the mid-oesophagus. Biopsy of this area confirms a squamous-cell carcinoma.

Answers to **2.46**

1.   E   Heller's cardiomyotomy

This patient has the features of achalasia of the cardia. This is due to failure of integration of the parasympathetic impulses so that oesophageal peristalsis is disorganized and there is failure of relaxation of the cardia. The treatment is essentially to disrupt the constricting fibres of the cardia, which can usually be achieved with hydrostatic dilatation. In this patient, this procedure has failed and so the operative treatment now is Heller's procedure (oesophagocardiomyotomy).

2.   G   Nissen's fundoplication

In patients who have severe gastro-oesophageal reflux, the symptoms may progress to dysphagia due to peptic stricture of the oesophagus. Patients who are refractory to medical treatment will need an antireflux operation and the commonest procedure performed is fundoplication, where the fundus of the stomach is wrapped around the lower oesophagus combined with tightening of the diaphragmatic hiatus. This operation is designed to restore the cardio-oesophageal angle thus preventing reflux.

3.   D   Dilatation of the oesophagus and correction of nutritional deficiency

This patient has Plummer–Vinson syndrome. The dysphagia yields readily to dilatation of the stricture but this patient also needs iron replacement together with vitamins. Once the anaemia is under control and the patient can swallow an adequate diet, rapid improvement occurs and is usually maintained.

4.   A   Cervical oesophagomyotomy

This patient has the classic features of a pharyngeal pouch. The surgical approach is by cervical oesophagomyotomy after resection of the pouch. This gives a fairly good result.

5.   J   Radiotherapy

This patient has a squamous-cell carcinoma of the mid-oesophagus. This could be treated either with radiotherapy or by an oesophagectomy. Since this patient has multiple medical problems, it is preferable to treat with a non-surgical approach. Oesophagectomy carries high morbidity and mortality, so radiotherapy would be the preferred option in this patient.

Management of a scrotal swelling

A Antibiotics
B Epidydimectomy
C Estimation of alpha-fetoprotein/BHCG levels
D Eversion of the tunica vaginalis
E Excision of the lump
F Excision of the scrotum
G Exploration of the scrotum
H High ligation of the testicular vein
I Orchidectomy
J Orchidopexy
K Repair of the inguinoscrotal hernia

For each of the presentations below choose the SINGLE most appropriate method of management from the above list. Each option may be used once, more than once, or not at all.

1. A 7-year-old boy presents with sudden onset of left testicular pain. On examination, the testis is high-riding, very tender to touch and with minimal swelling.

2. A 35-year-old man presents with a 6-month history of left testicular swelling and a feeling of heaviness. On examination, the testis is found to be enlarged, firm, smooth and heavy. His serum beta human chorionic gonadotrophin and alpha-fetoprotein levels are raised.

3. A 30-year-old man comes in for investigations of infertility. He is found to have an extratesticular swelling on the left side of his scrotum. The swelling appears when the patient stands up and disappears on lying down. On palpation, it is soft and feels like a bag of worms.

4. A 50-year-old diabetic man presents with sudden pain in the scrotum. On examination, he is pale and pyrexial, and has a tachycardia and hypotension. The scrotum is found to be severely inflamed bilaterally with some areas of gangrene.

5. A 20-year-old male develops a painless swelling of the right testis. The swelling is confined to the scrotum and seems cystic. There is fluctuation and the transillumination test is positive.

Answers to **2.47**

1.   **G**   **Exploration of the scrotum**

This patient has symptoms suggestive of torsion of the testis. It is imperative that the scrotum be urgently explored because of the danger of the testis becoming non-viable. At the time of exploration, if the testis is torted and is viable then this can be untwisted and fixed to the scrotum. Similar fixation needs to be done on the opposite side. If the testis is non-viable, then an orchidectomy is needed.

2.   **I**   **Orchidectomy**

This patient has a malignant tumour of the testis. After initial staging, the testis needs to be removed. Following this, radiotherapy to the para-aortic and external iliac lymphatic chains may be required. This should give a good result.

3.   **H**   **High ligation of the testicular vein**

This patient has a varicocele. The veins of the testis and epididymis form an anastomosing plexus – the pampiniform plexus. In symptomatic patients, the treatment is to ligate the testicular vein above the inguinal ligament.

4.   **F**   **Excision of the scrotum**

This patient has the signs and symptoms of Fournier's gangrene. This is a vascular condition with an infective origin and is usually seen in diabetics. It has been known to follow minor injuries or procedures in the perineum. The haemolytic streptococcus, associated with other organisms such as *E. coli*, *Cl. welchii*, sets up a fulminating inflammation within the scrotal subcutaneous tissues that results in an obliterative arteritis of the arterioles supplying the overlying skin. Treatment is by wide excision of the scrotum and antibiotics.

5.   **D**   **Eversion of the tunica vaginalis**

This patient has a hydrocele. There are many operations for this and the Lord's procedure is one in which the hydrocele fluid is drained and the tunica vaginalis is totally everted.

Surgical management decisions

A Antibiotics and intravenous (i.v.) fluids
B Do not operate and discharge patient
C Do not operate but arrange to be seen by a physician
D No operation but review later in the surgical clinic
E Operate immediately (next hour)
F Operate on the next available elective list
G Operate within 6 h
H Operate within 24 h
I Palliative care
J Place patient on the routine waiting list
K Reassurance

For each of the following presentations, choose the SINGLE most likely plan of management from the above list of options. You may use each option once, more than once, or not at all.

1. An 89-year-old woman presents with symptoms of subacute intestinal obstruction. She had a laparotomy 6 months prior to this admission when she had an ileotransverse bypass anastomosis for an inoperable caecal tumour.

2. A fit 78-year-old man presents with a 6-hour history of severe, left-sided loin-to-groin pain. On examination, he is cold and clammy with a blood pressure of 70/40 mmHg and he has a thready pulse of 110/min. Palpation of his abdomen reveals a large pulsatile mass.

3. A 20-year-old man presents with a 2-hour history of severe, left-sided testicular pain. On examination, he is apyrexial and his left testis is found to be elevated and exquisitely tender to touch.

4. A 69-year-old woman presents to her doctor with a 2-day history of colicky, left iliac fossa pain. This has worsened considerably by the time she is seen in the A&E department. Her temperature is now 39°C. Examination of the abdomen reveals marked tenderness with rebound in the left iliac fossa. Bowel sounds are present. Erect chest and abdominal X-rays are unremarkable.

5. A 58-year-old man presents with a painful lump in his groin. He has had this lump intermittently over the past 12 months. On examination, he is found to have a tender, left inguinal hernia, which was initially irreducible but later reduced spontaneously with analgesics.

Answers to **2.48**

1. **I**   Palliative care

This lady has an inoperable carcinoma of the caecum for which she has already had a palliative operation to relieve the intestinal obstruction. Further surgery is futile and so the most appropriate management would be for her to receive palliative care.

2. **E**   Operate immediately

This man has a life-threatening condition in the form of a leaking abdominal aortic aneurysm. Every minute is vital and his only chance for survival is an immediate laparotomy to position a clamp on the neck of the aortic aneurysm.

3. **G**   Operate within 6 h

This man has symptoms suggestive of testicular torsion. A torted testis can become non-viable if it is left for more than 6 hours. However, it is not a life-threatening condition so there is time to complete the standard preoperative procedures, and then to proceed to exploration of the testis.

4. **A**   Antibiotics and i.v. fluids

This lady has the signs and symptoms of acute diverticulitis. She does not need surgery at this time and conservative management in the form of i.v. fluids and i.v. antibiotics will suffice. The symptoms usually improve with this treatment.

5. **H**   Operate on the next available elective list

This man has a left inguinal hernia, which at the time of presentation is irreducible. This fact and the presence of tenderness suggest that it may have become strangulated. Fortunately for him it reduced spontaneously. However, there is a high risk of this situation recurring so it is appropriate to operate on the next available operating list.

Acute paediatric surgical emergencies

A Appendicitis
B Duodenal atresia
C Inguinal hernia
D Intussusception
E Meckel's diverticulum
F Meconium ileus
G Mesenteric adenitis
H Oesophageal atresia
I Pyloric stenosis
J Testicular torsion
K Volvulus

For each of the following presentations, choose the SINGLE most likely cause from the above list of options. You may use each option once, more than once, or not at all.

1. A 6-year-old boy presents with a 1-day history of colicky abdominal pain. On examination, he is pyrexial with a temperature of 40°C and he has tenderness in the right iliac fossa which shifts to the midline when he lies on his left side.

2. A 10-year-old girl presents with a 16-hour history of constant abdominal pain, which initially was periumbilical but at presentation has moved to the right iliac fossa. On examination, she is pyrexial at 37.6°C, has a pulse of 100 per minute and has maximum tenderness in the right iliac fossa with guarding and rebound.

3. A 3-year-old boy presents with a 6-hour history of severe, colicky abdominal pain. During each attack, the boy screams with pain and draws up his legs. In between attacks he looks withdrawn. On examination, there seems to be a lump in the right iliac fossa.

4. An 8-week-old male infant is brought to the hospital with a 1-week history of projectile vomiting occurring soon after a feed. The vomitus is not bile-stained. On examination, the baby looks emaciated and there is a suggestion of a mass in the upper abdomen.

5. A 12-year-old boy is brought to the hospital with symptoms and radiological findings of an acute small bowel obstruction, which requires a laparotomy. At surgery, it is found that a loop of small bowel has twisted around a congenital band which was arising from an antimesenteric abnormality situated 60 cm from the ileocolic junction.

Answers to **2.49**

1. G Mesenteric adenitis

This condition is often mistaken for acute appendicitis. The colicky pain with a high temperature and shifting abdominal tenderness are useful clues to the diagnosis, but sometimes the distinction is difficult and the appendix is explored.

2. A Appendicitis

This is one of the most common causes for an acute surgical admission. The patient is usually below the age of 30 and has a low-grade pyrexia and pain. The pain typically originates as a diffuse visceral pain in the periumbilical area and then shifts to the point where the inflamed appendix irritates the parietal peritoneum. Rebound tenderness and guarding are usually present at this stage.

3. D Intussusception

This is due to one section of intestine becoming invaginated into another, immediately adjacent, section of bowel. The typical patient is a male child below the age of 3 years. The onset of pain is sudden with paroxysms of abdominal pain, which make the child scream with pain, drawing up his legs. In between attacks the child remains listless. Sometimes, there is passage of blood and mucus per rectum, which is well described as the 'redcurrant jelly stool'.

4. I Pyloric stenosis

This is a congenital condition in which the pyloric antrum is hypertrophied, resulting in a very narrow lumen causing obstruction. The patient is usually a male neonate who presents with forcible and projectile non-bilious vomiting, occurring soon after a feed. The baby is usually hungry soon after the vomiting. Lack of nutrition leads to weight loss and on examination a lump is usually felt below the liver.

5. E Meckel's diverticulum

This occurs in 2% of the population and is present on the antimesenteric border of the ileum about 60 cm proximal to the ileocolic junction. Bleeding is the most common complication but sometimes it may present as intestinal obstruction, as a result of intussusception when a diverticulum is inverted into the ileum. Sometimes a loop of bowel may pass under the band that runs from the base of the mesentery to the tip of the diverticulum and becomes trapped.

Congenital childhood surgical conditions

A   Cystic hygroma
B   Duodenal atresia
C   Gastroschisis
D   Hirschsprung's disease
E   Hydrocele
F   Imperforate anus
G   Inguinal hernia
H   Oesophageal atresia
I   Omphalocele
J   Pyloric stenosis
K   Undescended testis

For each of the following presentations, choose the SINGLE most likely cause from the above list of options. You may use each option once, more than once, or not at all.

1. A 2-year-old boy is brought to the doctor when his mother had noticed a swelling in the right side of the scrotum while she was bathing him. On examination, this swelling is separate from the testis, and could be reduced quite easily into the abdominal cavity.

2. A 6-week-old baby boy is brought to the hospital with a history of not being able to tolerate his feeds with subsequent bilious vomiting. On examination, the baby is very thin and a plain abdominal X-ray shows a bubble of air in the stomach and another in the duodenum.

3. A 15-day-old baby is brought in with a history of abdominal distension and bilious vomiting. The baby had not passed meconium until quite late after delivery and now has severe constipation, with occasional diarrhoea. Abdominal X-rays show a grossly distended small and large bowel.

4. A 60-day-old female baby is brought to the doctor with a swelling predominantly on the right side of the neck and extending from the lower third of the neck to the ear. On examination, the swelling is soft, compressible and is brilliantly translucent.

5. A new-born infant is referred with evisceration of the bowel. On examination, there is a defect of the anterior abdominal wall on the right side of an intact umbilicus.

Answers to **2.50**

1. G Inguinal hernia

This is one of the more common congenital conditions. The history of the appearance of a reducible swelling suggests that this is a hernia. The fact that this swelling is separate from the testis differentiates it from that of a congenital hydrocele.

2. B Duodenal atresia

This usually occurs in early intrauterine life and can be complete (atresia) or incomplete (stenosis). Most atresias are distal to the ampulla of Vater, hence the bilious vomiting. Plain X-rays of the abdomen will show the double bubble sign with one air bubble in the stomach and the second in the duodenum, proximal to the obstruction.

3. D Hirschsprung's disease

Ganglionic megacolon is a neurogenic form of intestinal obstruction in which there is an absence of ganglion cells. Most infants with Hirschsprung's disease are symptomatic at birth. They present with a delayed passage of meconium, which can be differentiated from an imperforate anus where meconium is not passed at all. There is marked distension of the abdomen with vomiting and constipation. Diarrhoea may occur due to the enterocolitis of Hirschsprung's disease.

4. A Cystic hygroma

This condition usually presents at birth. Sequestration of a portion of the jugular lymph sac accounts for the appearance of these swellings. Typically, the swelling occupies the lower third of the neck. Due to intercommunication of its many compartments, the swelling is softly cystic and is partially compressible. The characteristic feature that distinguishes it from all other cervical swellings is that it is brilliantly translucent.

5. C Gastroschisis

This is a defect of the anterior abdominal wall and is situated usually to the right of an intact umbilical cord. The anomaly is probably the result of a defect that occurs at the site where the umbilical vein involutes. Unlike an omphalocele there is no peritoneal sac, hence evisceration of the bowel occurs through the defect. Prompt surgery is required after adequate resuscitation.

Investigation of paediatric surgical conditions

A   Abdominal X-ray
B   Barium enema
C   Barium swallow
D   Bronchoscopy
E   Colonoscopy
F   Computerized tomography (CT)
G   Gastrograffin enema
H   Laparoscopy
I   Rectal biopsy
J   Ultrasound scan of abdomen
K   Tc-pertechnetate scintiscan

For each of the following presentations, choose the SINGLE most appropriate investigation from the above list of options. You may use each option once, more than once, or not at all.

1. A 4-week-old boy is brought in with a history of projectile, non-bilious vomiting following every feed. On examination, the baby is found to be underweight with visible gastric peristalsis. On abdominal palpation, an olive-shaped mass is felt between the xiphoid and umbilicus.

2. A 2-year-old boy has recurrent attacks of severe colicky abdominal pains. During attacks the boy screams and draws up his legs. In between attacks the boy is listless. On examination of the abdomen, a sausage-shaped mass is felt on the right of the mid-abdomen. Abdominal X-rays showed dilated loops of small bowel.

3. A 3-week-old girl is brought in with failure to thrive, intolerance to attempted feeding and bilious vomiting. The mother had polyhydramnios when she was carrying this baby. Duodenal atresia is suspected.

4. A 4-year-old-boy presents with an absent left testis. On examination, the left hemiscrotum is smaller than the right side where a normal sized testis is felt. The left testis is not felt in the external ring or in the inguinal canal. Computerized tomography failed to localize it as well.

5. A 14-year-old girl presents with painless, dark rectal bleeding. Physical examination of the abdomen and rectum is normal. A colonoscopy failed to localize the source of bleeding. At this point a bleeding Meckel's diverticulum was suspected.

Answers to **2.51**

1.   **J**   Ultrasound scan of the abdomen

This baby has the classic signs and symptoms of a pyloric stenosis. An ultrasound scan of the abdomen is preferred because it is not invasive and the diagnosis is confirmed if a pyloric mass is found. Only if this is inconclusive will a barium contrast study be required.

2.   **B**   Barium enema

This child has the typical signs and symptoms of an intussusception. Abdominal X-rays show signs of small bowel obstruction. Confirmatory diagnosis can be achieved with a barium enema, which may reveal the claw sign at the point of bowel invagination. Also, hydrostatic barium enema is the mainstay of non-operative treatment, whereby reduction can be achieved.

3.   **A**   Abdominal X-ray

Duodenal atresia occurs in intrauterine life. Polyhydramnios may be present in the mother. These babies are usually quite sick and require urgent surgical intervention. A plain X-ray of the abdomen will demonstrate the double bubble sign with one bubble in the stomach and the other in the duodenum.

4.   **H**   Laparoscopy

Undescended testes are observed in 1–2% of full-term babies. In most of these patients a thorough physical examination will reveal the testis to be in the external ring or in the inguinal canal. Computerized tomography can also be used to find it. If this fails a retroperitoneal laparoscopy can locate the testis if it is present.

5.   **J**   Tc-pertechnetate scintiscan

Meckel's diverticulum is the most common form of persistent vitelline duct remnant. Usually they are silent but they can present as painless bleeding per rectum, which can be recurrent. Diagnostic evaluation of a patient with a suspected bleeding Meckel's diverticulum should have a 99 Tc-pertechnetate scintiscan. This isotope is picked up by the ectopic gastric mucosa, which is sometimes present in the Meckel's diverticulum.

Obstetrics and Gynaecology

Complications during early pregnancy

A Complete molar pregnancy
B Definite blighted ovum
C Ectopic (tubal) pregnancy
D Heterotopic pregnancy
E Incomplete miscarriage
F Inevitable miscarriage
G Intrauterine pregnancy (but not possible to confirm viability)
H Intrauterine pregnancy (but very likely to be blighted ovum)
I Intrauterine pregnancy with dermoid cysts
J Intrauterine pregnancy with hyperstimulated ovaries
K Partial molar pregnancy

For each scenario below, choose the SINGLE most appropriate diagnosis from the above list of options. Each option may be used once, more than once, or not at all.

1. A 38-year-old woman in her first pregnancy at 6 weeks' gestation presents with minimal vaginal bleeding and some lower abdominal discomfort. The transvaginal ultrasound shows a 12-mm intrauterine gestational sac with a yolk sac but with no fetal pole or fetal heart.

2. A 22-year-old woman is admitted with right iliac fossa pain and an 8-week history of amenorrhoea. A transvaginal ultrasound (TVS) shows a 17-mm sac-like structure (without fetal pole, yolk sac or 'double ring') in the uterine cavity with some free fluid in the pelvis. No adnexal masses are noted. Her serum beta-HCG is elevated at 1500 IU/L.

3. You are asked to see a woman in her third pregnancy, who has had a scan, which shows an intrauterine sac measuring 35 mm but with no evidence of a yolk sac or fetal pole.

4. A 41-year-old woman has a routine transvaginal ultrasound scan following recent in-vitro fertilization (IVF) treatment which shows a single live fetus (equivalent to 8 weeks' gestation) within the uterus with a further two multicystic masses, without any solid areas, on either side of the uterus.

5. An 18-year-old woman presents with amenorrhoea for the last 10 weeks and a brownish vaginal discharge for the last 2 weeks. A pelvic ultrasound scan shows an area of mixed echogenicity within the uterine cavity without a demonstrable fetal pole or fetal heart. Her serum beta-HCG is 40 000 IU/L.

Answers to **3.1**

1. G   Intrauterine pregnancy (but not possible to confirm viability)

The gestational sac diameter increases in size from 2–4 mm by 5 weeks' gestation. A gestational sac size of 2, 10, 20 and 25 mm corresponds to a pregnancy of about 4, 6, 7 and 8 weeks' gestation respectively from the last menstrual period (LMP). Therefore, in this case it is simply too early to confirm viability and most scans have a cut-off of 20-mm gestational sac diameter before accepting non-viability with intrauterine pregnancies. Also, the presence of a yolk sac makes it very unlikely to be a tubal pregnancy.

2. C   Ectopic (tubal) pregnancy

A normal intrauterine pregnancy can usually be visualized using transvaginal ultrasound (TVS) if the beta-HCG is ≥ 1500 IU/L. The intrauterine sac-like structure may be a pseudosac as the 'double ring' sign, normally present in an intrauterine pregnancy sac is absent. The diagnosis is further strengthened by the presence of unilateral abdominal pain and free fluid in the pelvis, which may be blood.

3. B   Definite blighted ovum

A fetal heart should always be present in a normally developing pregnancy where the gestational sac diameter is ≥ 30mm (~ 6+ weeks from LMP).

4. J   Intrauterine pregnancy with hyperstimulated ovaries

Although it is possible to have a heterotopic pregnancy (one in the tube and one in the uterine cavity) following assisted reproduction, the likelihood of this happening is low (1:3000 or more). As she has recently had IVF the ovaries are still likely to appear hyperstimulated and resemble dermoid cysts (which also tend to have solid components within them).

5. A   Complete molar pregnancy

The diagnosis of molar pregnancy is suggested by the presence of the following: 'snowstorm appearance' of mixed echogenicity of the hydropic villi with areas of haemorrhage, serum beta HCG of >20 000 IU/L or passage of the 'grape-like' material (hydropic vesicles). A complete molar pregnancy has no identifiable fetal tissue as opposed to fetal development in a partial mole.

Management of labour

A   Artificial rupture of membranes and oxytocin infusion
B   Augment labour with oxytocin
C   Continuous electronic fetal heart-rate monitoring for the rest of labour
D   Emergency classic caesarean section
E   Emergency lower segment caesarean section
F   Epidural analgesia
G   Fetal scalp sampling
H   Immediate induction of labour
I   Induction of labour if not in spontaneous labour after 24–48 h
J   Internal podalic version and breech extraction
K   No action needed

For each scenario below, choose the SINGLE most appropriate course of action from the above list of options. Each option may be used once, more than once, or not at all.

1.   A 32-year-old primigravida presents with spontaneous rupture of membranes at 39 weeks' gestation. The admission cardiotocograph is normal, and the fetus is of cephalic presentation. Fresh meconium is draining and the cervix is partially effaced admitting a fingertip. There are no palpable uterine contractions.

2.   A multiparous woman at 42 weeks' gestation is in active labour. The cervix is 8 cm dilated, having dilated 4 cm in 3 hours, and the fetal vertex is at maternal ischial spines. The liquor is now stained with meconium. The fetal heart rate is 120/min with accelerations noted on Pinnard auscultation. The uterus contracts strongly every 3 minutes.

3.   A 38-year-old primigravida is currently 9 cm dilated and the cardiotocograph shows late decelerations with a fetal heart rate of 160/min. The liquor draining is clear and the fetal vertex is just above the maternal ischial spines. Uterine contractions are moderate to strong occurring every 3–4 minutes.

4.   A 25-year-old woman at 36 weeks' gestation presents with rupture of her membranes and regular uterine contractions. An ultrasound scan reveals virtual anhydramnios with the fetus lying transversely and the fetal spine facing inferiorly in the lower segment.

5.   A primigravida at 36 weeks' gestation is in the second stage of labour to deliver a twin pregnancy. The first twin is delivered by spontaneous vertex presentation. The second twin in clinically 'well grown' and lying transversely with the membranes being intact. The uterine contractions are strong and occurring every 3 minutes and she already has an epidural sited for pain relief in labour.

Answers to **3.2**

1.   H   Immediate induction of labour

Meconium-staining of the amniotic fluid is noted in 10% of all pregnancies. Aspiration occurs in 5% of these cases and meconium aspiration syndrome contributes to neonatal mortality in 10% of these babies (1:2000 of all pregnancies). It is generally accepted that when there is meconium-staining of the liquor, the delivery should be expedited by means of induction of labour rather than conservative management for 24 hours or so.

2.   C   Continuous electronic fetal heart-rate monitoring for the rest of labour

The incidence of meconium passage during labour increases with gestational age reaching 30% at 40 weeks' and up to 50% at 42 weeks' gestation. It has been suggested that this is a reflection of fetal gastrointestinal maturity (gut motility increases with gestational age). However, the sudden presence of meconium could be a sign of fetal hypoxia. In this case however, the woman is progressing well in labour (therefore no need to augment) and the fetal heart rate is satisfactory. Therefore the only course of action is to monitor the fetal heart rate using the cardiotocograph rather than a fetal scalp sampling in the absence of any other indicators of fetal distress.

3.   G   Fetal scalp sampling

Late decelerations are associated with fetal hypoxia and it is worth knowing the fetal pH in order to plan further management especially as she is already almost fully dilated. If the fetal pH is >7.21 then it is acceptable to wait.

4.   D   Emergency classic caesarean section

An emergency caesarean section is indicated due to the transverse lie and anhydramnios and also to avoid a possible cord prolapse. The reason to consider a classic caesarean section is due to the fact that the fetal back is lying inferiorly in the lower segment. This makes it more difficult to deliver the fetus through a transverse incision on the uterus (although one could consider extending this in the midline, i.e. 'inverted T', or laterally upwards, i.e. 'J' incision).

5.   J   Internal podalic version and breech extraction

Once the first twin has delivered, the birth canal is more than likely to accommodate the passage of the second twin. Here, internal podalic version and breech extraction is a viable option, rather than opting for an emergency caesarean section, as there is no evidence that the latter option is safer in twin pregnancies. The Canadian Breech Study (2000) applies to term, breech presentation and singleton pregnancies only.

Causes of subfertility

A Androgen-secreting tumour of the adrenal gland
B Anovulatory subfertility
C Cervical mucus hostility
D Connective tissue disease
E Endometriosis
F Oligoasthenospermia
G Oligospermia
H Polycystic ovary syndrome
I Premature ovarian failure
J Prolactinoma
K Resistant ovary syndrome

For each presentation below, choose the SINGLE most likely cause from the above list of options. Each option may be used once, more than once, or not at all.

1. A couple present with a 3-year history of primary subfertility. In the female partner the serum level of luteinizing hormone is 4.6 IU/L, follicular stimulating hormone 3.2 IU/L, prolactin 440 mmol/L and luteal phase progesterone 12 nmol/L. Hysterosalpingogram shows bilateral patent fallopian tubes. Semen analysis shows a volume of 2.5 mL with a sperm count of 40×10^6/mL, normal forms greater than 50%, 50% forward progression with motility and no evidence of agglutination, white blood cells or organisms.

2. The male partner of a couple with a history of secondary subfertility returns to clinic to find out the results of his semen analysis. The volume is 3 mL, sperm count 10×10^6/mL, 20% forward progression with motility, normal forms greater than 50% and no agglutination, white blood cells or organisms are seen.

3. A 29-year-old woman presents with a 3-year history of menstrual irregularity and difficulty conceiving her first child. She has noticed that milk oozes intermittently from her nipples.

4. A 25-year-old woman presents with a 12-month history of primary subfertility. Her body mass index is 31. She has noticed irregular periods over the last year and a recent increase in facial hair.

5. A 32-year-old woman has been amenorrhoeic for the last 2 years. Her serum biochemical profile is as follows: luteinizing hormone and follicular stimulating hormone levels are elevated (greater than 90 IU/L), oestradiol level is low but androgen and prolactin levels are normal. Thyroid function is normal.

Answers to 3.3

1. B   Anovulatory subfertility

    Ovulation is followed by the luteal phase during which progesterone is the main hormone produced by the corpus luteum. The progesterone levels are usually greater than 30nmol/L. Anovulatory subfertility (ovulatory failure) is more common in older, obese women.

2. F   Oligoasthenospermia

    Oligospermia is defined as a sperm count of less than 20×10^6 per mL. Asthenospermia is defined as motility with less than 50% forward progression. Zoospermia is defined as normal sperm forms of less than 50%. This diagnosis is therefore a combination of low sperm count and motility.

3. J   Prolactinoma

    Hyperprolactinaemia in women causes galactorrhoea in up to 80% of cases, menstrual irregularity and infertility. It may be associated with oestrogen deficiency resulting in decreased libido, vaginal dryness and dyspareunia. A benign pituitary microadenoma is the commonest cause of hyperprolactinaemia in premenopausal women. Treatment is with a dopamine agonist drug such as bromocriptine, which can reduce hormone hypersecretion and tumour size. Surgery and/or radiotherapy may be needed for larger tumours.

4. H   Polycystic ovary syndrome

    Polycystic ovary syndrome is characterized by menstrual disturbance, subfertility (failure of ovulation), hyperandrogenism (hirsuitism and alopecia), recurrent miscarriages and obesity. There is hypersecretion of luteinizing hormone (LH) and androgens with normal follicular stimulating hormone (FSH), prolactin and thyroxin levels. The serum LH:FSH ratio is elevated. Pelvic ultrasound reveals enlarged ovaries, increased stromal volume and numerous cysts (ten or more) up to 8 mm in diameter arranged around the circumference. Significantly elevated androgens could also be secondary to an androgen-secreting tumour of the ovary or adrenal gland.

5. I   Premature ovarian failure

    Premature ovarian failure is characterized by secondary amenorrhoea due to ovarian atresia and failure in women less than 40 years of age. The luteinizing and follicular stimulating hormones are elevated. The ovaries appear small and atrophic in contrast to the normal appearance of the ovaries in the resistant ovary syndrome (amenorrhoea, elevated LH and FSH and elevated oestradiol). Treatment of premature ovarian failure includes hormone replacement therapy (HRT).

Causes of hypertension in pregnancy

A   Cushing's syndrome
B   Eclampsia
C   Essential hypertension
D   Gestational hypertension
E   Glomerulonephritis
F   HELLP syndrome
G   Phaeochromocytoma
H   Polycystic kidneys
I   Pre-eclampsia
J   Renal artery stenosis
K   Systemic lupus erythematosus

For each presentation below, choose the SINGLE most likely cause from the above list of options. Each option may be used once, more than once, or not at all.

1. A 25-year-old primigravida presents at 34 weeks' gestation with frontal headaches. Her blood pressure is 145/95 mmHg and urinalysis shows moderate proteinuria. The serum aspartate transaminase level is 80 IU/L and her platelet count is 100×10^6/mL. A blood film shows signs of rouleaux formation.

2. A 28-year-old woman is found to have hypertension at the booking clinic at 13 weeks' gestation. She complains of difficulty getting up from a chair and walking upstairs. On examination, she is obese with moon-like facies.

3. A 23-year-old primigravida woman presents at 36 weeks' gestation with a history of convulsions at home. On examination, she appears disorientated and her blood pressure is 160/110 mmHg with urinalysis showing 3+ proteinuria.

4. A 40-year-old woman presents at the booking clinic at 12 weeks' gestation with a blood pressure of 160/90 mmHg. She is otherwise asymptomatic and urinalysis is unremarkable.

5. A 22-year-old woman's blood pressure is consistently elevated at 150/100 mmHg at 26 weeks into her twin pregnancy. Her booking blood pressure was 110/60 mmHg. Urinalysis is unremarkable.

Answers to **3.4**

1. **F** **HELLP syndrome**

The presentation is typical of HELLP syndrome, which is a severe form of pre-eclampsia. It is characterized by *h*aemolysis, *e*levated *li*ver enzymes and *l*ow *p*latelets. There is hypertension and proteinuria and the blood film shows signs of haemolysis with elevated liver enzymes and thrombocytopenia. It affects up to 4% of women with pre-eclampsia and is associated with fetal loss in about 60% and a maternal mortality of about 25%. Prompt delivery is the treatment of choice.

2. **A** **Cushing's syndrome**

The presence of hypertension, obesity with moon-like facies and proximal muscle weakness is suggestive of Cushing's syndrome. Conception is uncommon in untreated Cushing's syndrome and for those who do get pregnant, there is a significant risk of preterm delivery and stillbirth. Magnetic resonance imaging of the adrenal and pituitary glands is required in the presence of cortisol hypersecretion.

3. **B** **Eclampsia**

The presence of marked hypertension, proteinuria and convulsion during pregnancy is highly suggestive of eclampsia. Risk factors for pre-eclampsia or eclampsia are diabetes mellitus, first pregnancy, multiple pregnancy, chronic renal disease and chronic hypertension. The definitive treatment involves urgent delivery.

4. **C** **Essential hypertension**

Hypertension at such an early stage of her pregnancy (before 16 weeks' gestation) in the absence of proteinuria is suggestive of essential hypertension. The development of pre-eclampsia in chronic hypertension may be difficult to diagnose but there is usually worsening of the hypertension with proteinuria.

5. **D** **Gestational hypertension**

This is a pregnancy-induced hypertension with elevated blood pressure in the second half of the pregnancy (after 20 weeks' gestation) in the absence of proteinuria and it resolves after delivery. It has no adverse effects on maternal or fetal wellbeing.

Management of contraception

A   Coitus interruptus
B   Combined oral contraceptive pill
C   Intrauterine contraceptive device
D   Intrauterine progesterone-only contraceptive (Mirena)
E   Laparoscopic sterilization
F   Levonorgestrel
G   Medroxyprogesterone acetate (Depo Provera)
H   Oral progesterone-only contraceptive (Minipill)
I   Parenteral progesterone-only contraceptive (Implanon)
J   Sheath
K   Too late, nothing can be done

For each scenario below, choose the SINGLE most appropriate
contraceptive method from the above list of options. Each option may be
used once, more than once, or not at all.

1. A 16-year-old girl presents with a history of having had unprotected
intercourse for the first time 2 days ago.

2. A 37-year-old woman has requested advice about contraception. She is a
company director and is currently nulliparous. She plans to start a
family in 6–12 months' time. She smokes 20 cigarettes a day.

3. A 32-year-old woman who has three children aged between 1 and 5
years is seeking advice on the most effective form of contraception. She
is still unsure if she has completed her family. She is not keen on any
kind of hormonal treatment and her husband has a latex allergy.

4. A 27-year-old single woman is seeking advice to avoid pregnancy as she
has had unprotected intercourse 6 days ago. Her last menstrual period
was 19 days ago and she has a regular 28-day cycle.

5. A 20-year-old woman attends the practice for contraception advice. She
has no children but has had two terminations of pregnancy over the last
12 months. She is positive for factor V Leiden and has a poor record of
attending follow-up appointments.

Answers to **3.5**

1.   F   Levonorgestrel

The safest option for this young girl for emergency contraception is
levonorgestrel, which has fewer side effects than a combined hormonal
contraceptive. It is effective in reducing the risk of pregnancy from 8% to
1% if the first dose is taken within 72 hours of unprotected intercourse
(two doses 12 hours apart).

2.   H   Oral progesterone-only contraceptive (Minipill)

The oral progesterone-only contraceptive (Minipill) is suitable for this
older woman (age-associated lower fertility) who is nulliparous and a
smoker. Other indications include hypertension, diabetes mellitus,
migraine and breastfeeding. However, the failure rate is greater than with
the combined oral contraceptive pill. As she plans to start a family soon,
long term solutions are not viable options.

3.   C   Intrauterine contraceptive device

There is little option but to consider the intrauterine contraceptive
device (IUCD). It prevents implantation in the endometrium and the
copper-wire in the IUCD has a toxic effect on sperm. A progesterone-
releasing IUCD prevents endometrial proliferation and causes changes
in the cervical mucus.

4.   C   Intrauterine contraceptive device

The intrauterine contraceptive device (IUCD) is more effective than
hormonal methods of emergency contraception. It can be inserted up
to 5 days after the calculated date of ovulation even if this is more than
5 days after intercourse.

5.   I   Parenteral progesterone-only contraceptive (Implanon)

This is probably the best option as there is no need for concern about
her compliance for taking any oral preparations or attending the surgery
for regular Depo-injections or follow-up. The implant is inserted into
the upper arm and is effective for up to 3 years. Barrier methods alone
would be insufficient and she would be at risk of a thromboembolic
event with any oestrogen-containing preparations.

Drug treatment during pregnancy

A   Aspirin
B   Aspirin and heparin
C   Corticosteroids
D   Cyclogest
E   Folic acid 0.4 mg per day
F   Folic acid 5 mg per day
G   Heparin
H   Human chorionic gonadotrophin
I   Nifedipine
J   Non-steroidal anti-inflammatory drugs (NSAIDs)
K   Stop drugs

For each scenario below, choose the SINGLE most appropriate treatment from the above list of options. Each option may be used once, more than once, or not at all.

1.   A couple that have already had a child with a neural tube defect, attend a clinic for prepregnancy counselling. They would like to know of any prophylaxis to reduce the risk of recurrence in future pregnancies.

2.   A 30-year-old woman presents with a history of having had four first trimester miscarriages. She has a positive test for serum anticardiolipin antibodies and is currently at 6 weeks' gestation.

3.   A 29-year-old woman is now 12 weeks pregnant. She is anxious because of her last pregnancy, which ended in an intrauterine death at 26 weeks' gestation associated with severe pre-eclampsia presenting 2 weeks earlier. She would like advice on how to avoid a recurrence of these events.

4.   A 39-year-old obese woman, who has been on antiepileptics for the last 5 years, is keen to start a family. She presents for prepregnancy counselling.

5.   A 40-year-old woman presents at 26 weeks' gestation with a threatened preterm labour. She had corticosteroids to improve fetal lung maturity last week when she was admitted with a similar episode.

Answers to **3.6**

1. **F** **Folic acid 5 mg per day**

The usual dose for folic acid supplements in pregnancy to prevent neural tube defects is 0.4 mg per day but in women with a history of a previously-affected child, or if they are on antiepileptic medication, the recommended dose is 5 mg/day. Supplementation should continue until week 12 of the pregnancy.

2. **B** **Aspirin and heparin**

This patient has a history of recurrent miscarriages and studies have shown that a combination of aspirin and heparin would increase the live birth rates rather than aspirin alone. There is no proven benefit of either human chorionic gonadotrophins or progestogens in these cases.

3. **A** **Aspirin**

Low-dose aspirin has been shown not to be effective for prevention of pre-eclampsia in subsequent pregnancies except in cases of early onset pre-eclampsia with a very poor perinatal outcome as in this case.

4. **F** **Folic acid 5 mg per day**

There is an increased risk of neural tube defects in babies born to mothers who are on antiepileptic treatment (especially valproate, carbamazepine and phenytoin) and this can be reduced with folic acid 5 mg per day. There is also a risk of neonatal bleeding which can be counteracted with prophylactic vitamin K injections given to the mother prior to the delivery. Women who plan to become pregnant should receive counselling and should be offered antenatal screening.

5. **I** **Nifedipine**

Nifedipine is a calcium-channel blocker, which is an effective tocolytic (reduces uterine contractility) and is used in preference to ritodrine (beta-agonist) and non-steroidal anti-inflammatory drugs (NSAIDs) due to the side effect profile of the latter. It may inhibit premature delivery. Steroids are used to promote fetal lung maturation and reduce the risk of respiratory distress syndrome.

Gestational age for tests in pregnancy

A   6–8 weeks' gestation
B   10–12 weeks' gestation
C   15 weeks' gestation
D   16–18 weeks' gestation
E   19–20 weeks' gestation
F   22–24 weeks' gestation
G   26 weeks' gestation
H   28 weeks' gestation
I   32 weeks' gestation
J   36–40 weeks' gestation
K   Not necessary to have a test

For each patient below, choose the SINGLE most appropriate gestational age to perform the indicated investigation from the above list of options. Each option may be used once, more than once, or not at all.

1.   A mother with a twin pregnancy at booking wishes to know about the possibility of her 'babies sharing one placenta', as she has heard that this can be 'dangerous' for the babies. She is keen to have this checked using any means possible.

2.   A 40-year-old woman is concerned about the risk of Down's syndrome in this pregnancy and she is at 12 weeks' gestation at present. The woman is keen to have an amniocentesis at the earliest and safest gestation with respect to miscarriage rates.

3.   A 28-year-old woman inquires about the 'nuchal translucency' test, as she is keen to have this done to exclude Down's syndrome in this pregnancy.

4.   A woman who suffers from epilepsy has been diligently taking her folic acid in order to reduce the risk of neural tube defects. She is currently 6 weeks pregnant and wants to know the earliest gestation when she can have serum screening for neural tube defects.

5.   A primigravid woman who is O Rhesus-negative is seen in the booking clinic at 12 weeks' gestation. The father of the child is also O Rhesus-negative. She has no detectable anti-D titres at present. She wishes to know when she should return to have her antibody status rechecked.

Answers to **3.7**

1.   **B**   10–12 weeks' gestation

The best method to check for dichorionicity is by ultrasonography to look for the λ sign which is best done towards the end of the first trimester. Complications of monochorionic twin pregnancies include early miscarriage, premature delivery, growth restriction and fetal defects.

2.   **D**   16–18 weeks' gestation

Although amniocentesis can be done under 16 weeks the risk of miscarriage is greatly increased. The usual earliest recommended gestation to carry out this procedure is around 16 weeks. Amniotic fluid with fetal fibroblasts can be obtained through a fine needle passed into the amniotic cavity under ultrasound guidance. The risk of miscarriage is about 1%.

3.   **B**   10–12 weeks' gestation

The test for nuchal translucency is a relatively new screening test for Down's syndrome, which involves ultrasonographic measurement of the translucent space on the neck of the fetus at 10–12 weeks' gestation. It is possible to predict the risk of Down's syndrome based on this measurement of nuchal translucency, and maternal age at this stage of gestation.

4.   **C**   15 weeks' gestation

Serum alpha-fetoprotein levels are used to screen for neural tube defects. This is usually commenced from 15 weeks' up until 18 weeks' gestation. These are measured in multiples of median (MOM) and levels greater than 2.2 MOM will usually detect 90% of cases with these abnormalities.

5.   **K**   Not necessary to have a test

There is no risk of the baby being Rhesus-positive as both parents are Rhesus-negative. There is therefore no need to recheck antibody status. Normally, Rhesus-negative women with Rhesus-positive partners are recalled to have their antibody status checked at 24–32 weeks' gestation. However, if they are known to have been sensitized in the past and have detectable anti-D antibodies, then they need to be seen every 2–4 weeks from booking.

Intervention in obstetrics

A   Await spontaneous onset of labour and aim for vaginal delivery
B   Breech extraction
C   Classic caesarean section
D   Episiotomy followed by spontaneous vertex delivery
E   Hysterotomy
F   Induction of labour and aim for vaginal delivery
G   Lovset's manoeuvre for delivery
H   Lower segment caesarean section
I   Neville–Barnes forceps
J   Rotational ventouse delivery
K   Spencer–Wells forceps

For each presentation below, choose the SINGLE most appropriate intervention from the above list of options. Each option may be used once, more than once, or not at all.

1. A 28-year-old woman at 39 weeks' gestation has a cardiorespiratory arrest during the second stage of labour. Fetal monitoring until this moment has been normal.

2. A 34-year-old primigravid woman has been in the second stage of labour for the last 2 hours. There was no delay in the first stage of labour and she has an epidural in situ. The cardiotocograph is normal and uterine contractions are occurring once every 2 minutes. Vaginal examination shows the fetal head to be 1 cm below the maternal ischial spines, the position being direct occipitotransverse with minimal caput or moulding. The liquor is clear.

3. A 39-year-old multiparous women presents with a transverse lie (fetal back lying superiorly in the uterine cavity) at 41 weeks' gestation but is not yet in labour.

4. A 20-year-old woman presents with an intrauterine death due to placental abruption at 36 weeks' gestation in her second pregnancy. Her observations and haematological parameters are stable. She delivered a 3.4-kg infant at 40 weeks' gestation by forceps in her first pregnancy.

5. A 36-year-old multiparous woman has been in the second stage of labour for the last 3 hours. The cardiotocograph is normal and uterine contractions are occurring once every 5 minutes. She has an epidural sited for pain relief. The anterior fontanelle, supraorbital ridges and nose are palpable on vaginal examination. The liquor draining is clear.

Answers to **3.8**

1. C Classic caesarean section

A classic caesarean section involves midline skin and uterine incisions and is only rarely done (less than 1% cases). In this situation, a classic caesarean section (so-called post-mortem caesarean section) allows rapid delivery to save the baby and more effective resuscitation for the mother by reducing the intra-abdominal pressure and improving venous return. Other possible indications for a classic caesarean section are a poorly formed lower uterine segment, placenta praevia in the lower segment and large cervical fibroids.

2. J Rotational ventouse delivery

As there is no obvious sign of an obstructed labour, rotating the fetal head and an attempt at ventouse delivery should be made. The ventouse is indicated in delay or fetal distress in the second stage of labour, and is preferable to the forceps as it is less likely to cause injuries to the mother. Contraindications include a face presentation and a gestation of less than 34 weeks.

3. H Lower segment caesarean section

Lower segment caesarean section is the safest mode of delivery in this case, as she is at risk of developing a cord prolapse if she labours and her membranes rupture, especially as her pregnancy is post-date. Complications of a caesarean section include haemorrhage, infection and thromboembolism. Classic caesarean section is indicated only when the fetal back is lying inferiorly with ruptured membranes.

4. F Induction of labour and aim for vaginal delivery

In cases of intrauterine death, especially due to abruption, induction of labour usually results in the rapid delivery of the dead fetus. The only exception to this case may be a primigravid woman who is clinically unstable where immediate delivery by caesarean section is indicated in maternal interests. Psychological support and pain relief should be offered.

5. H Lower segment caesarean section

In this case, the woman has been in the second stage of labour for 3 hours, which is too long for a multiparous woman and is a sign of obstructed labour. The brow presentation is a midway position between face and vertex, which is associated with a presenting diameter of 13 cm. It is not compatible with vaginal delivery and a caesarean section is essential for delivery.

Causes of antepartum haemorrhage

A Abruptio placenta
B Cervical ectropion
C Grade II placenta praevia
D Grade IV placenta praevia
E Intramembranous haematoma
F Placenta accreta
G Placenta secreta
H Threatened miscarriage
I Unexplained antepartum haemorrhage
J Uterine scar rupture
K Vasa praevia

For each scenario below, choose the SINGLE most appropriate cause from the above list of options. Each option may be used once, more than once, or not at all.

1. A 25-year-old primigravid woman at 32 weeks' gestation presents with painless vaginal bleeding. The fetal movements are normal and the uterine size is equivalent to her gestation and is not tender on palpation. An ultrasound scan reveals the placenta to be completely covering the internal os.

2. A 19-year-old cocaine addict at 28 weeks' gestation is admitted with a history of sudden onset of abdominal pain with minimal vaginal bleeding. The uterus feels hard on palpation and the fetal parts are difficult to palpate. Fetal heart activity is detectable on Doppler ultrasound.

3. A midwife has just done an artificial rupture of membranes on a woman at 41 weeks' gestation in her third pregnancy. Shortly after this, the midwife notices a moderate amount of 'bright red' vaginal bleeding and fetal bradycardia.

4. A 30-year-old woman at 39 weeks' gestation is concerned about the risk of bleeding and hysterectomy at delivery because of the anterior placenta praevia, diagnosed on ultrasound 2 weeks previously. She has had two previous caesarean sections.

5. A 25-year-old woman experiences a sudden onset of severe suprapubic pain despite having an epidural in situ. Her cervix is 6 cm dilated with the fetal head at the maternal ischial spines. This is followed by fetal bradycardia with some fresh vaginal bleeding. The uterine contractions, occurring every 3 minutes, have ceased abruptly. She had a caesarean section for her previous delivery.

Answers to **3.9**

1.   **D**   Grade IV placenta praevia

Recurrent painless vaginal bleeding is very suggestive of placenta praevia. The bleeding is from the maternal circulation and is more likely to compromise the mother than the fetus. The grade of praevia relates to the distance of the placenta from the internal os as it implants in the lower uterine segment. The internal os is completely covered by the placenta in Grade IV. Risk factors for developing placenta praevia generally include previous caesarean section, multiple gestation and a structural uterine abnormality.

2.   **A**   Abruptio placenta

Abruptio placenta is the premature separation of the placenta, which presents with dark vaginal bleeding (in about 70% cases), abdominal pain and uterine contractions. The cause is not known in most cases but there is a significant association with cocaine abuse and the characteristic finding is a 'woody' hard uterus due to uterine hypertonicity. Other associations include abdominal trauma, smoking, uterine overdistension and pre-eclampsia.

3.   **K**   Vasa praevia

This is a rare cause of antepartum haemorrhage, which tends to occur when the membranes are ruptured and there is a velamentous (eccentric) insertion of the umbilical cord. This is fetal, as opposed to maternal, bleeding which causes acute fetal distress and bright red bleeding. It is possible to test for fetal blood by the Kleihauer test (resistant to denaturation by acid or alcohol). Treatment is with immediate delivery by caesarean section.

4.   **F**   Placenta accreta

The risk of placenta accreta (retained placenta morbidly adherent to uterus) increases with a low-lying placenta in a woman who has had a previous caesarean section. Hysterectomy is the treatment of choice in those who do not wish to have any more children. Otherwise a simple excision with oversewing may be adequate.

5.   **J**   Uterine scar rupture

Uterine scar rupture occurs in 1:200 deliveries amongst those with a pre-existing uterine scar usually from a previous caesarean section. Placenta praevia is unlikely in this case because the fetal head is deeply engaged. Those with two or more previous caesarean sections would generally not be allowed to proceed to normal labour, as they would need an elective caesarean section. The clinical features include acute abdominal pain, fetal distress and cessation of uterine contractions with or without bleeding. The risk of rupture increases with a large baby and induced or accelerated labour.

Causes of infection in obstetrics   3.10

A Chlamydia
B Cytomegalovirus
C Group B haemolytic streptococcus
D Group C haemolytic streptococcus
E Herpes simplex II virus
F Human immunodeficiency virus
G *Listeria monocytogenes*
H *Neisseria gonorrhoea*
I Parvovirus
J Rubella
K *Staphylococcus aureus*

For each scenario below, choose the SINGLE most likely infection from the above list of options. Each option may be used once, more than once, or not at all.

1. A 23-year-old woman at 20 weeks' gestation wishes to breastfeed her baby in due course but has been advised against it.

2. A 30-year-old primigravida who is O Rhesus-positive and currently at 26 weeks' gestation has had a scan, which shows polyhydramnios, fetal ascites and subcutaneous skin oedema. She had a flu-like illness 4 weeks ago.

3. A 38-year-old woman returns from the ultrasound department after her 18-week detailed scan, looking extremely upset. She has been told that the fetus has microcephaly, cardiac lesions and hepatosplenomegaly.

4. A 25-year-old mother is informed that her 1-day-old baby has a purulent discharge from his eyes with corneal hazing. The swab of the left eye has grown Gram-negative organisms.

5. A 35-year-old multiparous woman presents with a vaginal discharge at 32 weeks' gestation. A high vaginal swab has grown Gram-positive cocci. She needs antibiotic cover whilst she is in labour.

Answers to **3.10**

1.   F   Human immunodeficiency virus

Avoiding breastfeeding, elective caesarean section and combination antiretroviral drugs reduce the risk of vertical transmission (infection transmitted from mother to neonate) of human immunodeficiency virus (HIV). Bottle feeding reduces the vertical transmission rate by up to 50%. The three interventions may reduce the risk of transmission from 40% to less than 2–3%.

2.   I   Parvovirus

Parvovirus B19 is an infective cause of non-immune hydrops fetalis (hepatosplenomegaly, oedema and cardiac failure) and haemolytic anaemia, which may require intrauterine blood transfusion. It usually presents as a flu-like illness in the mother and may cause arthralgia and a macular rash. There is no specific treatment for this infection.

3.   J   Rubella

The findings described are typical of rubella infection during the first trimester of pregnancy when the fetus is most at risk. Rubella causes severe congenital infections with cardiovascular defects, deafness, blindness, microcephaly, hepatitis and mental retardation. The majority of young adults are immune to rubella and parents are strongly advised to immunize their infants with the measles, mumps and rubella vaccine.

4.   H   *Neisseria gonorrhoea*

Neisseria gonorrhoea is sexually transmitted and may cause neonatal conjunctivitis (ophthalmia neonatorum) and eventually blindness from corneal scarring, if it is untreated. The other infective organism causing neonatal conjunctivitis is Chlamydia but it is an obligate intracellular bacterium and is not picked up on Gram staining.

5.   C   Group B haemolytic streptococcus

This is usually picked up incidentally if a woman presents with a vaginal discharge but 10% of women may be (healthy) carriers. This is probably the only infection when intravenous antibiotics are recommended in labour to reduce the risk of neonatal pneumonia and septicaemia.

Assessment of presenting diameters of the fetal skull at delivery

A   Bifemoral diameter
B   Bifrontal diameter
C   Biparietal diameter
D   Bitrochanteric diameter
E   Mentobregmatic diameter
F   Mentovertical diameter
G   Occipitobregmatic diameter
H   Occipitofrontal diameter
I   Suboccipitobregmatic diameter
J   Suboccipitofrontal diameter
K   Submentobregmatic diameter

For each scenario below, choose the SINGLE most appropriate presenting diameter of the skull from the above list of options. Each option may be used once, more than once, or not at all.

1. At vaginal examination the midwife feels fetal buttocks and the anal ridge.

2. A 25-year-old woman has had a 2-hour second stage of labour to deliver a potentially macrocosmic baby. A vaginal examination performed to assess suitability for assisted vaginal delivery reveals the anterior fontanelle and supraorbital ridges.

3. The midwife is concerned about a cardiotocograph. She felt the eyes and nose of the fetus at the last vaginal examination.

4. A 32-year-old woman has just had a spontaneous vertex delivery. The midwife reports that the fetal head was well-flexed.

5. Findings of a vaginal examination on a 31-year-old woman with a prolonged second stage are as follows: anterior fontanelle at 6 o'clock position and posterior fontanelle at 12 o'clock position. There is minimal caput and moulding and the fetal head feels well-flexed.

Answers to **3.11**

1. D   Bitrochanteric diameter

This is a breech presentation, which occurs in less than 5% of term pregnancies. About one-third of babies in breech presentation are delivered by an elective caesarean section.

2. F   Mentovertical diameter

This is a brow presentation, which is associated with a large fetus. It is the greatest longitudinal diameter (13 cm) measured from the chin to the vertex. It is not possible to pass through the pelvis.

3. K   Submentobregmatic diameter

This is a face presentation. It is measured from the chin to the anterior fontanelle (9.5 cm).

4. I   Suboccipitobregmatic diameter

This is the diameter of a well-flexed occipitoanterior position. It is measured from the suboccipital region to the centre of the bregma (anterior fontanelle), which is 9.5 cm.

5. H   Occipitofrontal diameter

This is an occipitoposterior position. It is measured from the suboccipital region to the prominence of the forehead (10 cm).

Management of pain in obstetrics

A   Epidural anaesthesia
B   General anaesthesia
C   Halothane
D   Nitrous oxide in 20% oxygen
E   Midazolam
F   Morphine
G   Nitrous oxide in 50% oxygen
H   Non-steroidal anti-inflammatory drugs (NSAIDs)
I   Pudendal block
J   Spinal anaesthesia
K   Transcutaneous electric nerve stimulator (TENS)

For each scenario below, choose the SINGLE most appropriate management from the above list of options. Each option may be used once, more than once, or not at all.

1. A 30-year-old woman has just delivered a 3.5-kg infant by spontaneous vertex delivery but has a retained placenta. She has not had any analgesia during labour.

2. A 27-year-old woman at 37 weeks' gestation develops HELLP syndrome (*h*aemolysis, *e*levated *l*iver enzymes and *l*ow *p*latelets) with a platelet count of 70×10^6/L. She needs to be delivered as soon as possible by caesarean section.

3. A 25-year-old primigravid woman whose cervix is now 6 cm dilated requests pain relief. Although she has an occipitoposterior position labour has progressed well until now.

4. A 32-year-old woman is admitted in the early stages of labour and the cervix is less than 2 cm dilated and not yet fully effaced. She is requesting some pain relief which will not affect her mobility.

5. A 24-year-old primigravid mother has asked for inhalational anaesthesia during her labour.

Answers to **3.12**

1. J Spinal anaesthesia

Spinal anaesthesia is preferable to general anaesthesia in pregnancy because of the risks particularly of aspiration with the latter. It is quick to administer and relatively short acting. Local anaesthetic is injected into the subarachnoid space to provide the anaesthetic for manual exploration with or without curettage of the uterine cavity. Antibiotic prophylactic cover is needed to prevent postpartum endometritis.

2. B General anaesthesia

Regional anaesthesia is generally contraindicated in women with thrombocytopenia because of the risk of bleeding when the spinal needle penetrates through the epidural space, dura and into the subarachnoid space. General anaesthesia is the only other anaesthetic for caesarean section.

3. A Epidural anaesthesia

As the fetus is in an occipitoposterior position, labour especially in the second stage, is likely to be prolonged and the woman is likely to suffer from significant backache and perineal discomfort. Epidural anaesthesia is ideal because it is longer lasting than a spinal one and the epidural can be topped up every 2 hours or so. It is particularly useful in a prolonged labour as in this case and where there is a high risk of possible surgical intervention.

4. K Transcutaneous electric nerve stimulator (TENS)

Electrodes are placed on the back and emit electrical pulses that block the pain fibres in the posterior ganglia by stimulating the small afferent fibres. It is under maternal control and is very effective for the early part of the first stage of labour and allows the woman to be freely mobile.

5. G Nitrous oxide in 50% oxygen

Nitrous oxide in 50% oxygen (Entonox) is used extensively in labour and is self-administered using a demand valve. It provides quick onset, short-lasting and effective analgesia without causing loss of consciousness. It may cause nausea and light-headedness.

Pharmacological intervention in obstetrics

A Atenolol
B Betamethasone
C Broad-spectrum antibiotics
D Dinoprostone (Prostin)
E Ergometrine
F Hydralazine
G Magnesium sulphate
H Methyldopa
I Midazolam
J Nifedipine
K Oxytocin

For each scenario below, choose the SINGLE most appropriate intervention from the above list of options. Each option may be used once, more than once, or not at all.

1. A 22-year-old woman develops a severe headache and visual disturbance 6 hours after her delivery by emergency lower segment caesarean section for pre-eclampsia. Her blood pressure measures 150/100 mmHg and urinalysis shows 3+ proteinuria. Her reflexes are brisk and there is demonstrable clonus.

2. A 40-year-old woman in her third pregnancy presents at 12 weeks' gestation with a booking blood pressure of 150/105 mmHg. Urinalysis is normal. She has a history of essential hypertension and was on atenolol 50 mg once daily before this pregnancy.

3. A 30-year-old primigravid woman develops a primary postpartum haemorrhage (approximately 800 ml) following delivery of twins and blood is still trickling per vaginum. She has a history of well-controlled pre-eclampsia prior to delivery.

4. A 23-year-old woman is admitted with preterm ruptured membranes at 29 weeks' gestation and is feverish with a temperature of 38°C. The uterus is tender and contracting every 3 minutes. On speculum examination, her cervix is long and uneffaced.

5. A 26-year-old primigravid woman is admitted at 42 weeks' gestation and requests induction of labour. Her membranes are intact and the fetal heart rate is normal. Her Bishop's score is 3.

Answers to **3.13**

1.   G   Magnesium sulphate

This woman is likely to have a fit or develop eclampsia. The best drug in this instance is magnesium sulphate, which has been shown to reduce the likelihood of seizures in eclampsia (by relaxation of cerebral vasospasm or by blocking the neuronal damage associated with cerebral ischaemia) and to control blood pressure. Side effects include hypotension, arrhythmias, respiratory depression and toxicity from over-dosage (e.g. drowsiness, diplopia, slurring of speech and confusion).

2.   H   Methyldopa

Methyldopa is the antihypertensive treatment of choice because it is safe, long-acting and well-tested in pregnancy. Atenolol is associated with an increased risk of intrauterine growth retardation and poor perinatal outcome in pregnancy. Calcium channel antagonists are teratogenic in animals. Hydralazine is most commonly used during labour and should be avoided before the third trimester.

3.   K   Oxytocin

This woman has most likely an atonic uterus, which accounts for 90% of postpartum haemorrhages. Oxytocin infusion causes uterine contraction, which may stop the bleeding. Ergometrine is best avoided in women with pre-eclampsia as it causes marked peripheral vasoconstriction. Carboprost (not on the list of options) may be used in postpartum haemorrhage unresponsive to oxytocin or ergometrine.

4.   C   Broad-spectrum antibiotics

This woman has chorioamnionitis, which presents with uterine contractions and delivery following rupture of the membranes. Corticosteroids and tocolytics are probably best avoided. The best option for the moment is antibiotic cover.

5.   D   Dinoprostone (prostin)

Dinoprostone (prostin) is a prostaglandin E_2 that is routinely used as vaginal tablets, pessaries or gels for induction of labour especially if cervical ripening is required with a Bishop's score (scoring based on extent of cervical dilatation, consistency and position of cervix, length of cervical canal and distance of presenting part above the ischial spines) of less than 7.

Prenatal investigations

A Amniocentesis
B Amniotic fluid index
C Anomaly scan
D Biophysical profile
E Chorionicity scan
F Chorionic villus sampling
G Cordocentesis
H Maternal serum alpha-fetoprotein
I Nuchal translucency test
J Triple test
K Umbilical artery Doppler estimation

For each scenario below, choose the SINGLE most appropriate investigation from the above list of options. Each option may be used once, more than once, or not at all.

1. A 40-year-old woman is 10 weeks pregnant. Her sister had a child with Down's syndrome and she is very sure that she will opt for a termination of pregnancy if this child has Down's syndrome.

2. A 28-year-old primigravid woman who is 32 weeks pregnant has been scanned for being large for dates. The scan confirms severe fetal hydrops. The woman is O Rhesus-negative.

3. A 30-year-old woman at 36 weeks' gestation reports a 2-day history of reduced fetal movements.

4. A 32-year-old woman at 12 weeks' gestation and who is taking antiepileptic medication is concerned about the risk of 'hare-lip' in the baby.

5. A 22-year-old woman with a 14-week twin pregnancy is concerned about the risk of Down's syndrome. She may consider termination of pregnancy if one or either of the twins is affected.

Answers to **3.14**

1.   **F**   Chorionic villus sampling

Chorionic villus sampling will give a rapid diagnosis. It involves aspiration or a biopsy of the chorionic villi in the placenta under ultrasound guidance at 10 or more weeks' gestation. The miscarriage rate is about 1%. Termination of pregnancy can be facilitated by surgical means under a general anaesthetic, as she will be at less than 12 weeks' gestation by the time the diagnosis is confirmed.

2.   **G**   Cordocentesis

The aim here is to establish the extent of fetal anaemia, which is likely to be the cause of the hydrops fetalis (marked oedema from a severe form of haemolytic anaemia). Rhesus incompatibility is unlikely as the patient is a primigravid woman. A needle is passed transabdominally into the umbilical cord to sample the fetal blood. The miscarriage rate is about 1%.

3.   **D**   Biophysical profile

A biophysical profile involves assessing fetal movements, breathing, qualitative amniotic fluid and fetal tone ultrasonographically and monitoring the fetal heart rate with the cardiotocograph. It has been shown to reduce perinatal death but it does not reduce morbidity in terms of mental or physical handicap.

4.   **C**   Anomaly scan

An anomaly scan is a detailed study of the fetus at 20–22 weeks' gestation to screen for congenital abnormalities. The most common abnormalities seen are central nervous system and cardiac defects.

5.   **C**   Anomaly scan

The only logical option here is to consider anomaly scanning. The likelihood of Down's syndrome in one or both fetuses is extremely unlikely in view of her young age. This has to be borne in mind when considering invasive tests and biochemical markers, which are of little value in multiple pregnancies.

Diagnosis in pregnancy

A Antepartum haemorrhage
B Asymmetrical intrauterine growth retardation
C Early intrauterine death
D Early neonatal death
E Fresh stillbirth
F Incomplete miscarriage
G Inevitable miscarriage
H Late neonatal death
I Macerated stillbirth
J Symmetrical intrauterine growth retardation
K Threatened miscarriage

For each scenario below, choose the SINGLE most appropriate diagnosis
from the above list of options. Each option may be used once, more than
once, or not at all.

1. A baby delivered at 40 weeks' gestation has been pronounced dead by
   the paediatrician. The fetal skin is peeling.

2. A 29-year-old woman who is now at 23 weeks' gestation is admitted
   with lower abdominal pain and vaginal bleeding. An ultrasound scan
   confirms a single live fetus of appropriate size for the gestation and the
   placenta is not low-lying.

3. A 32-year-old woman has an uneventful delivery at 38 weeks' gestation.
   However her baby is admitted to the neonatal unit 2 days later with a
   seizure and dies 9 days after birth.

4. A 34-year-old primigravid woman encounters severe fetal shoulder
   dystocia in the second stage of labour, which results in her 4.3-kg infant
   being admitted to the neonatal unit. The baby suffers severe hypoxic
   ischaemic encephalopathy and dies 4 days later.

5. A 32-year-old woman has delivered an infant who shows no signs of life.
   A fetal heart rate of 160/min was recorded 5 minutes prior to delivery.

Answers to **3.15**

1. I Macerated stillbirth

Any fetus that is delivered after 24 weeks' gestation without cardiac pulsations is called a stillbirth. The fact that the fetal skin was beginning to peel suggests that the fetus had died in utero and this is called a macerated stillbirth.

2. K Threatened miscarriage

Bleeding <24 weeks' gestation is still defined as a threatened miscarriage; antepartum haemorrhage is when bleeding occurs >24 weeks' gestation.

3. H Late neonatal death

This refers to late neonatal death, which can be at any time between 7 and 28 days after delivery.

4. D Early neonatal death

This refers to early neonatal death that occurs during the first 7 days after delivery.

5. E Fresh stillbirth

This is obviously a fresh stillbirth as a fetal heart rate was recorded just prior to delivery.

Causes of pelvic pain

A   Acute appendicitis
B   Acute diverticulitis
C   Acute pelvic inflammatory disease
D   Adenomyosis
E   Chronic pelvic inflammatory disease
F   Endometriosis
G   Inflammatory bowel disease
H   Irritable bowel syndrome
I   Torted ovarian cyst
J   Tubal pregnancy
K   Uterine perforation

For each presentation below, choose the SINGLE most likely cause from
the above list of options. Each option may be used once, more than once,
or not at all.

1.   A 19-year-old woman presents with lower abdominal pain worse in
      both iliac fossae. On examination, she looks flushed with a temperature
      of 39°C and a pulse rate of 100 beats/min. Urinalysis is unremarkable
      and a pregnancy test is negative. Speculum examination reveals a
      yellowish, offensive discharge.

2.   A 24-year-old nulliparous woman has a 12-month history of worsening
      dysmenorrhoea. She is on the combined oral contraceptive pill and
      presents on the second day of her period with severe lower abdominal
      pain. Vaginal examination reveals mild cervical excitation, a normal
      sized uterus with no palpable adnexal masses and mild fornicial
      tenderness. Urinalysis is unremarkable and a pregnancy test is negative.

3.   A 30-year-old woman presents with a 3-day history of right iliac fossa
      pain. Her last menstrual period was 6 weeks ago and her pregnancy test
      is positive. Her observations are within normal limits and a full blood
      count taken in the A&E department has been reported to be normal.

4.   A 45-year-old woman with three young children presents with an
      8-month history of cyclical lower abdominal pain, worse 3 days
      premenstrually and unrelieved by oral analgesia. She also has worsening
      deep dyspareunia and heavy periods. Examination, high vaginal and
      Chlamydia swabs, full blood count and pelvic ultrasound scan are all
      normal.

5.   A 20-year-old woman presents with a 24-hour history of right iliac fossa
      pain, deep central dyspareunia and vomiting. There is rebound
      tenderness and her temperature is 37°C. Her pregnancy test is negative.
      She has been using the minipill as contraception.

Answers to **3.16**

1. C Acute pelvic inflammatory disease

This patient is toxic and has bilateral lower abdominal pain, which is likely to be pelvic inflammatory disease because of the presence of a vaginal discharge. There may be deep dyspareunia and tenderness on cervical motion. Infections are often caused by Chlamydia, gonorrhoea, bacterial vaginosis and trichomoniasis. Complications include tubal damage with subsequent ectopic pregnancy and infertility.

2. F Endometriosis

Cyclical dysmenorrhoea that is not relieved by the combined oral contraceptive pill is most likely to be due to endometriosis. Other pathognomonic symptoms include cyclical haematuria, haemoptysis and rectal bleeding. Laparoscopy is the investigation of choice, which allows direct visualization and biopsy of the lesions.

3. J Tubal pregnancy

Tubal pregnancy is the most likely diagnosis in this woman with unilateral abdominal pain and a positive pregnancy test. Risk factors for ectopic pregnancies include chronic pelvic inflammatory disease, previous pelvic surgery, use of an intrauterine contraceptive device and age. The absence of an intrauterine gestation sac may indicate tubal pregnancy.

4. D Adenomyosis

Although the diagnosis is usually made histologically on hysterectomy specimens, adenomyosis is the most likely diagnosis in a multiparous woman presenting with the above symptoms in her late thirties or early forties. Endometrial tissue is found within the myometrium and this causes menorrhagia (heavy menstrual bleeding) and dysmenorrhoea. Hysterectomy is the definitive treatment.

5. I Torted ovarian cyst

Acute abdominal pain with vomiting and signs of peritonism in a young woman is likely to be due to an ovarian cyst accident. The minipill is associated with a higher incidence of ovarian cyst formation. Ovarian cysts are unlikely to be malignant in those less than 35 years of age, especially if they are less than 10 cm in diameter.

Risk factors for gynaecological malignancy

A   Anorexia nervosa
B   BRCA1 and 2 genes
C   BRCA6 and 8 genes
D   Combined oral contraceptive pill
E   Human papillomavirus (HPV) 10, 12 infection
F   Human papillomavirus (HPV) 16, 18 infection
G   Hypothyroidism
H   Lichen sclerosis
I   No identifiable risk factor
J   Progestogen therapy
K   Unopposed oestrogen therapy

For each scenario below, choose the SINGLE most appropriate risk factor from the above list of options. Each option may be used once, more than once, or not at all.

1. A 30-year-old woman has a cervical smear which shows severe dyskaryosis.

2. A 53-year-old woman's pipelle biopsy shows severe atypical hyperplasia of the endometrium.

3. A 74-year-old woman presents with vulval irritation and itching. The skin of the vulva appears red and thickened.

4. A 44-year-old woman is recently diagnosed with ovarian carcinoma. Her mother and aunt have been similarly affected.

5. A 50-year-old woman is incidentally found to have a primary fallopian tube carcinoma at hysterectomy.

Answers to 3.17

1. F   Human papillomavirus (HPV) subtype 16, 18 infection

These human papillomavirus (HPV) subtypes are associated with an increased risk of cervical carcinoma. Up to a third of sexually active women will have had HPV infection of the genital tract by the age of 30 years. The risk of infection increases with smoking, the number of sexual partners and an early age of starting intercourse.

2. K   Unopposed oestrogen therapy

Unopposed oestrogen therapy increases the risk of endometrial hyperplasia and subsequent carcinoma. This effect is both dose- and duration-dependent. The addition of progestogens for 12–14 days per month reduces this risk. Other risk factors for endometrial carcinoma include diabetes, nulliparity, late menopause, obesity and a family history of carcinoma of the breast, colon or ovary. Cigarette smoking and the use of oral contraceptive or progesterone reduce the risk of endometrial carcinoma.

3. H   Lichen sclerosis

Vulval carcinoma is associated with lichen sclerosis (thickened, red appearance) in older women but is associated with vulval intraepithelial neoplasia in younger women.

4. B   BRCA1 and 2

Familial ovarian cancer accounts for less than 10% of ovarian tumours. The defective genes are BRCA1 (about 80% of cases) and less commonly BRCA2 (about 15% of cases). A woman with a family history of breast or colorectal carcinoma and a BRCA1 gene defect has an 80% risk of developing breast cancer and a 40% risk of developing ovarian cancer.

5. I   No identifiable risk factor

No risk factors have been identified for the development of primary carcinoma of the fallopian tube, which is rare. However, about half the patients are nulliparous and infertility is reported in about three-quarters of such patients. It is usually unilateral and diagnosed at laparotomy. It may present with postmenopausal bleeding, vaginal discharge or lower abdominal pain.

Diagnosis of ovarian tumours

A Arrhenoblastoma
B Benign mature teratoma
C Choriocarcinoma
D Dysgerminoma
E Endodermal sinus tumour
F Functional ovarian cyst
G Granulosa cell tumour
H Immature (malignant) teratoma
I Mucinous cystadenocarcinoma
J Serous cystadenocarcinoma
K Serous cystadenoma

For each scenario below, choose the SINGLE most appropriate diagnosis from the above list of options. Each option may be used once, more than once, or not at all.

1. A 19-year-old girl has had a laparotomy followed by a left salpingo-oophorectomy for a 7-cm semi-solid and semi-cystic ovarian mass. The rest of the pelvis, omentum, right ovary and uterus are all macroscopically normal. Histology shows evidence of well-formed teeth, muscle and hair in the ovarian mass.

2. A 68-year-old woman presents with abdominal distension and discomfort. Examination reveals shifting dullness. The serum CA 125 level is elevated at 1200 IU/L and computerized tomography (CT) of the abdomen shows bilateral solid ovarian cysts.

3. A 30-year-old woman is found to have a 5-cm ovarian mass of mixed echogenicity. Her serum alpha-fetoprotein level is elevated but the serum CA 125, beta-human chorionic gonadotrophin and CA 19–9 levels are all normal.

4. A 59-year-old woman has a total abdominal hysterectomy for recurrent postmenopausal bleeding. Histology shows simple endometrial hyperplasia and an ovarian tumour.

5. A 40-year-old woman presents with all the symptoms of pregnancy with a positive pregnancy test despite not being in a sexual relationship. She is found to have a 6-cm left ovarian mass. Her serum beta-human chorionic gonadotrophin is 20 000 IU/L and all other tumour markers are normal.

Answers to **3.18**

1. **B** **Benign mature teratoma**

Benign mature teratomas tend to be cystic and contain well-differentiated tissue, e.g. hair and teeth arising from primitive germ cells. They are more common in younger women between the ages of 30 and 50. Immature teratomas are usually unilateral, malignant solid masses, which contain poorly-differentiated tissue.

2. **J** **Serous cystadenocarcinoma**

These papillary tumours tend to be solid and rapidly growing, metastasizing to the peritoneum and omentum with marked ascites and typically with a markedly elevated serum level of CA 125.

3. **E** **Endodermal sinus tumour**

An endodermal sinus (yolk sac) tumour is a malignant germ cell tumour of the ovary. It secretes alpha-fetoprotein.

4. **G** **Granulosa cell tumour**

A granulosa cell tumour is a sex-cord tumour, which is rare. It is usually of low-grade malignancy and secretes oestrogen, which in turn causes endometrial hyperplasia and irregular bleeding. They can occur at the extremes of reproductive life with postmenopausal bleeding in older women and sexual precocity in prepubertal girls.

5. **C** **Choriocarcinoma**

A choriocarcinoma originates from placental trophoblastic epithelium and is a malignant tumour. It may follow a molar pregnancy, miscarriage or normal pregnancy (metastases from an intraplacental choriocarcinoma). It may also occur as a non-gestational tumour. Symptoms include vaginal bleeding, uterine enlargement, breathlessness (if there are lung metastases) and abdominal pain. The plasma human chorionic gonadotrophin is usually markedly elevated and this is useful in diagnosis and monitoring the response to treatment.

Drugs used in gynaecology

A Antimuscarinic drugs
B Combined oral contraceptive pill (oestrogen and progestogen)
C Cyproterone acetate
D Danazol
E Dianette (cyproterone acetate and oestradiol)
F Ferrous sulphate
G Gonadotrophin-releasing hormone analogue
H Norethisterone (progestogen)
I Oral progesterone-only contraceptive (Minipill)
J Spironolactone
K Tranexamic acid

For each presentation below, choose the SINGLE most appropriate or matching drug from the above list of options. Each option may be used once, more than once, or not at all.

1. A 35-year-old woman complains of increased facial hair, acne and a hoarse voice after she started to take a drug recently prescribed for menorrhagia.

2. A 21-year-old woman requests some contraceptive advice. She has recently been diagnosed as having polycystic ovaries and is noted to have acne and hirsutism.

3. A 31-year-old woman presents with significant dysmenorrhoea and a laparoscopy has revealed endometriosis. She admits to being very forgetful with oral medication and she is not keen for any surgical treatment.

4. A 53-year-old woman has recently developed urinary urgency and urge incontinence. She has no evidence of a vaginal prolapse or any demonstrable stress incontinence and a recent mid-stream urine specimen is normal.

5. A 37-year-old woman presents with menorrhagia. Her periods are regular and she is not keen to have the 'pill' as she has been sterilized. She is also a smoker. What is your first line of therapy?

Answers to 3.19

1. D Danazol

This 19-nortestosterone derivative is used in the treatment of menorrhagia, endometriosis and gynaecomastia. It inhibits pituitary gonadotrophins and has anabolic and androgenic side effects such as acne, hirsutism and voice changes if used in high doses.

2. E Dianette

Dianette is useful as a contraceptive (oestradiol valerate) and in treating hirsutism and acne (cyproterone acetate – antiandrogen). Spironolactone may be used in treating hirsutism although it does not provide the contraception needed in this case. The polycystic ovarian syndrome, however, is associated with menstrual disturbance and anovulatory subfertility.

3. G Gonadotrophin-releasing hormone analogue

Gonadotrophin-releasing hormone analogues, e.g. buserelin and goserelin are used in endometriosis, fibroids and infertility. They are usually given in depot form on a monthly basis (up to 6 months) and are associated with significant ovarian suppression. Side effects include menopausal-like symptoms (hot flushes and night sweats), osteoporosis, hypertension and palpitations. Low-dose hormone replacement therapy may be started as an add-back therapy to reduce the risk of osteoporosis.

4. A Antimuscarinic drugs

Antimuscarinic drugs such as tolterodine and oxybutynin are used to treat detrusor instability by diminishing unstable detrusor contractions and therefore increasing bladder capacity. Side effects include a dry mouth, blurring of vision, drowsiness and confusion.

5. K Tranexamic acid

Tranexamic acid is an antifibrinolytic which is the first line oral treatment for menorrhagia. It is prescribed for use only during the menses and it can reduce menstrual flow by up to 80%. The combined oral contraceptive pill is relatively contraindicated in this patient because of her smoking and her age (greater than 35 years), as these factors are associated with an increased risk of thromboembolism.

Causes of gynaecological problems in adolescents

A   Constitutional delay in puberty
B   Hypogonadotrophic hypogonadism
C   Imperforate hymen
D   Kallmann's syndrome
E   McCune–Albright syndrome
F   Polycystic ovarian syndrome
G   Primary ovarian failure
H   Sheehan's syndrome
I   Testicular feminization syndrome
J   True hermaphrodite
K   Turner's syndrome

For each scenario below, choose the SINGLE most likely cause from the above list of options. Each option may be used once, more than once, or not at all.

1. A 16-year-old girl presents with a 12-month history of cyclical lower abdominal pain. She has yet to start menstruating and she is not sexually active. She has normal secondary sexual characteristics and her serum gonadotrophin and oestradiol levels are normal. A pelvic ultrasound scan shows a 10-cm mass in the midline extending into the vagina.

2. The mother of a 13-year-old girl is concerned that her daughter is short and is not showing any sign of breast development or starting her periods. On examination, there is some webbing of the neck and an increased carrying angle.

3. A 17-year-old girl is concerned that she has not started her periods. On examination, she has normal breast development and the vulva looks normal but there is sparse pubic hair. She has bilateral swellings in her groins. Her serum luteinizing and follicular stimulating hormones are elevated and her serum oestradiol is low.

4. A 14-year-old girl has not started her periods. She runs 6 miles three times a week and her body mass index is 20. On examination, there is no obvious abnormality. Her serum gonadotrophin and oestradiol levels are low.

5. A 16-year-old girl presents with a history of an impaired sense of smell and primary amenorrhoea. Examination shows poor secondary sexual characteristic development and her serum gonadotrophin levels are low.

Answers to **3.20**

1. C   Imperforate hymen

The mass is likely to be old blood in the uterine cavity extending into the vagina as the menstrual blood is trapped behind the imperforate hymen.

2. K   Turner's syndrome

The main features of Turner's syndrome include a short stature, an increased carrying angle of the arms, widely spaced nipples and a webbed neck. It is associated with markedly elevated gonadotrophins and low levels of oestradiol because of ovarian failure (streak ovaries). The karyotype is 45XO.

3. I   Testicular feminization syndrome

The testicular feminization syndrome is due to a deficiency of androgen intracellular receptors resulting in end-organ resistance to testosterone. Those affected are genetic males with testes but develop as phenotypic females with normal breast development and vulva. However there is an absent uterus, vagina (or blind vagina) and ovarian tissue as the development of the Müllerian duct is suppressed by Müllerian inhibiting factor produced by the testes. The gonads need to be removed, as there is a 20% risk of malignancy.

4. B   Hypogonadotrophic hypogonadism

Hypothalamic hypogonadotrophic hypogonadism may be functional (as in this case of exercise-related amenorrhoea) or organic and leads to a reduction of serum gonadotrophin and oestradiol levels. Menstrual irregularities including amenorrhoea are commonly seen in high performance athletes with low body weight and low body fat content.

5. D   Kallmann's syndrome

The presence of anosmia (characteristically unable to tell the difference by smelling between tea and coffee) together with delayed puberty and amenorrhoea is highly suggestive of Kallmann's syndrome. It may occur sporadically or can be inherited as an X-linked recessive condition. Synthesis of gonadotrophin-releasing hormone (GnRH) by the hypothalamus is impaired resulting in low serum gonadotrophins and oestradiol.

Surgical interventions in gynaecology

A Anterior colporrhaphy
B Manchester repair
C Posterior colporrhaphy
D Radical trachelectomy and lymph node dissection
E Subtotal hysterectomy with conservation of the ovaries
F Total abdominal hysterectomy and bilateral salpingo-oophorectomy
G Total abdominal hysterectomy with conservation of the ovaries
H Transcervical endometrial resection of the endometrium
I Transvaginal tension free tape
J Vaginal hysterectomy
K Wertheim's hysterectomy

For each scenario below, choose the SINGLE most appropriate surgical intervention from the above list of options. Each option may be used once, more than once, or not at all.

1. A 57-year-old woman presents with a 2-year history of 'something coming down her front passage'. On examination, she has a second-degree uterovaginal prolapse with no demonstrable stress incontinence.

2. A 29-year-old woman is found to have a second-degree uterovaginal prolapse with no incontinence. She is unsure about whether she has completed her family but is adamant for the prolapse to be corrected.

3. A 32-year-old mother of three presents with increasing vaginal discharge. She is later diagnosed as having stage 1A (microinvasive) carcinoma of the cervix.

4. A 46-year-old woman wishes to have a permanent solution to her menorrhagia. She has a strong family history of ovarian cancer.

5. A 40-year-old woman presents with urinary incontinence, which she finds distressing. It usually occurs when she is coughing or straining and also when she cannot get to the toilet in time. Urodynamic studies show urodynamic stress incontinence with no detrusor overactivity.

Answers to **3.21**

1. J   Vaginal hysterectomy

Vaginal hysterectomy is the best surgical procedure for uterovaginal prolapse. An anterior repair may suffice for a cystourethrocele with minimal or no uterine descent as posterior repair is for a rectocele.

2. B   Manchester repair

A Manchester repair is reserved for women with a uterovaginal prolapse who wish to preserve their fertility. It involves shortening the transverse cervical ligaments, amputation of the cervix and an anterior and posterior repair.

3. K   Wertheim's hysterectomy

Invasive cervical carcinoma is treated with surgery and radiotherapy if it is confined to the cervix. Wertheim's hysterectomy involves radical hysterectomy and removal of the upper one-third of the vagina, parametrial tissue and pelvic lymph nodes. Radical trachelectomy involves conserving the body of the uterus, which is reserved for women who have not had any children. Radiotherapy is the mainstay of treatment if the disease has spread beyond the cervix.

4. F   Total abdominal hysterectomy and bilateral salpingo-oophorectomy

A hysterectomy is reserved for those unresponsive to medical therapy (hormonal, antifibrinolytics or antiprostaglandins) or more conservative surgical intervention (e.g. endometrial resection or ablation). The only option available on the list provided is a hysterectomy. As this woman is close to her menopause and she has a family history of ovarian carcinoma, a bilateral salpingo-oophorectomy is also indicated.

5. I   Transvaginal tension free tape

This is one of the more effective solutions for urodynamic stress urinary incontinence other than colposuspension. It involves inserting a self-retaining prolene tape under the midurethra under local anaesthetic.

Investigations in gynaecology

A   Cervical smear
B   Culdoscopy
C   Hysteroscopy, dilatation and curettage
D   Laparoscopy
E   Magnetic resonance imaging (MRI) scan
F   Pipelle biopsy
G   Serum CA125
H   Serum beta-human chorionic gonadotrophins
I   Serum inhibin
J   Transvaginal ultrasonography
K   Urodynamic studies

For each presentation below, choose the SINGLE most appropriate investigation from the above list of options. Each option may be used once, more than once, or not at all.

1. A 29-year-old woman presents with intermenstrual bleeding. Speculum examination reveals a 2-cm fungating mass at the cervix.

2. A 76-year-old woman presents with ascites and an ultrasound scan of the abdomen confirms bilateral ovarian masses.

3. A 49-year-old woman presents with mixed urge and stress incontinence for 2 years following a hysterectomy.

4. An 18-year-old woman presents with left iliac fossa pain and a weakly-positive pregnancy test. She has been amenorrhoeic for the last 2 months. An ultrasound scan shows an empty uterus with no free fluid or adnexal masses.

5. A 52-year-old woman presents with several episodes of postmenopausal bleeding for the last 3 months. She is not on hormone replacement therapy.

Answers to 3.22

1.   E   Magnetic resonance imaging (MRI) scan

This woman has stage 1b (invasive carcinoma confined to the cervix) or stage 2 (tumour extending into the upper third of the vagina or parametrium) carcinoma of the cervix at the very least. In order to determine the extent of lateral spread the MRI is probably the best option.

2.   G   Serum CA125

Serum CA125 is the first line investigation of ovarian carcinoma. A raised serum CA125 especially in a postmenopausal woman is highly suggestive of an ovarian carcinoma.

3.   K   Urodynamic studies

In cases of mixed incontinence, urodynamic studies are essential before proceeding any further especially if there is a history of a previous hysterectomy. This is to detect the presence of an overactive bladder, which may worsen after surgical correction of urodynamic stress urinary incontinence.

4.   D   Laparoscopy

The likely diagnosis is an ectopic pregnancy and laparoscopy will help confirm the diagnosis. Although the serum beta-human chorionic gonadotrophins may be relevant it will not necessarily add to the management of this patient.

5.   J   Transvaginal ultrasonography

Whilst a pipelle biopsy or hysteroscopy and dilatation and curettage are important, the first line investigation for postmenopausal bleeding ought to be transvaginal ultrasonography. This is because if the endometrial thickness is less than 5 mm, then no further investigations are needed especially if the patient is asymptomatic.

Management of the menopause 3.23

A Bisphosphonates
B Clonidine
C Continuous combined hormone replacement therapy (HRT)
D Cyclical hormone replacement therapy
E Low dose aspirin
F Oestrogen implants
G Oestrogen pessaries
H Progestogen pessaries
I Tamoxifen
J Tibolone
K Transdermal oestrogen patches

For each patient below, choose the SINGLE most appropriate management from the above list of options. Each option may be used once, more than once, or not at all.

1. A 56-year-old woman recently underwent a total abdominal hysterectomy and bilateral salpingo-oophorectomy for recurrent postmenopausal bleeding. Histology confirms a small focus of endometrial carcinoma within the uterine cavity with no stromal invasion. She would like to consider hormone replacement therapy (HRT).

2. A 49-year-old woman is experiencing hot flushes, which she finds very uncomfortable. She is keen to start HRT. However, she has had two deep vein thromboses in the past.

3. A 77-year-old woman presents with some vaginal discomfort. A transvaginal scan reveals an endometrial thickness of 3 mm and a speculum examination shows marked atrophic vaginitis.

4. A woman in her mid 50s presents with reduced libido and hot flushes. Her periods stopped about 12 months ago and she does not wish to have any further menstrual bleeding.

5. A 51-year-old woman is keen to consider HRT as she has a strong family history of osteoporosis. However, she was diagnosed with breast cancer last year.

Answers to **3.23**

1. **C   Continuous combined hormone replacement therapy (HRT)**

    This form of HRT is more acceptable, as the progestogen will negate any unopposed effects of oestrogen, which could possibly increase the risk of a recurrence in this case. It is reasonable to prescribe HRT in patients with early stage, well-differentiated tumours, as the quality of life in these women is an important consideration. It should, however, be used cautiously and for a short term (2–3 years) for relief of menopausal symptoms, as per the latest recommendations.

2. **B   Clonidine**

    Clonidine is an alpha-blocker which is effective for vasomotor symptoms in women who cannot tolerate HRT. She would be at high risk of further venous thromboembolism (VTE) with any oestrogen preparation. The risk of VTE is increased by 3 per 1000 women (aged 50 to 69 years) on HRT, and is higher in those taking it for the first time.

3. **G   Oestrogen pessaries**

    This is the best management for the local effects of hypo-oestrogenism especially in women who do not require HRT on a regular basis. Symptoms of menopausal vaginal atrophy include vaginal dryness, dyspareunia, frequency and urgency of micturition.

4. **J   Tibolone**

    Tibolone has androgenic effects in addition to oestrogenic and progestogenic activity. It is given continuously so that 80% of patients are free from cyclical bleeding. It should only be used when women have been menopausal for at least 12 months, or those older than 55 years. The main reason for choosing tibolone over continuous combined hormone replacement therapy, which is also free from cyclical bleeding, is its potential beneficial effect on libido, which is applicable to this patient.

5. **A   Bisphosphonates**

    Bisphosphonates are used in treating osteoporosis in postmenopausal women particularly if they are unable to tolerate HRT or if HRT is relatively contraindicated because of a history of breast carcinoma (as in this case) or VTE. An alternative (not on the list) would be raloxifene, which is a selective oestrogen receptor modulator. It is used for the prevention and treatment of osteoporosis but it has no effect on vasomotor symptoms.

Treatment of menorrhagia

A   Combined oral contraceptive pill
B   Cone biopsy
C   Danazol
D   Gonadotrophin-releasing hormone analogues
E   Intrauterine contraceptive device
F   Mirena (intrauterine progesterone-only contraceptive)
G   Prempak C
H   Progestogens
I   Thermal balloon ablation of the endometrium
J   Total abdominal hysterectomy
K   Tranexamic acid

For each presentation below, choose the SINGLE most appropriate treatment from the above list of options. Each option may be used once, more than once, or not at all.

1. A 16-year-old girl presents with a 6-month history of heavy periods. She suffers from frequent migraines, which are beginning to affect her schooling.

2. A 39-year-old mother of two presents with a 2-year history of secondary dysmenorrhoea and menorrhagia. Her husband has had a vasectomy and she is a company executive who cannot afford to take time off work. She has tried a number of medical preparations, which have not helped.

3. A 26-year-old woman presents with a 7-month history of heavy periods. She has been prescribed the 'pill', which has only partially relieved her symptoms. She has one child, aged 3 years.

4. A 44-year-old woman presents with increasingly heavy and irregular periods. She also complains of hot flushes.

5. A 38-year-old woman complains that her periods are very heavy and unbearable. She has one child and has had a sterilization. An ultrasound scan shows a 9-cm intramural uterine fibroid.

319

Answers to **3.24**

1. **K** Tranexamic acid

As she suffers from migraines, the combined oral contraceptive pill is contraindicated. Antifibrinolytics such as tranexamic acid used during menstruation may reduce menstrual flow by up to 80%. Danazol inhibits gonadotrophins and may be used to treat menorrhagia but its androgenic effects are often unacceptable.

2. **I** Thermal balloon ablation of the endometrium

As medical treatment has had limited effect, surgical intervention should be considered. Although a hysterectomy may be considered, it is often reserved for those who have not responded to more conservative surgical interventions such as endometrial ablation. This is performed as a day case with few postoperative complications. However, up to one-third of patients may have no improvement in their excessive menstrual bleeding.

3. **F** Mirena (intrauterine progesterone-only contraceptive)

This is a parous woman with menorrhagia who will probably want to preserve her fertility. Mirena (intrauterine progesterone-only contraceptive) may be used effectively both as a contraceptive and to reduce blood loss. Fertility returns soon after its withdrawal.

4. **G** Prempak C

This is a form of cyclical hormone replacement therapy (conjugated oestrogens with progesterone), which should regulate her bleeding and may make it lighter. It will also help her vasomotor perimenopausal symptoms but should only be used for a short duration of 2–3 years, and reviewed annually.

5. **J** Total abdominal hysterectomy

Total abdominal hysterectomy is the treatment of choice as she has completed her family. Endometrial ablation is less successful in the presence of such a large uterine fibroid.

Causes of menstrual disorders 3.25

A Adenomyosis
B Asherman's syndrome
C Cervical ectropion
D Dermoid cyst of the ovary
E Dysfunctional uterine bleeding
F Endometriosis
G Hyperthyroidism
H Hypothyroidism
I Pituitary adenoma
J Polycystic ovary syndrome
K Sheehan's syndrome

For each presentation below, choose the SINGLE most appropriate cause from the above list of options. Each option may be used once, more than once, or not at all.

1. A 39-year-old woman presents with a 2-year history of oligomenorrhoea, weight gain and acne. Her serum oestradiol is low with a raised level of serum luteinizing hormone level.

2. A 22-year-old woman has noticed several episodes of postcoital bleeding. Her periods are regular and she is otherwise fit and well. She uses the combined pill for contraception.

3. A 27-year-old woman presents with amenorrhoea, lethargy and vaginal dryness. Three months ago she had a spontaneous vertex delivery followed by a primary postpartum haemorrhage. Since then she has not been able to breastfeed due to poor milk production.

4. A 30-year-old woman presents with light periods and a 12-month history of subfertility. She has had one child followed by two miscarriages for which she had a dilatation and curettage. Her serum progesterone is ovulatory.

5. A 29-year-old woman presents with a 6-month history of heavy periods. Her recent pelvic scan is normal and a full blood count shows a mild microcytic anaemia. She is parous and suffers minimal dysmenorrhoea. Speculum examination of the cervix is normal.

Answers to **3.25**

1. J   Polycystic ovary syndrome

This patient exhibits many of the symptoms of this syndrome, which include oligomenorrhoea, subfertility, obesity, hirsutism and recurrent miscarriage. The luteinizing hormone (LH): follicular stimulating hormone (FSH) ratio is elevated. A transvaginal ultrasound of the ovaries reveals increased ovarian stromal volume and the 'string of pearls' sign (numerous peripheral cysts).

2. C   Cervical ectropion

Cervical ectropion occurs in women on the oral contraceptive pill and may present with postcoital bleeding or persistent intermenstrual discharge (due to an increased area of columnar epithelium with mucus-secreting glands). Treatment involves discontinuing the oral contraceptive pill or ablative therapy with a thermal probe under local anaesthetic.

3. K   Sheehan's syndrome

This is now very rare but is associated with necrosis of the pituitary gland from prolonged periods of hypotension during delivery and is commonly due to postpartum haemorrhage. This results in hypopituitarism, which may present with poor lactation and failure to recommence menstruation.

4. B   Asherman's syndrome

Asherman's syndrome is due to dilatation and curettage usually following a miscarriage that results in intrauterine fibrosis and synecheia. If very severe, it may be associated with secondary amenorrhoea and infertility due to an inadequately vascularized endometrium for implantation. Other causes include tuberculosis and schistosomiasis.

5. E   Dysfunctional uterine bleeding

Dysfunctional uterine bleeding occurs in about half of women with menorrhagia and accounts for 10% of all new gynaecology outpatient referrals. The diagnosis is made by exclusion of organic disease. The primary cause is not known.

SECTION 4

Paediatrics

Diagnosis of inherited neurological disorders

4.1

A	Ataxia telangiectasia
B	Friedreich's ataxia
C	Hypomelanosis of Ito
D	Leber's disease
E	Linear naevus syndrome
F	Neurofibromatosis 1
G	Neurofibromatosis 2
H	Sturge–Weber syndrome
I	Tuberous sclerosis
J	Von Hippel–Lindau disease
K	Werdnig–Hoffmann disease

For each presentation below, choose the SINGLE most likely diagnosis from the above list of options. Each option may be used once, more than once, or not at all.

1. On a routine check-up by the school doctor a 10-year-old girl is found to have multiple, hyperpigmented patches over the trunk and limbs with axillary freckling. On questioning, her mother has similar skin lesions and is under follow-up by the adult neurologists.

2. A 10-month-old infant is brought to the A&E department with right-sided focal seizures and is noted to have a port-wine stain on the left side of his face over the upper face and eyelids, which has been present since birth.

3. An 8-year-old boy presents with a seizure. He has had mild developmental delay and attends a special school. He has skin lesions consisting of hypopigmented patches over his trunk and extremities with fleshy, tiny, red nodules over the nose and cheeks.

4. A 5-year-old girl is seen in the paediatric clinic with a history of progressive clumsiness over the past 18 months and prominent blood vessels seen over the bulbar conjunctiva.

5. A 3-month-old girl is brought in with severe weakness with marked hypotonia, limb weakness, poor feeding and a cough. The tendon reflexes are absent and her tongue is fasciculating with some wasting.

Answers to **4.1**

1. F   Neurofibromatosis 1

Neurofibromatosis (NF) is an autosomal dominant disorder. The two main forms are type 1 NF (peripheral) and type 2 NF (central and characterized by bilateral acoustic neuromas and other intracranial tumours such as meningioma and ependymoma). The NF-1 gene is located on chromosome 17 and NF-2 on chromosome 22.

2. H   Sturge–Weber syndrome

The Sturge–Weber syndrome (mostly sporadic)consists of a constellation of symptoms and signs. These can include a port-wine stain (capillary haemangioma) involving the area supplied by the 1st and/or 2nd divisions of the trigeminal nerve (often with an associated ipsilateral intracranial capillary haemangioma of the pia arachnoid with tramline calcification seen on a skull X-ray), seizures, hemiparesis and, in many cases, mental retardation.

3. I   Tuberous sclerosis

Tuberous sclerosis is inherited as an autosomal dominant trait. It may present during infancy with infantile spasms, and careful examination of the skin on the trunk and extremities reveals typical hypopigmented skin lesions (ash-leaf macules). During childhood, it most often presents with generalized seizures and the pathognomonic skin lesions include shagreen patches (roughened, raised lesions in the lumbosacral area) angiofibromas (tiny, red, fleshy nodules over the nose and cheeks) and subungual or periungual fibromas.

4. A   Ataxia telangiectasia

Ataxia telangiectasia (the Louis–Bar syndrome) is an autosomal recessive condition characterized by slowly progressive cerebellar ataxia starting at about 2 years of age and there is usually loss of ambulation by adolescence. Patients also have telangiectasia over the conjunctiva, pinnae and face, chronic sinopulmonary disease, a higher incidence of malignancy (leukaemia and lymphoma) and immunodeficiency.

5. K   Werdnig–Hoffmann disease

Werdnig–Hoffmann disease (spinal muscular atrophy type I) is characterized by degeneration of the anterior horn cells resulting in progressive muscle weakness. It is an autosomal recessive inherited disorder. Mothers may notice a lack of fetal movements and the infants may be floppy and weak at birth. Muscle fasciculation, especially of the tongue, is an important feature but this can be difficult to elicit. There is also loss of the deep tendon reflexes. Symptoms are always present before 6 months.

Diagnosis of failure to thrive in childhood

A   Chronic renal failure
B   Coeliac disease
C   Cystic fibrosis
D   Diabetes insipidus
E   Diabetes mellitus
F   Growth hormone deficiency
G   Human immunodeficiency virus (HIV) infection
H   Hypothyroidism
I   Inflammatory bowel disease
J   Lactose intolerance
K   Psychosocial disorder

From the options above choose the SINGLE most likely diagnosis for each clinical scenario described below. Each option may be used once, more than once, or not at all.

1. A 6-year-old girl, who has stopped growing for a year, has recently developed lethargy and constipation of 3 months' duration.

2. A 1-year-old boy presents with diarrhoea and on examination is fair, has long eyelashes and is noted to have abdominal distension. His appetite is poor and he is often miserable.

3. A 2-year-old girl presents with a chronic cough, repeated chest infections and diarrhoea. Her stools are bulky and greasy.

4. A 12-year-old boy who has not grown for the last year presents with a 1.5-kg loss of weight. More recently he has developed abdominal pain. Rectal examination reveals a skin tag.

5. A 7-year-old boy presents with fatigue, lethargy, polyuria, polydipsia and growth failure. His BM stix test is normal. On examination, he is slightly pale and has hypertension.

Answers to **4.2**

1.   H   Hypothyroidism

Acquired hypothyroidism is commonly due to lymphocytic thyroiditis (autoimmune thyroid disease) and is typically seen in adolescence but can occur at any age. Deceleration of growth is usually the first clinical manifestation but this sign often goes unrecognized in the presence of normal school progress. Bone age is markedly delayed. Myxoedematous changes of the skin, constipation, cold intolerance, decreased energy and an increased need for sleep develop insidiously.

2.   B   Coeliac disease

Gluten-sensitive enteropathy (coeliac disease) is a disorder in which small bowel mucosal damage is the result of a permanent sensitivity to gluten. Typically, it presents when the child is introduced to cereals between 6 months and 2 years of age. Most patients present with diarrhoea but children can have failure to thrive or vomiting as the only manifestation. Many of the children have a fair complexion and long eyelashes. IgA gliadin and endomysial antibodies are useful screening tests. Jejunal biopsies are needed to confirm the presence of subtotal villous atrophy before treatment with a gluten-free diet.

3.   C   Cystic fibrosis

Cystic fibrosis is the major cause of severe chronic lung disease in children and is responsible for most cases of exocrine pancreatic insufficiency during early life. It presents as intestinal obstruction in the newborn, and as failure to thrive with fatty diarrhoea and recurrent respiratory infections in early childhood. It is inherited as an autosomal recessive trait. The sweat test remains the standard approach to diagnosis with the chloride content of the sweat being high in this condition.

4.   I   Inflammatory bowel disease

Crohn's disease is an idiopathic, chronic inflammatory disorder of the bowel which can involve any region of the alimentary tract. Children may present with recurrent abdominal pain, fever, malaise, fatigability, oral ulcers and perianal disease (anal tags, fissures and perianal ulcers/abscesses are common in colonic disease). Diarrhoea may be absent. Growth failure and delayed sexual development may precede other symptoms by 1–2 years.

5.   A   Chronic renal failure

Pallor and hypertension at such an early age in this child would favour the diagnosis of chronic renal failure rather than diabetes insipidus. The pallor is due to anaemia (nutritional, blood loss or reduced erythropoeitin production) and hypertension may be related to sodium retention and the underlying renal disease. Those with end-stage renal failure will require dialysis and renal transplantation.

Vaccinations in children

A   BCG (Bacillus Calmette-Guérin) vaccine
B   Diphtheria and tetanus (DT)
C   *Haemophilus influenzae* B (Hib)
D   Hepatitis B
E   Japanese encephalitis
F   Measles/mumps/rubella (MMR)
G   Meningococcal C
H   Oral polio (Salk) vaccine
I   Pneumococcal
J   Rabies
K   Triple vaccine (diphtheria, tetanus, pertussis) (DTP)

From the options above choose the SINGLE best answer for each question below. Each option may be used once, more than once, or not at all.

1. An infant aged 2 months is due for his routine primary course of vaccinations. Which vaccine is given along with DTP, polio and meningococcal C?

2. A baby girl aged 13 months has completed her primary course of vaccinations. For which vaccine is she due now?

3. A 4-year-old boy has completed his primary course of vaccinations and has received his second MMR vaccine. For which vaccine is he due now along with polio?

4. A 6-year-old Afro-Caribbean boy with homozygous sickle cell disease has severe splenic dysfunction. Which vaccine is recommended along with *Haemophilus influenzae* B (Hib)?

5. Which vaccine listed above, other than the MMR vaccine, contains live attenuated microorganisms?

Answers to 4.3

1. C *Haemophilus influenzae* B (Hib)

2. F Measles/mumps/rubella (MMR)

3. B Diphtheria and tetanus (DT)

4. I Pneumococcal

5. A BCG (Bacillus Calmette-Guérin) vaccine

Immunization provides protection against infectious diseases. Live, attenuated vaccines such as MMR, BCG, yellow fever and poliomyelitis (Sabin) are contraindicated in those with immunodeficiency (including those on corticosteroids and chemotherapy). Inactivated poliomyelitis vaccine (Salk) may be used for those unable to take the live vaccine. Extracts of, or detoxified, exotoxins from the microorganism, e.g. diphtheria and tetanus may also be used for immunization.

Immunization Schedule

Vaccine	Age	Notes
DTP and Hib	1st dose 2 months	Primary course
Polio	2nd dose 3 months	
Meningococcal C	3rd dose 4 months	
MMR	12–15 months	
Booster DT and Polio	3–5 years	Three years after completion of primary course
MMR 2nd dose		
BCG	10–14 years or infancy	
Booster DT and Polio	13–18 years	

Physical signs in paediatric cardiology

4.4

A   Absent femoral pulse
B   Apical thrill
C   Central cyanosis
D   Ejection click
E   Fixed splitting of 2nd heart sound
F   Irregular pulse
G   Opening snap
H   Pulsus alternans
I   Reversed splitting of 2nd heart sound
J   Splinter haemorrhages
K   Wide pulse pressure

For each of the following scenarios, select the SINGLE most likely additional physical sign you would expect to find. Each option may be used once, more than once, or not at all.

1. A 1-year-old boy is referred by his GP because of a heart murmur. His blood pressure in the right arm is 140/70 mmHg and the murmur is heard loudest at the back between the scapulae.

2. A 14-year-old boy presents with tiredness and breathlessness on exertion. He has a soft ejection systolic murmur at the left upper sternal border and a prominent right ventricular impulse. His electrocardiogram shows right ventricular hypertrophy with an rSR pattern in the right ventricular leads and his chest X-ray reveals cardiomegaly with pulmonary plethora.

3. A 2-year-old girl presents with exercise intolerance, recurrent chest infections and weight loss. She has a loud, harsh continuous murmur at the left upper sternal edge. Her chest X-ray shows cardiomegaly and prominent pulmonary vessels.

4. A 5-year-old boy, who is known to have aortic stenosis, presents with a 12-day history of an intermittent high temperature, night sweats, malaise and lethargy.

5. A 3-day-old baby on the postnatal ward is not feeding well and has an oxygen saturation of 65% on air. There are no murmurs. The chest X-ray shows an egg-shaped heart with a narrow pedicle and the electrocardiogram (ECG) shows right ventricular hypertrophy.

Answers to **4.4**

1. A   Absent femoral pulse

The signs described in this child fit with coarctation of the aorta, and the absent femoral pulses would be consistent with the diagnosis. There is narrowing of the descending aorta usually distal to the left subclavian artery. Large collateral arteries develop to bypass the obstruction over which a loud flow murmur can be heard.

2. E   Fixed splitting of 2nd heart sound

Atrial septal defects can be missed in early childhood and they may present later with failure to thrive and exercise intolerance. Symptoms occur in middle life with the onset of atrial fibrillation. In most patients the 2nd heart sound is characteristically widely split with no variation in all phases of respiration. This is because it takes longer for the volume overloaded right ventricle to empty, and the pulmonary valve closure is delayed.

3. K   Wide pulse pressure

The symptoms and signs described are consistent with a patent ductus arteriosus. A wide pulse pressure and a collapsing pulse, due to the sudden leak of blood from the aorta to the pulmonary artery (through the patent ductus), are the characteristic signs. If the duct is small there is a risk of bacterial endoarteritis. There may be problems with heart failure, pulmonary hypertension and shunt reversal with larger ducts. Ligation or catheter occlusion may be required.

4. J   Splinter haemorrhages

Subacute bacterial endocarditis should be actively looked for in any child with underlying heart disease who presents with fever and lethargy. Many of the classic skin manifestations develop much later in the course of the disease. They include Osler's nodules (tender, pea-sized intradermal nodules in the pulp of the fingers and toes), Janeway lesions (painless, small, erythematous or haemorrhagic lesions on the palms, ankles and soles) and splinter haemorrhages (linear lesions beneath the nails). These lesions may represent vasculitis produced by circulating antigen–antibody complexes.

5. C   Central cyanosis

Central cyanosis is associated with low oxygen saturations. It is not corrected by breathing 100% oxygen if there is an underlying cardiac defect that allows deoxygenated venous blood to bypass the lungs. The appearance of the cyanosis on the first day of life together with the X-ray and ECG findings suggest that this baby has transposition of the great arteries. Unless urgent treatment with balloon septostomy is performed, the baby will die.

Diagnosis of the common childhood viral illnesses

A Erythema infectiosum
B Hand, foot and mouth disease
C Herpes simplex
D Measles
E Molluscum contagiosum
F Mumps
G Respiratory syncytial virus (RSV)
H Roseola infantum (exanthem subitum)
I Rotavirus
J Rubella
K Varicella

Choose from the options above the SINGLE most appropriate diagnosis for each clinical situation given below. Each option may be used once, more than once, or not at all.

1. A 10-month-old infant is brought in with a 1-day history of mild fever, vomiting and watery diarrhoea (10 to 20 times a day) and on examination is moderately dehydrated.

2. A 4-year-old girl is brought to the A&E department with a 2-day history of fever and malaise. She has now developed swellings behind and below both ears.

3. A 7-month-old infant is admitted with a low-grade intermittent fever, cough for 3 days and intermittent respiratory distress for 1 day. Her older brother aged 11 years also has a fever and cough.

4. An 18-month-old child with a low-grade fever for 3 days has developed a papulovesicular rash over her trunk during the last 24 hours.

5. A 3-year-old boy, who is mildly unwell having had a low-grade fever for 2 days, has developed vesicles on the palms and soles over the last 12 hours.

Answers to **4.5**

1. I Rotavirus

In early childhood, the single most important cause of severe dehydrating diarrhoea is rotavirus (RNA virus) infection. The vomiting and fever typically abate during the second day of the illness but the diarrhoea continues for 5–7 days. The incubation period is less than 48 hours. Early diagnosis is important for the prevention or speedy correction of electrolyte disturbance and metabolic acidosis.

2. F Mumps

Mumps is caused by a paramyxovirus. In children, prodromal manifestations are rare with mumps but may be manifested by fever, muscular pain (especially in the neck), headache and malaise. They then develop painful swelling of the parotids, unilateral at first and becoming bilateral in 70%. Parotid swelling peaks in 1–3 days and subsides by 3–7 days. The incubation period is between 14–21 days. Complications include meningoencephalitis, orchitis, pancreatitis, uveitis and myocarditis.

3. G Respiratory syncytial virus (RSV)

Respiratory syncytial virus (RSV) is the major cause of bronchiolitis and pneumonia in children younger than 1 year, and is the most important respiratory tract pathogen of early childhood. Breastfeeding may protect against the more severe RSV infections. Maternal smoking impairs the development of the bronchioles, which increases the risk of airways obstruction. Management is mainly supportive and conservative. Infection is usually imported into the family by an older child at school.

4. K Varicella

Varicella (chickenpox) is highly infectious. It starts as a low-grade fever with the rash appearing 2 days later. The rash is seen mainly on the trunk and consists of macular, papular and vesicular lesions. Crops of lesions at different stages are seen. The incubation period is between 12–21 days. After recovery, the virus remains latent in the dorsal root ganglia and may reactivate in the future as shingles (herpes zoster). Usually, varicella is benign but complications such as varicella pneumonia (more common in adults) and encephalitis may occur.

5. B Hand, foot and mouth disease

Hand, foot and mouth disease is caused by the Coxsackie A16 virus and usually occurs in epidemics. The child is usually mildly unwell and develops vesicles in the mouth and on the palms and soles of the feet. They may cause some discomfort but they heal without crusting. Mild cases are often unnoticed. The incubation period is between 5–7 days.

Investigation of a febrile illness in childhood

A   Blood culture
B   Chest X-ray
C   Computerized tomography (CT) of the head
D   Echocardiogram
E   Full blood count
F   Lumbar puncture
G   Radionucleotide bone scan
H   Stool culture
I   Throat swab
J   Ultrasound scan of the abdomen
K   Urine microscopy and culture

For each presentation below, choose the SINGLE most discriminative investigation from the above list of options. Each option may be used once, more than once, or not at all.

1. An 8-month-old infant is rushed to the A&E department with a 4-hour history of fever, drowsiness and a petechial rash over the legs.

2. A 4-month-old infant is seen in the Children's Emergency Assessment Unit with a 1-day history of fever and poor feeding. On examination, he is irritable and has a slightly bulging anterior fontanelle. Neck stiffness is not detected.

3. A 7-year-old boy presents with a cough and a high spiking temperature over the last 2 days. Examination reveals mild tachypnoea.

4. A 4-year-old girl presents to the GP with a fever, vomiting for 3 days and discomfort during micturition.

5. A 3-year-old boy presents to the GP with fever and a sore throat for 2 days. Examination reveals enlarged tonsils with an overlying yellowish-white exudate.

Answers to **4.6**

1. A Blood culture

The history is suggestive of meningococcal septicaemia with *Neisseria meningitidis*. Groups B and C predominate in the industralized countries. The disease is rapidly progressive and can be fatal in 12 hours from the onset of fever (mortality rate is between 10–20%). The child should receive intravenous antibiotics (cefotaxime or benzyl penicillin) as soon as possible, preferably after obtaining a blood culture and PCR (polymerase chain reaction) for meningococci. If seen in the community the patient should receive intramuscular benzyl-penicillin before being transferred urgently to the nearest hospital.

2. F Lumbar puncture

The history and examination are suggestive of meningitis and a lumbar puncture is the most discriminating investigation. Lumbar puncture is contraindicated in children with focal neurological signs, papilloedema, a significant bulging fontanelle, signs of cerebral herniation or disseminated intravascular coagulation.

3. B Chest X-ray

The history and examination suggest a lower respiratory tract infection and a chest X-ray is the investigation of choice. There may be evidence of lobar collapse, consolidation or pleural effusion.

4. K Urine microscopy and culture

Urine culture is necessary to confirm a urinary tract infection (UTI) in this child. Microscopy, or dipstick of the urine, is inadequate for the diagnosis. Only 50% of children with a UTI have a pyuria which, even if present, does not confirm UTI. Urine should be cultured for microbial identification.

5. I Throat swab

Most cases of pharyngitis and tonsillitis are caused by viruses. Group A beta-haemolytic streptococcus is the only significant bacterial cause. It can be extremely difficult to distinguish a viral from a bacterial infection, although streptococcal infection is less likely in preschool children. It is usual to treat symptomatically with paracetamol and to ensure adequate fluid intake. Antibiotics should be reserved for those with bacterial infection confirmed by the throat swab.

Diagnosis of jaundice in the newborn period

A ABO haemolytic disease
B Biliary atresia
C Breast milk jaundice
D Galactosaemia
E Glucose-6-phosphodehydrogenase deficiency
F Hereditary spherocytosis
G Hypothyroidism
H Intrauterine infection (TORCH infection)
I Neonatal sepsis
J Physiological jaundice
K Rhesus haemolytic disease

Choose from the options above the SINGLE most appropriate diagnosis for each clinical situation given below. Each option may be used once, more than once, or not at all.

1. A baby born to a group B-positive mother is jaundiced at 24 hours of age. The baby's blood group is A positive. The baby is otherwise handling well.

2. A baby born to a group A-positive mother is found to be mildly jaundiced at 3 days of age. He is bottle-feeding and handling well. His blood group is A positive.

3. A 3-week-old infant is referred to the hospital with progressively worsening jaundice. He is passing dark urine and light-coloured stools. On examination, he seems reasonably well apart from the jaundice and minimal hepatomegaly. Blood tests reveal a conjugated hyperbilirubinaemia.

4. A baby boy born to a group O-negative mother is found to be jaundiced at 18 hours of age. He is feeding and handling well. His blood group is B positive. DCT (Direct Coomb's test) is positive.

5. A baby born to a group B-positive mother is jaundiced at 2 days of age. The baby's blood group is also B positive, and the direct Coomb's test (DCT) is negative. A blood film reveals many small red cells, some oval and spherical in shape.

Answers to **4.7**

1.   A   ABO haemolytic disease

Jaundice apparent within the first 24 hours is *never* physiological and strongly suggests excessive haemolysis. Incompatibility of the ABO system may arise if the mother is group B, and the baby A. Type A_1 is more antigenic than A_2. This form of haemolytic disease is usually mild.

2.   J   Physiological jaundice

Physiological jaundice affects up to 40% of normal babies. It usually appears at 2–3 days of age and resolves by the end of the first week. After birth, there is increased bilirubin production following breakdown of fetal red blood cells, transient limitation in bilirubin uptake and conjugation (hepatic immaturity), and a relatively poor fluid intake.

3.   B   Biliary atresia

Biliary atresia causes extrahepatic or, less commonly, intrahepatic obstructive jaundice (conjugated hyperbilirubinaemia). A high success rate from surgical intervention for extrahepatic atresia can be achieved if surgery is performed before 2 months of age. Failure to re-establish biliary drainage will lead to progressive liver failure.

4.   K   Rhesus haemolytic disease

Rhesus incompatibility occurs when the Rhesus-negative mother is sensitized by Rhesus-positive (inherited from the father) fetal blood entering her circulation during pregnancy at the end of labour and delivery. After birth, there may be a rapid rise in unconjugated bilirubin in the first 24 hours. Fortunately, this condition is much less common because administration of anti-D antibodies to mothers immediately after birth destroys any fetal red cells which may have escaped into the maternal circulation.

5.   F   Hereditary spherocytosis

Hereditary spherocytosis is an autosomal dominant inherited disorder resulting in fragile spherocytes which are destroyed prematurely in the spleen. It may present as neonatal jaundice and can be confused with ABO incompatibility as spherocytes are present in both conditions. However, osmotic fragility is increased and the direct Coomb's test is negative.

Diagnosis of seizures in infancy and childhood

A   Absence seizure (petit mal)
B   Complex partial seizure
C   Febrile convulsion
D   Grand mal epilepsy
E   Infantile spasms
F   Meningitis
G   Photosensitive epilepsy
H   Secondary to hypocalcaemia
I   Secondary to hypoglycaemia
J   Secondary to hyponatraemia
K   Simple partial seizure

Choose from the options above the SINGLE most appropriate diagnosis for each clinical situation given below. Each option may be used once, more than once, or not at all.

1. An 11-year-old boy has an episode of stiffening of the limbs followed by jerking of all four limbs lasting 3 minutes. During this episode he became unconscious for 5–6 minutes and on recovery he felt extremely tired and sleepy. He has had two similar episodes within the past 6 months.

2. A 4-year-old girl is referred with a 3-month history of recurrent, brief vacant episodes lasting for about 5 seconds. Her development is normal except that she gets episodes of day-dreaming. Examination is unremarkable.

3. An 8-month-old infant is referred with a history of repeated jerks, involving flexion of the head and arms, for the past 2–3 weeks. His parents say that his development may have regressed particularly with sitting and crawling.

4. An infant weighing 4.2 kg born to a poorly controlled diabetic mother has a multifocal clonic seizure at 8 hours of age. There is no obvious sepsis.

5. A 3-year-old boy is rushed by ambulance to the A&E department with a history of a generalized tonic–clonic seizure lasting 2 minutes. He woke up with a runny nose and fever in the morning and had the seizure just after lunch. An hour later in A&E department he was alert and was starting to play.

Answers to **4.8**

1.   D   Grand mal epilepsy

The event described is a generalized tonic–clonic seizure and, as they are recurrent, the diagnosis is of grand mal epilepsy. There is loss of consciousness, cessation of respiration and generalized rigidity (tonic phase) with extension of the limbs and arching of the back. This is followed by a clonic phase with generalized coarse rhythmic jerking during which the tongue may be bitten and incontinence may occur.

2.   A   Absence seizure (petit mal)

Typical absence seizures usually start between the ages of 5–10 years (rare before the age of 3 years). They cause impaired consciousness and sudden cessation of activity for 5–20 seconds before the child recommences activity as though nothing has happened. There may be blinking and upward deviation of the eyes but posture is maintained. Attacks can be precipitated by hyperventilation. There is an associated characteristic EEG pattern of generalized three-per-second spike and wave discharges.

3.   E   Infantile spasms

Infantile spasms usually start between 3–8 months of age. Sudden flexion of the neck and limbs (salaam or jack-knife spasms) lasting a few seconds may occur several hundred times a day. The attacks are often difficult to control and there is often regression of development and severe mental disability. About half the infants may have an underlying cause such as phenylketonuria, hypoglycaemia, encephalitis, tuberous sclerosis and Tay–Sachs' disease.

4.   I   Secondary to hypoglycaemia

Children born to diabetic mothers are at risk of hypoglycaemia in the immediate newborn period. The maternal hyperglycaemia causes fetal hyperglycaemia and this leads to fetal hyperinsulinaemia. At birth, the glucose supply through the placenta is suddenly interrupted without a proportional effect on the hyperinsulinism resulting in hypoglycaemia.

5.   C   Febrile convulsion

Febrile convulsions occur between 6 months and 3 years of age. They consist of tonic–clonic generalized seizures lasting a few minutes and resulting from the body temperature rising rapidly in a febrile illness. There is often a family history of febrile convulsions. Recurrences are common but can be minimized by antipyretics (paracetamol) and tepid sponging when febrile. About 3% of children with febrile convulsions develop epilepsy.

Diagnosis of respiratory distress in the neonatal period

A Cerebral hypoxia
B Choanal atresia
C Coarctation of the aorta
D Congenital diaphragmatic hernia
E Meconium aspiration syndrome
F Persistent pulmonary hypertension of a newborn (PPHN)
G Pneumonia
H Pneumothorax
I Respiratory distress syndrome (RDS)
J Tracheo-oesophageal fistula
K Transient tachypnoea of the newborn

Choose from the options above the SINGLE most appropriate diagnosis for each clinical situation below. Each option may be used once, more than once, or not at all.

1. A male infant is born at 29 weeks' gestation by caesarean section to a diabetic mother. He develops respiratory distress 30 minutes later.

2. A full-term infant born by normal vaginal delivery develops respiratory distress and poor feeding several hours after delivery. A high vaginal swab from the mother has grown Group B beta-haemolytic streptococci.

3. A female full-term infant born after an uneventful antenatal period by normal vaginal delivery needed frequent aspiration of secretions from the oesophagus, and has developed respiratory distress immediately after her first feed.

4. A male infant born at 38 weeks' gestation by normal vaginal delivery develops respiratory distress with persistent cyanosis at birth and on examination has a scaphoid abdomen and his apex beat is felt on the right side.

5. A female infant born at term develops poor feeding and respiratory distress on the 4th day. On examination, the infant has a tachycardia, an enlarged liver and poor pulses in the lower limbs.

Answers to **4.9**

1. **I   Respiratory distress syndrome (RDS)**

   Respiratory distress syndrome (RDS), also known as hyaline membrane disease, occurs primarily in premature infants and is due to surfactant deficiency. Its incidence is inversely proportional to gestational age. An increased frequency is associated with infants of diabetic mothers, male sex, caesarean birth, precipitous delivery, asphyxia and multifetal pregnancies. Administration of corticosteroids to women 48 hours before a preterm delivery significantly reduces the incidence, morbidity and mortality of RDS. Clinical manifestations include worsening tachypnoea in the hours after birth, grunting, flaring of the ala nasae, intercostal recession and cyanosis. The chest X-ray shows a ground-glass appearance (diffuse granular patterns) with an air bronchogram.

2. **G   Pneumonia**

   Intrauterine pneumonia is usually due to aspiration of amniotic fluid and is associated with prolonged rupture of fetal membranes, amnionitis and fetal hypoxia. It manifests within hours or days after birth and the chest X-ray is indistinguishable from that of RDS though the early symptoms may be non-specific (poor feeding, apnoea, lethargy).

3. **J   Tracheo-oesophageal fistula**

   A tracheo-oesophageal fistula should be suspected if a newborn baby needs repeated aspiration of accumulated secretions in the pharynx, and develops respiratory distress after feeds. Feeding is followed by immediate regurgitation and choking due to inhalation of feeds. With choanal atresia there is an inability to pass a nasogastric tube and the respiratory distress improves when the baby cries.

4. **D   Congenital diaphragmatic hernia**

   A scaphoid abdomen occurs with congenital diaphragmatic hernia (CDH) due to the abdominal contents lying in the chest cavity. The heart can be displaced to the opposite side. This herniation of abdominal contents causes hypoplasia or compression of the lung. If CDH is suspected in an infant needing resuscitation then the infant should be intubated as bagging is contraindicated. A chest X-ray will show loops of bowel in the chest.

5. **C   Coarctation of the aorta**

   Examination of the femoral pulses is a mandatory part of the routine examination of the newborn and absent femorals and/or radiofemoral delay is the classic sign of coarctation of the aorta.

Causes of meningitis and respiratory infections

A   Group B beta-haemolytic streptococci
B   *Haemophilus influenzae*
C   Herpes simplex virus
D   *Legionella pneumophila*
E   *Listeria monocytogenes*
F   *Mycobacterium tuberculosis*
G   *Mycoplasma pneumoniae*
H   *Pneumocystis carinii*
I   Respiratory syncytial virus
J   *Staphylococcus aureus*
K   *Streptococcus pneumoniae*

For each presentation below, choose the SINGLE most likely causative organism from the above list of options. Each option may be used once, more than once, or not at all.

1. A neonate is born at term by normal vaginal delivery following prolonged (70 hours) rupture of the membranes. At 2 days of age the infant becomes very lethargic and feeds poorly. He is noted to have a bulging anterior fontanelle. A lumbar puncture produces cloudy cerebrospinal fluid with a raised protein and polymorph count.

2. A 9-year-old boy has a 4-day history of a high spiking temperature, cough and right-sided chest pain. The chest X-ray shows right lower lobe consolidation.

3. An 8-month-old infant presents in the winter with a low-grade fever and a cough for 4 days with increasing respiratory distress for 1 day. A chest X-ray shows hyperinflated lungs.

4. An 11-year-old, previously well boy has a 6-day history of a high fever and a cough. A chest X-ray shows a well-circumscribed lesion in the right lung with an air/fluid level.

5. A 4-year-old boy presents with a fever and headache for 12 days and a generalized tonic–clonic seizure 6 hours ago, which lasted for 2 minutes. Since then he has been drowsy and examination reveals neck stiffness and a right facial nerve palsy. A computerized tomography (CT) scan shows basilar enhancement and acute hydrocephalus.

Answers to **4.10**

1.   **A**   **Group B beta-haemolytic streptococci**

Group B beta-haemolytic streptococci is the commonest cause of sepsis/meningitis/pneumonia in the newborn period. It is usually acquired from the mother and the risk factors are a very low birth weight, prolonged rupture of membranes (>24 hours), prolonged labour and, most importantly, maternal chorioamnionitis.

2.   **K**   *Streptococcus pneumoniae*

Lobar consolidation on a chest X-ray along with the classic symptoms described is almost always due to *Streptococcus pneumoniae*. The treatment of choice is penicillin.

3.   **I**   **Respiratory syncytial virus**

Respiratory syncytial virus (RSV) is the most important respiratory pathogen in childhood and causes bronchiolitis. RSV infection usually peaks in winter.

4.   **J**   *Staphylococcus aureus*

The abnormality described on the X-ray is a lung abscess and, in a previously well person, it is usually due to *Staphylococcus aureus*.

5.   **F**   *Mycobacterium tuberculosis*

The prolonged course of the illness, the focal neurological deficit and the CT scan findings are highly suggestive of tuberculous meningitis which is most common in children less than 5 years of age. There may not be a history of contact with TB. A rapid diagnosis may be reached with a polymerase chain reaction (PCR) of DNA within the CSF.

Normal motor development of a child

A	3 months
B	6 months
C	9 months
D	12 months
E	24 months
F	36 months
G	48 months
H	60 months
I	5 years
J	7 years
K	10 years

For each motor milestone below, choose the SINGLE most probable normal age at which it is likely to be accomplished. Each option may be used once, more than once, or not at all.

1. Hop on one foot.

2. Walk with one hand held/unsupported.

3. Able to roll over.

4. Walk up and down stairs.

5. Able to pull to standing position and sit up alone.

Answers to **4.11**

1. G   48 months

2. D   12 months

3. B   6 months

4. E   24 months

5. C   9 months

Motor development

3 months: Early head control (complete by 4 months). Holds objects placed in hand with a palmar grasp.

6 months: Rolls prone to supine and lifts head when pulled to sitting.

9 months: Starting to crawl, sits unsupported, develops pincer grip.

12 months: Walks with one hand held or unsupported and has a mature pincer grip.

24 months: Climbs up and down stairs with two feet to a step, runs well, opens doors, climbs on furniture, and jumps, kicks ball without overbalancing.

36 months: Rides tricycle, stands momentarily on one foot, walks upstairs one foot per step.

48 months: Hops on one foot, throws ball overhand, climbs well, uses scissors to cut out pictures.

60 months: Skips.

Causes of acute abdominal pain in children

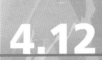

A Acute appendicitis
B Acute gastritis
C Acute pancreatitis
D Constipation
E Henoch–Schönlein purpura
F Intussusception
G Lower lobe pneumonia
H Obstructed inguinal hernia
I Renal colic
J Torsion of testis
K Urinary tract infection

For each presentation below, choose the SINGLE most likely cause from the above list of options. Each option may be used once, more than once, or not at all.

1. A 7-year-old girl presents with a 3-day history of fever, suprapubic pain and enuresis. She is normally happy and active but more recently has become lethargic and withdrawn.

2. A 2-year-old boy presents with a sudden onset of lower abdominal pain together with a swollen, painful scrotum.

3. A 6-year-old boy presents with abdominal pain, a swollen and tender right ankle and melaena. His urine shows microscopic haematuria.

4. A 9-year-old girl presents with a mild temperature and nausea for a day with increasing abdominal pain in the right lower quadrant.

5. An 11-year-old girl presents with a spiking temperature, cough and abdominal pain.

Answers to **4.12**

1. **K   Urinary tract infection**

    Any child presenting with frequency and/or painful micturition should have the urine tested to rule out a urinary tract infection (UTI). However, the symptoms will be less specific in a younger child. Neonates and infants may present with poor feeding, failure to thrive, irritability, fever, vomiting, diarrhoea, jaundice and septicaemia. Normal bowel organisms (particularly *E. coli*) are responsible for the majority of cases of UTI. During the school years a UTI is 25 times commoner in girls than boys.

2. **J   Torsion of testis**

    Testicular torsion is a common cause of an acute painful swelling of the scrotum. Prompt surgical exploration is required to avoid ischaemic damage to the testis. Both testes should be fixed to the scrotum during surgery. Differential diagnosis includes torsion of the hydatid of Morgagni (less severe pain), epididymo-orchitis (unusual, most common in the first year of life and usually associated with urinary tract abnormalities), mumps orchitis (rare before puberty) and a neoplasm.

3. **E   Henoch–Schönlein purpura**

    Henoch–Schönlein purpura has four main features: a palpable purpuric rash (mainly over the legs and buttocks), arthritis (mainly knees and ankles), gastrointestinal tract involvement (abdominal pain and melaena) and renal involvement (nephritis with haematuria and/or proteinuria). It is mainly diagnosed clinically.

4. **A   Acute appendicitis**

    Acute appendicitis is the commonest abdominal emergency in childhood. The classic features are low-grade fever, anorexia and/or vomiting, change in bowel habit (usually constipation) and central abdominal pain shifting to the right iliac fossa. The differential diagnosis includes mesenteric adenitis, Meckel's diverticulitis, renal colic, pyelonephritis and constipation. A right lower lobe pneumonia can also mimic appendicitis.

5. **G   Lower lobe pneumonia**

    Symptoms usually include breathlessness, cough and fever, although early symptoms and signs are not specific. Pneumonia can cause abdominal pain. It is important to exclude an empyema.

Diagnosis of childhood pyrexial illnesses

A   Bacterial meningitis
B   Bronchopneumonia
C   Connective tissue disorder
D   Encephalitis
E   Factitious fever
F   Infective endocarditis
G   Septic arthritis
H   Suppurative otitis media
I   Tonsillitis
J   Upper respiratory tract infection
K   Urinary tract infection

For each presentation below, choose the SINGLE most likely underlying illness from the above list of options. Each option may be used once, more than once, or not at all.

1.   A 6-month-old infant is admitted with a 1-day history of pallor, fever, poor feeding and vomiting. She is lethargic and has a bulging anterior fontanelle but there is no obvious neck stiffness.

2.   A 2-year-old child has a 2-day history of a high fever and screaming on moving the right lower limb.

3.   A 9-year-old boy is admitted with a 5-day history of lethargy, fever, drowsiness and hallucinations. He is pyrexial with a mild left-sided weakness but there is no evidence of meningism.

4.   A 4-year-old girl presents with a 3-day history of a runny nose, fever and pulling at her right ear lobe. She is also irritable and has lost her appetite.

5.   A 4-month-old infant with a known underlying ventricular septal defect has had a fever for 1 week. Examination reveals a palpable spleen together with a loud pansystolic murmur heard all over the precordium.

Answers to **4.13**

1. **A   Bacterial meningitis**

    Palpating the anterior fontanelle is part of the routine examination in an infant and a tense, bulging fontanelle implies increased intracranial pressure. Detection of neck stiffness in an infant is often difficult, whilst meningism is much more obvious in children over the age of 3 years. Given the history of fever and poor feeding, a diagnosis of bacterial meningitis is the most likely possibility. If dehydration is present from persistent vomiting then the fontanelle tension may be normal or even reduced.

2. **G   Septic arthritis**

    Acute septic arthritis usually occurs in the presence of bacteraemia or septicaemia but occasionally may be due to a penetrating wound. The associated signs include fever, swelling, a restricted range of movement and tenderness. The pain is acute in onset and is worse at rest. *S. aureus* is the commonest cause of septic arthritis. Aspiration under sterile conditions (and general anaesthesia) is an important diagnostic procedure. Surgical drainage is often required as the definitive therapeutic intervention together with antibiotics, as a septic arthritis will not be adequately managed only with repeated aspiration.

3. **D   Encephalitis**

    Herpes simplex virus may cause meningoencephalitis, which has a high mortality rate. It may present with fever, meningism, drowsiness, behavioural changes, seizures and a focal neurological defect. Early treatment with acyclovir reduces the mortality to 20% but it does not reduce the high risk of subsequent severe neurological or behavioural problems. PCR (polymerase chain reaction – gene amplication technique) of the cerebrospinal fluid is the investigation of choice.

4. **H   Suppurative otitis media**

    Acute suppurative otitis media presents with fever, otalgia (child may be pulling at the ear lobe) and malaise. The main organisms involved include *Streptococcus pneumoniae* and *Haemophilus influenzae*. On otoscopy, the tympanic membrane may be red, bulging and the malleus obscured. There will be a purulent discharge if the membrane ruptures. Glue ear (persistent middle-ear effusion) may develop causing conductive deafness, which can affect language development. Viral infection is usually bilateral and associated with pharyngitis.

5. **F   Infective endocarditis**

    Infective endocarditis should be actively looked for as a cause of a febrile illness in any child known to have a structural heart defect. Investigations include repeated blood cultures and an echocardiogram. The main organisms involved include *Streptococcus viridans*, *Staphylococcus aureus* and *Staphylococcus albus*.

Diagnosis of joint pain and/or limp in a child

A   Henoch–Schönlein purpura
B   Inflammatory bowel disease
C   Juvenile chronic arthritis
D   Non-accidental injury
E   Osteomyelitis
F   Rheumatic fever
G   Septic arthritis
H   Slipped capital femoral epiphysis
I   Systemic lupus erythematosus
J   Transient synovitis
K   Trauma

For each presentation below, choose the SINGLE most likely underlying illness from the above list of options. Each option may be used once, more than once, or not at all.

1. A 1-year-old Caucasian boy is brought to the A&E department by his mother with a history of not moving his right arm. He is found to have some bruising of his right arm and a spiral fracture of the shaft of the right humerus. His mother thinks he sustained the injury after a fall at the playground.

2. A 5-year-old Afro-Caribbean girl presents to the A&E department with a low-grade fever, a limp and pain in the left hip for the last 2 days. She had cold-like symptoms 10 days ago and her erythrocyte sedimentation rate (ESR) and white blood count (WBC) are normal.

3. A 12-year-old Caucasian boy presents with diarrhoea, weight loss for 4 weeks and a swollen left elbow and right wrist for the past few days. He also has a limp and is unable to play football.

4. A 14-year-old Afro-Caribbean girl has developed aching knees and wrists for the last 2 weeks. She also complains of lethargy and patchy alopecia. Examination reveals a facial rash with scaling and follicular plugging. She has previously tried a number of facial creams and emollients with little benefit.

5. A 7-year-old girl of Indian origin presents with a 5-week history of a high intermittent fever, an evanescent rash and hepatosplenomegaly. For the last week she has developed swelling of both knees.

Answers to **4.14**

1. **D   Non-accidental injury**

   The features of child abuse include frequent accidents with gripping injuries, bony injuries (fractures of the long bones, skull and ribs), bite or scald marks, previous injury/abuse of other siblings, inconsistent histories and inappropriate parental concern. Shaking of a child may tear the superficial veins over the brain and cause a subdural haematoma. The safety and protection of the abused child must be ensured.

2. **J   Transient synovitis**

   Transient synovitis of the hip occurs predominantly in the 3–8-year-old age group and is characterized by an acute onset of unilateral pain, limp and mild restriction of movement, especially abduction and internal rotation. It usually follows an upper respiratory tract infection. Normally WBC, ESR and hip X-rays are normal. The condition is self-limiting and resolves within a few weeks. Septic arthritis and osteomyelitis of the hip must be excluded.

3. **B   Inflammatory bowel disease**

   Inflammatory bowel disease may present with recurrent abdominal pain, diarrhoea, growth failure, anorexia and extraintestinal manifestations (oral ulcers, peripheral arthritis, erythema nodosum, pyoderma gangrenosum, uveitis, cholangitis and rarely glomerulonephritis and cerebral thromboembolic disease).

4. **I   Systemic lupus erythematosus**

   Systemic lupus erythematosus (SLE) is rare in children. It tends to occur in adolescent girls, particularly of Afro-Caribbean origin. It is associated with a photosensitive rash over sun-exposed areas, Raynaud's phenomenon, alopecia, lethargy, and anorexia and arthralgia (common). There is also involvement of the central nervous system with convulsions, chorea, polyneuropathy, mononeuritis multiplex and psychoses. There may be renal (glomerulonephritis), lung and cardiac involvement. Haematological problems include autoimmune haemolytic anaemia, thrombocytopenia and antiphospholipid syndrome. Double-stranded DNA antibodies are present.

5. **C   Juvenile chronic arthritis**

   The history given is typical of systemic onset juvenile chronic arthritis (JCA – Still's disease) where the arthritis appears at a variable period (2–6 weeks) after a spiking fever, rash and associated visceral involvement (hepatosplenomegaly, lymphadenopathy and serositis).

Causes of wheezing in childhood

A   Allergic bronchopulmonary aspergillosis
B   Bronchial asthma
C   Bronchiectasis
D   Bronchiolitis
E   Bronchopneumonia
F   Carcinoid syndrome
G   Cystic fibrosis
H   Foreign body aspiration
I   Gastrooesophageal reflux
J   Laryngotracheobronchitis
K   Lymphoma

The following children all present with difficulty in breathing. For each presentation, choose the SINGLE most likely underlying illness from the above list of options. Each option may be used once, more than once, or not at all.

1. A 6-month-old girl with a 3-day history of a runny nose and a low-grade fever presents to the A&E department during the winter, with increasing difficulty in breathing over the last day. Examination reveals widespread crackles and expiratory wheezes.

2. A 7-year-old boy presents with unilateral wheezing and prominent veins over the neck and face. He has a mild spiking temperature and generalized itching.

3. A 4-year-old girl has a 2-day history of progressive shortness of breath and wheezing with a history of eczema. She has had two previous similar episodes.

4. A 3-year-old boy presents with recurrent chest infections, diarrhoea and failure to thrive. His siblings and parents are fit and well.

5. A 1-year-old previously well girl is brought to the A&E department by her father with a sudden onset of breathlessness and a unilateral wheeze whilst playing with her older brother.

Answers to **4.15**

1. **D** **Bronchiolitis**

Acute viral bronchiolitis (50% are due to the respiratory syncytial virus) is the commonest disease of the lower respiratory tract in infants. It results in inflammatory obstruction of the airways. It occurs during the first 3 years of life with a peak incidence at around 6 months. The incidence is highest during the winter. Maternal smoking during pregnancy (retards development of the bronchioles) is a risk factor.

2. **K** **Lymphoma**

Beware of unilateral wheeze! Think of internal or external obstruction of a large bronchus. With enlarged veins in the neck it is most probably due to external compression (superior vena cava syndrome). Non-Hodgkin's lymphoma is more common than Hodgkin's lymphoma. It can present with generalized painless lymphadenopathy. Mediastinal involvement may cause superior vena caval obstruction and airway obstruction. Other features include night sweats, fever, pruritus, hepatosplenomegaly and weight loss (>10%).

3. **B** **Bronchial asthma**

Clues to the diagnosis of asthma are the history of atopy (e.g. eczema, hay fever) and recurrent episodes of wheeze. One-third of children over the age of 3 years with recurrent wheezing have asthma. There is overlap in presentation between acute viral bronchiolitis and asthma. Those over the age of 3 years, particularly with a history of eczema and hay fever and a family history of asthma, are more likely to have asthma.

4. **G** **Cystic fibrosis**

Cystic fibrosis (CF) is an autosomal recessive inherited disorder characterized by failure of chloride transport (defect of CF transmembrane conductance regulator), such that secretions from the exocrine glands become dry and viscid. Complications include meconium ileus, bronchiectasis, respiratory failure, failure to thrive, rectal prolapse, infertility, cirrhosis and diabetes mellitus. Screening involves the detection of raised immunoreactive trypsin on a dried blood spot sample, before confirmation by sweat test and defective deltaF508 gene.

5. **H** **Foreign body aspiration**

A diagnosis of a foreign body should be considered if there is a sudden onset of respiratory distress and a unilateral wheeze in a previously well child. The most common foreign bodies are peanuts.

Diagnosis of altered or loss of consciousness in children

A Arrhythmia
B Bacterial meningitis
C Concussion
D Diabetic ketoacidosis
E Hypoglycaemia
F Hypovolaemia
G Poisoning
H Post-ictal state
I Reye's syndrome
J Vasovagal faint
K Viral encephalitis

For each presentation below, choose the SINGLE most likely underlying illness from the above list of options. Each option may be used once, more than once, or not at all.

1. A 10-year-old boy fell off his bike and lost consciousness for several minutes before being brought to the A&E department with headache and vomiting.

2. A 7-year-old girl presents with loss of weight for about a month, together with abdominal pain, persistent vomiting, drowsiness and confusion. In the week before she started vomiting she was eating and drinking very well.

3. A 15-year-old, previously fit girl is found unconscious at home by her mother. She was due to sit her end of year examinations, but had not been unduly worried about them.

4. A 5-month-old boy is brought to the A&E department with a history of diarrhoea and vomiting for 3 days and altered consciousness for a couple of hours. On examination, his fontanelle and eyes are deeply sunken. He has a tachycardia with a weak pulse.

5. A 12-year-old boy with learning difficulties is brought to an A&E unit in an unresponsive state, following an episode of jerking of all four limbs lasting 5 minutes and which occurred while out shopping with his mother. On arrival in hospital he starts to recover slowly.

Answers to **4.16**

1. **C Concussion**

   A common result of a head injury is concussion which is characterized by immediate and transient alteration of consciousness, disturbance of vision and equilibrium and later followed by headaches and vomiting (from vagal stimulation). It is essential to protect the airway and avoid hypovolaemia and hypoxia. In children, death from head injury is usually due to the primary brain injury or cerebral oedema.

2. **D Diabetic ketoacidosis**

   Any patient presenting with an altered sensorium should have a BM stix test for blood sugar. The clinical scenario here is quite typical of diabetic ketoacidosis but usually there is also a history of polyuria, weight loss (breakdown of fat/protein and dehydration) and polydipsia. As insulin deficiency worsens, metabolic acidosis develops due to the overproduction of ketone bodies.

3. **G Poisoning**

   Another common cause of an altered sensorium is ingestion of drugs either accidental in infants and small children or deliberate in older children, especially in girls. This girl is emotionally disturbed and may have resorted to taking an overdose because of stress associated with her school examinations.

4. **F Hypovolaemia**

   The dehydration associated with gastroenteritis can place considerable stress on an infant with a high loss of body water, high metabolic rate and large surface-to-volume ratio. Those with moderate to severe dehydration may have signs of circulatory failure. The skin may be mottled with poor capillary return, with tachycardia and a poor volume pulse. Urgent intravenous fluids are required and the underlying cause of the diarrhoeal illness should be sought and treated accordingly.

5. **H Post-ictal state**

   Following a seizure, children are initially semi-comatose and typically remain in a deep sleep from 30 min to 2 hours. The post-ictal phase is often associated with vomiting and an intense bifrontal headache. The majority of children seem to grow out of their epilepsy and anti-epileptic treatment may be stopped after 2–3 years of being seizure-free.

Paediatric pharmacology (1)

A Adrenocorticotrophic hormone (ACTH)
B Aspirin
C Gentamicin
D Lorazepam
E Paracetamol
F Penicillin V
G Phenobarbital (phenobarbitone)
H Prednisolone
I Prostaglandins
J Sodium valproate
K Trimethoprim

From the options above choose the SINGLE most appropriate drug for
each clinical scenario given below. Each option may be used once, more
than once, or not at all.

1. A 10-year-old girl is brought to the A&E department by the paramedics
   because of a fit which has lasted for the past 5 minutes. She is a known
   epileptic and is on carbamazepine. Which is the next drug of choice you
   would use for her current seizure?

2. A 6-year-old boy is seen in the paediatric outpatients having been
   referred by his general practitioner for brief vacant spells. In clinic, on
   hyperventilation he has an absence seizure and the
   electroencephalogram (EEG) is consistent with childhood petit mal
   epilepsy. What is the first line of treatment for his seizures?

3. A 2-year-old girl who had a coliform urinary tract infection has had
   antibiotic treatment for 1 week and is now due for further investigation.
   What drug would you start as prophylaxis?

4. A 4-year-old boy has developed generalized oedema over a 2-week
   period. His urine has 4+ protein and his serum albumin is low. What is
   the drug of choice as the definitive treatment for this boy's condition?

5. A 10-month-old girl has been brought to her GP with a history of a
   runny nose, cough and fever for 2 days. He has diagnosed a viral upper
   respiratory tract infection. What is the one drug that will give her
   symptomatic relief?

Answers to **4.17**

1. **D Lorazepam**

   As per the Advanced Paediatric Life Support (APLS) guidelines the first-line treatment for a convulsion is lorazepam. The second line is paraldehyde.

2. **J Sodium valproate**

   For generalized seizures (tonic–clonic, absence, myoclonic, atonic), sodium valproate is the first-line drug of choice and for partial seizures (simple or complex partial, secondarily generalized) carbamazepine is the first choice drug. Ethosuximide (not on the list) is also very effective in petit mal epilepsy.

3. **K Trimethoprim**

   Any child less than 5 years old with a proven urinary tract infection should be investigated to rule out an anomaly of the urinary tract, the most common one being vesicoureteric reflux. They should also be on prophylactic antibiotics to prevent further urinary tract infections and the risk of scarring of the kidneys. The drug commonly used is trimethoprim given once daily at night.

4. **H Prednisolone**

   This boy is likely to have the nephrotic syndrome and as most cases in this age group are of the minimal change type they respond favourably to prednisolone.

5. **E Paracetamol**

   Paracetamol will provide symptomatic relief and as it is a viral upper respiratory tract infection there is no need for antibiotics. Aspirin must never be given as an antipyretic or analgesic to children under the age of 12 years for fear of developing Reye's syndrome.

Paediatric pharmacology (2)

4.18

A Adrenaline (epinephrine)
B Benzylpenicillin (penicillin G)
C Ceftazidime
D Diazepam
E Flucloxacillin
F Nebulized ipratropium bromide (Atrovent)
G Nebulized salbutamol
H Oral or nebulized corticosteroids
I Phenoxymethylpenicillin (penicillin V)
J Surfactant
K Vancomycin

For each patient below, choose the SINGLE most appropriate drug as first line of treatment from the options given above. Each option may be used once, more than once, or not at all.

1. A 4-year-old girl is brought to the A&E department with an acute exacerbation of asthma. She is not cyanosed but her pulse is 110 beats/min and her oxygen saturation by pulse oximetry is 90%. There are bilateral expiratory wheezes heard over the chest.

2. An 18-month-old infant with a 2-hour history of mild stridor is referred to the paediatric admissions unit by his GP. He has had a barking cough for the past 2 days with a runny nose and hoarseness.

3. A GP is called to see a 13-month-old infant with fever. He notices a couple of petechial spots around the ankles and suspects meningococcal septicaemia. What drug should be given to the child by the GP before referring him urgently to hospital?

4. A newborn infant, born preterm at 27 weeks, weighs 800 g. Which drug should be given as soon as possible after birth that will have a positive impact on the infant's survival?

5. A 6-year-old boy has developed a blistering rash on his extremities and is thought to have bullous impetigo. He is otherwise well.

Answers to **4.18**

1. G   Nebulized salbutamol

This child has an attack of bronchial asthma of moderate severity. As per the British Thoracic Society guidelines for the management of asthma, salbutamol is the first-line medical management in addition to oxygen. It is a beta agonist and produces bronchodilatation. Next line of management will be the addition of ipratropium bromide, steroids and aminophyline.

2. H   Oral or nebulized corticosteroids

This infant has laryngotracheobronchitis (croup) and steroids are indicated. It is a viral condition and in 75% of cases is due to the parainfluenza virus. Other viral causes include the adenovirus, respiratory syncytial virus, influenza and measles. Steroids reduce the inflammatory oedema that causes the cough and the difficulty in breathing and they also prevent destruction of the ciliated epithelium.

3. B   Benzylpenicillin (penicillin G)

Whenever meningococcal sepsis is suspected, penicillin should be given parenterally as soon as possible. In a surgery setting it is often given intramuscularly but in the A&E department the intravenous route is adopted. Pencillin V can only be administered orally and, because of its unpredictable absorption in the gut, has no role in serious infections.

4. J   Surfactant

Preterm babies are prone to the respiratory distress syndrome which is due to surfactant deficiency (decreased production and secretion). Multimode endotracheal instillation of exogenous surfactant has dramatically improved the survival of such babies.

5. E   Flucloxacillin

Bullous impetigo is a pyogenic skin infection caused by staphylococci and hence will respond best to penicillinase-resistant antibiotics. As the child is otherwise well, oral flucloxacillin is the appropriate antibiotic.

Diagnosis of congenital heart disease

A   Atrial septal defect
B   Coarctation of the aorta
C   Hypoplastic left heart
D   Patent ductus arteriosus
E   Pulmonary atresia
F   Pulmonary stenosis
G   Tetralogy of Fallot
H   Transposition of the great vessels
I   Tricuspid atresia
J   Truncus arteriosus
K   Ventricular septal defect

For each patient below choose the SINGLE most likely diagnosis from the above list of options. Each option may be used once, more than once, or not at all.

1. A 3-month-old infant is found incidentally to have a pansystolic murmur at the left sternal border. Pulse oximetry shows normal oxygen saturation.

2. A 6-month-old infant gets episodes of intermittent cyanosis and breathlessness which is worse during feeds. Examination shows minimal cyanosis around her lips. On auscultation, there is a single second sound and a grade III ejection systolic murmur heard maximally in the second and third left intercostal spaces. A chest X-ray shows a boot-shaped heart.

3. A 10-month-old infant with normal saturations on a pulse oximeter has a widely split and fixed second heart sound with a midsystolic murmur maximum at the second left intercostal edge.

4. A 6-week-old infant on a routine check-up was found to have absent foot pulses. His blood pressure (BP) in the right arm is 135/84 mm Hg.

5. A 2-year-old girl with normal saturations on a pulse oximeter has a grade IV ejection systolic murmur heard maximally at the upper left sternal border. The pulmonary component of the second heart sound is soft. She is otherwise a well and active child.

Answers to **4.19**

1.   K   Ventricular septal defect

Ventricular septal defects (VSD) are common and account for one-third of all cardiac defects. They are more likely to be small defects (with a loud pansystolic murmur) which often do not cause any symptoms and close spontaneously. Larger VSDs may be associated with failure to thrive, oedema and breathlessness due to cardiac failure.

2.   G   Tetralogy of Fallot

The tetralogy of Fallot has four components: pulmonary stenosis (infundibular), ventricular septal defect, an overriding aorta and right ventricular hypertrophy. Clinical features include intermittent cyanosis (gradual onset during the first few months of life), a systolic murmur at the left sternal edge and the pulmonary area (infundibular stenosis) and a single loud second heart sound (pulmonary sound inaudible). Squatting increases venous return and systemic vascular resistance which reduces the right-to-left shunt thus improving blood oxygenation. A chest X-ray shows a normal-sized heart with the apex uptilted and a concave left heart border (small pulmonary arteries) described as boot-shaped.

3.   A   Atrial septal defect

An atrial septal defect (ASD) can either be a foramen primum defect (low down in the septum) or, more commonly, a secundum defect (high in the septum). Small ASDs are often undetected. Larger lesions produce a high pulmonary blood flow (systolic pulmonary murmur) and wide fixed splitting of the second heart sound. An ECG shows right bundle branch block together with left axis deviation with the primum defects and right axis deviation with secundum defects.

4.   B   Coarctation of the aorta

An aortic stricture (distal aortic arch close to the site of the ductus arteriosus) leads to radiofemoral pulse delay, BP is raised in the arms and reduced in the legs with absent foot pulses. It may present in the newborn period with severe cardiac failure but presentation may be delayed even up to early adulthood.

5.   F   Pulmonary stenosis

Mild pulmonary valve stenosis (congenitally deformed and thickened) is usually benign but more severe lesions can cause right heart failure. There may be cyanosis in severe cases due to a right-to-left shunt through a patent foramen ovale.

Diagnosis of childhood malignancies

A   Acute lymphoblastic leukaemia
B   Acute myeloid leukaemia
C   Burkitt's lymphoma
D   Chronic myeloid leukaemia
E   Ewing's sarcoma
F   Hodgkin's lymphoma
G   Juvenile myelomonocytic leukaemia
H   Nephroblastoma (Wilms' tumour)
I   Neuroblastoma
J   Osteosarcoma
K   Retinoblastoma

For each patient below, choose the SINGLE most likely diagnosis from the above list of options. Each option may be used once, more than once, or not at all.

1. A 14-year-old boy is referred to the paediatric department by his GP because of a 2-month history of pain and swelling around his right knee. The pain has worsened recently and is now causing him to wake up during the night. An X-ray of the right knee and lower femur shows a sclerotic lesion with a sunburst pattern in the metaphyseal region of distal femur. His full blood count is normal.

2. A 4-year-old boy presents to his GP with a 3-week history of anorexia, painful limbs and lethargy. On examination, he is pale with some petechial lesions and has cervical lymphadenopathy. A full blood count reveals a haemoglobin level of 6 g/dl, platelets of 20 000 and a white cell count of 8000. A peripheral blood smear shows 75% lymphoid cells.

3. A newborn infant, on routine neonatal screening, has a unilateral white pupillary reflex (leukocoria). There is a positive family history of malignancy.

4. A 4-year-old girl is referred by the GP with a 1-month history of intermittent abdominal pain. On examination, there is an abdominal swelling which is smooth, mobile and firm. The mass is bimanually palpable and ballotable.

5. A 12-year-old boy has an unexplained fever and weight loss of 4 weeks' duration. Clinical examination reveals painless, firm cervical lymphadenopathy.

Answers to **4.20**

1. J Osteosarcoma

Osteosarcoma occurs most commonly during the adolescent growth spurt and usually affects the metaphyses of long bones. Over 50% of osteosarcomas arise in the lower femur or upper tibia. The radiological findings are usually of sclerotic destruction and, less commonly, lytic lesions can be seen. In contrast, a Ewing's sarcoma affects the diaphyses of long bones and flat bones and primarily shows a lytic, multilaminar periosteal reaction (onion skinning).

2. A Acute lymphoblastic leukaemia (ALL)

ALL accounts for 75% of all cases of leukaemia in childhood. The history and blood findings given here are quite typical of ALL. Most children with ALL have signs and symptoms of less than 4 weeks' duration and the initial symptoms are usually non-specific. Progressive bone marrow failure leads to pallor, bleeding, petechiae and fever.

3. K Retinoblastoma

Most cases are picked up during the routine newborn examination by finding an absent red reflex (cat's eye reflex). Strabismus is another common initial presentation, and orbital inflammation, hyphaema and pupillary irregularities can occur with advancing disease. About 40% of cases are hereditary and the retinoblastoma gene (RB1) is located on the long arm of chromosome 13.

4. H Nephroblastoma (Wilms' tumour)

The median age at diagnosis of a unilateral Wilms' tumour is 3 years and the most frequent sign is an abdominal or flank mass which is often asymptomatic. About half of affected children have abdominal pain, vomiting or both. Hypertension is reported in about 60% of patients and results from renal ischaemia due to pressure on the renal artery. Wilms' tumours are often associated with congenital anomalies of the genitourinary tract (4.4%) and aniridia (1%). Deletions involving one of two loci on chromosome 11 (11p13 and 11p15) have been noted in the cells of about 30% of cases. The differential diagnosis for an abdominal mass at this age is a neuroblastoma but these commonly present as a hard, fixed mass with discomfort.

5. F Hodgkin's lymphoma

Painless, firm, cervical or supraclavicular lymphadenopathy is the most common presenting sign. An anterior mediastinal mass is often present but this can quickly disappear with therapy. The systemic symptoms considered important for staging are unexplained fever, weight loss and drenching night sweats.

Diagnosis of anaemia in infancy and childhood

A Aplastic anaemia
B Diamond-Blackfan syndrome (congenital hypoplastic anaemia)
C G6PD deficiency
D Hereditary spherocytosis
E Iron deficiency anaemia
F Megaloblastic anaemia of infancy
G Physiological anaemia of infancy
H Pyruvate kinase deficiency
I Sickle cell anaemia
J Thalassaemia major (Cooley's anaemia)
K Transient erythroblastopenia of childhood

For each presentation below, choose the SINGLE most likely diagnosis from the above list of options. Each option may be used once, more than once, or not at all.

1. An 18-month-old Caucasian infant who is otherwise well but whose diet consists mainly of cow's milk is seen by his GP because of pallor. There is no lymphadenopathy or hepatosplenomegaly but his haemoglobin is 9 g/dl with a mean corpuscular volume (MCV) of 65 fl.

2. A 10-month-old Afro-Caribbean boy presents to the paediatric A&E department with painful swelling of the hands over the past 24 hours. He is afebrile and has no other abnormalities except for the presence of pallor. His haemoglobin is 8 g/dl and the peripheral blood smear shows a reticulocytosis with target cells.

3. A 6-year-old Caucasian girl is seen in clinic with abdominal pain. On examination, she is pale with a 2-cm splenomegaly. An ultrasound scan of the abdomen reveals gall stones. Her mother has a similar disorder.

4. A 3-month-old Caucasian infant is referred to the hospital with pallor. He is noted to have triphalangeal thumbs but has no hepatosplenomegaly. He is otherwise well although his haemoglobin is 6 g/dl with a reticulocyte count of 1.

5. A 7-year-old Chinese girl is referred with fatigue and lassitude. There is no lymphadenopathy, hepatomegaly or splenomegaly but she is pale with petechiae and bruises. Her full blood count shows a haemoglobin level of 7 g/dl, a white cell count of 1550 and platelets of 30 000. The peripheral blood smear shows a normochromic, normocytic anaemia with no blast cells. She is on no medication.

Answers to **4.21**

1. E Iron deficiency anaemia

Anaemia resulting from lack of sufficient iron for the synthesis of haemoglobin is the most common haematological disease of infancy and childhood. Iron is absorbed in the proximal small intestine and a deficiency could be due to poor intake (milk is a poor source), suboptimal absorption or excessive loss (blood loss). Iron deficiency results in a hypochromic, microcytic anaemia and the ferritin (an iron storage protein) level in the serum is low.

2. I Sickle cell anaemia

Sickle cell anaemia (homozygous Hb S) should be differentiated from sickle cell trait (heterozygous Hb S), which is asymptomatic. In sickle cell anaemia, pallor develops during the first 2–4 months of life and the other clinical manifestations are rare before 5–6 months of age. Diagnosis is made by Hb electrophoresis.

3. D Hereditary spherocytosis

Hereditary spherocytosis results in the presence of fragile spherocytes which are destroyed prematurely in the spleen. It may be a cause of haemolytic disease in the newborn period and presents as neonatal jaundice. The severity in infants and children is variable. Some children remain asymptomatic into adulthood, but others may have severe anaemia with pallor, icterus, fatigue, splenomegaly and exercise intolerance. Pigmentary gall stones may form as early as 4–5 years of age.

4. B Diamond-Blackfan syndrome

About 75% of children with the above condition present by 3 months of age. The most characteristic features are a macrocytic anaemia, reticulocytopenia and a deficiency, or absence, of red blood cell precursors in an otherwise normal cellular marrow. About one-third of affected children have congenital anomalies, most commonly craniofacial deformities or defects of the upper extremities.

5. A Aplastic anaemia

This clinical picture suggests an idiopathic form of aplastic anaemia due to primary stem cell failure, seen most commonly in the Chinese. The blood picture shows a pancytopenia. Careful history taking needs to exclude the secondary causes of aplastic anaemia such as drug toxicity (chloramphenicol, sulphonamides, phenylbutazone), viral illnesses (particularly hepatitis), chemicals (e.g. benzene toluene solvent abuse, insectides), post-radiation treatment and leukaemia.

Diagnosis of endocrine disorders in childhood

A   Acquired hypothyroidism
B   Acute Addison's disease
C   Congenital adrenal hyperplasia
D   Cushing's syndrome
E   Diabetes insipidus
F   Graves' disease
G   Hyperparathyroidism
H   Hypoparathyroidism
I   Isolated growth hormone deficiency
J   Phaeochromocytoma
K   Soto's syndrome

For each presentation below, choose the SINGLE most likely diagnosis from the above list of options. Each option may be used once, more than once, or not at all.

1. A 4-week-old baby boy born at term is referred with failure to regain his birth weight. He had been noted to have recurrent vomiting and on admission he was mildly dehydrated. The chemical profile reveals a serum sodium level of 124 mmol/L with a potassium of 6.5 mmol/L and a blood pH of 7.20.

2. A 6-year-old boy is referred to the paediatric clinic with a 6-month history of muscle cramps and two recent episodes of tonic seizures. Routine blood analysis reveals a low serum calcium level and an elevated phosphate level.

3. A 3-year-old girl is referred to the paediatric clinic as her parents are concerned about her height. She is now below the 4th centile for height but when born was on the 50th centile for both height and weight. Her development has otherwise been normal and she is an active, lively child.

4. A 5-year-old girl who has gained only 3 cm in height over the past 18 months has also been constipated for the last 4 months.

5. A 9-year-old boy presents with severe tiredness and muscle cramps following a recent viral illness. He has a tachycardia with a small volume pulse and a low blood pressure. His blood biochemistry tests show a serum sodium level of 128 mmol/L and a potassium level of 6.2 mmol/L.

Answers to **4.22**

1. C   Congenital adrenal hyperplasia

Congenital adrenal hyperplasia is a group of autosomal recessive disorders of adrenal steroidogenesis leading to a deficiency of cortisol. The deficiency of cortisol results in an increased secretion of corticotrophin which, in turn, leads to adrenocortical hyperplasia. Deficiency of 21-hydroxylase accounts for 90% of affected patients. Affected infants present with weight loss, vomiting and dehydration. Hyponatraemia, hyperkalaemia and acidosis are common.

2. H   Hypoparathyroidism

Any child referred with seizures should have their calcium, magnesium and phosphate levels checked to rule out hypoparathyroidism. This condition is frequently mistaken for epilepsy. Muscular pains and cramps are early manifestations.

3. I   Isolated growth hormone (GH) deficiency

Children with growth hormone deficiency are usually of normal size and weight at birth. Those with severe defects in GH production will fail to maintain normal growth and will fall more than four standard deviations below the mean by 1 year of age, whereas others with less severe deficiency may have regular but slow growth in height. The face is often short and broad and other facial characteristics can include a prominent frontal bone, small nose, depressed nasal bridge and underdeveloped mandible and chin, with crowded teeth. Intelligence is usually normal. Definitive diagnosis depends on the demonstration of absent or low levels of GH in response to stimulation (exercise, L-dopa, insulin, clonidine or glucagon).

4. A   Acquired hypothyroidism

Acquired hypothyroidism is commonly due to lymphocytic thyroiditis (autoimmune thyroid disease) and is typically seen in adolescence but can occur at any age. Deceleration of growth is usually the first clinical manifestation but it often goes unrecognized in the presence of normal progress at school. However, bone age is markedly delayed.

5. B   Acute Addison's disease

The presence of hyponatraemia with hyperkalaemia is strongly suggestive of Addison's disease. Acute presentations are common after an intercurrent infection or following surgery. Other symptoms include vomiting, diarrhoea, nausea and sometimes unexplained fever. Most often there is primary adrenal failure due to autoimmune adrenalitis.

Diagnosis of chronic diarrhoea

A   Amoebiasis (*Entamoeba histolytica*)
B   Coeliac disease
C   Cystic fibrosis
D   *Enterobius vermicularis* infection
E   Irritable bowel syndrome
F   Rota virus
G   Secondary lactose intolerance
H   Shigella dysentery
I   Toddler's diarrhoea (chronic non-specific diarrhoea)
J   Ulcerative colitis
K   Tropical sprue

For each patient described below choose the SINGLE most likely diagnosis
from the above list of options. Each option may be used once, more than
once, or not at all.

1. A 2-year-old boy is brought to clinic with a 6-month history of recurrent
    diarrhoea. The child appears well with normal appetite and normal
    milestones of development. Stool examination shows the presence of
    undigested vegetable particles with no blood or pus cells.

2. An 8-year-old girl complains of vulval irritation with no associated
    vaginal discharge. She has intermittent diarrhoea and on several
    occasions she has felt a crawling sensation in her anal region at night.

3. A 4-year-old boy presents with recurrent diarrhoea and failure to thrive.
    His mother gives a history of intermittent episodes of vomiting.
    Serological testing has shown the presence of antigliadin and
    antiendomysial antibodies.

4. A 10-month-old infant recovering from an acute, rota-viral diarrhoea
    develops watery diarrhoea after a week of remission. The parents report
    that the stools are explosive and there are perianal excoriations.

5. A 13-year-old boy presents with a 2-week history of passing bloody
    stools. He has not visited any foreign countries recently. On
    examination, he is found to have swollen and tender wrists with
    nodular, tender lesions on his shins.

Answers to **4.23**

1.   I   Toddler's diarrhoea (chronic non-specific diarrhoea)

Chronic non-specific diarrhoea in children is characterized by loose, brown, watery and slightly offensive stools. The onset is between 6 and 30 months of age. It usually resolves spontaneously by the age of 4. The patient is usually healthy and thriving. The stool may show mucus, undigested vegetable fibres and starch granules.

2.   D   *Enterobius vermicularis* infection

Enterobius vermicularis infection occurs world-wide and affects individuals of all ages and socioeconomic levels, but it is especially common in children. The most common presenting complaint is perianal and perineal irritation or pruritus. Tissue invasion does not occur in enterobiasis. *Enterobius vermicularis* are small (1 cm) white worms and the mature gravid females migrate at night from the caecum to the perianal region to deposit their eggs and this induces irritation.

3.   B   Coeliac disease

Coeliac disease ranges from severe intestinal malabsorption to normal health. The common symptoms are failure to thrive, diarrhoea, irritability, vomiting and anorexia. Serological testing often shows the presence of antigliadin, antireticulin and antiendomysial antibodies, but the definitive diagnosis requires a jejunal biopsy.

4.   G   Secondary lactose intolerance

Secondary lactose intolerance is one of the known complications of rota-viral diarrhoea and presents with explosive watery stools, abdominal distension, flatulence and an excoriated diaper area. Stoppage of lactose-containing feeds (mainly milk) for a few days allows for regeneration of the villi, the milk feeds can then be slowly reintroduced.

5.   J   Ulcerative colitis

This young patient's symptoms suggest an acute inflammatory diarrhoea with probable erythema nodosum affecting the lower limbs. Ulcerative colitis is usually characterized by recurrent, bloody diarrhoea associated with inflammation confined mainly to the colonic mucosa. The initial symptoms are diarrhoea with fresh blood and mucus, faecal urgency and lower abdominal cramps. Clinical signs of chronic ill-health are usually evident at the time of diagnosis. Extraintestinal manifestations are less common in children, but signs of arthritis are seen in 10%, erythema nodosum in 5% and rarely pyoderma gangrenosum.

Differential diagnosis of non-accidental injury

A   Acute lymphoblastic leukaemia
B   Emotional abuse
C   Haemophilia A
D   Henoch–Schönlein purpura
E   Immune thrombocytopenic purpura (ITP)
F   Neglect
G   Normal child with accidental injury
H   Osteogenesis imperfecta
I   Physical abuse
J   Sexual abuse
K   Thalassaemia minor

For each scenario below, choose the SINGLE most likely diagnosis from the above list of options. Each option may be used once, more than once, or not at all.

1. A 3-month-old infant is brought to the GP with bleeding from the mouth. On examination, the frenulum is torn and there are two bruises over the left cheek. The parents report that the child sustained the injuries after rolling off the cot.

2. An 11-year-old girl attends the hospital with her aunt because of generalized weakness. The girl lives with her stepmother. She is found to be thin, unkempt with matted hair, head lice and is smelly. There are no physical injuries seen on her.

3. A GP refers an 8-year-old boy to the hospital with multiple bruises over his arms and body. He develops epistaxis whilst awaiting a consultation and on questioning he reports that he had an upper respiratory infection 2 weeks ago. On examination, except for the bruises he is clinically well.

4. An 18-year-old mother brings her 8-week-old baby to the community paediatric doctor for immunization. The doctor notices that the right leg does not move well and so an X-ray is done which shows multiple fractures in both legs. The baby's sclerae appear blue.

5. A 5-year-old female child who lives with her mother and stepfather is brought to the A&E department with a 2-day history of bleeding per vagina. The paediatrician notices a couple of small bruises on the inner aspect of the thighs.

Answers to **4.24**

1. I **Physical abuse**

Bruises in young infants before they are fully mobile (7–8 months) should always raise the suspicion of physical abuse. Frenula tears are almost invariably due to forced attempts to feed or silence a screaming infant.

2. F **Neglect**

The given scenario is almost always due to neglect. The absence of external physical injuries usually rules out physical abuse although one must look carefully for them in this group of children.

3. E **Immune thrombocytopenic purpura (ITP)**

Not all bruises or purpura are due to non-accidental injury. One should be aware of other common conditions presenting with similar symptoms. ITP often appears to be related to sensitization following a recent viral infection. Bruising and a generalized petechial rash occur 1–4 weeks (average 2 weeks) after a viral infection (70%) or without an antecedent illness (30%). The platelet count is usually reduced to below 20×10^9/L. ITP has an excellent prognosis, even when no specific therapy is given. Gamma globulins and corticosteroids are used in selected cases.

4. H **Osteogenesis imperfecta (OI)**

Osteogenesis imperfecta in childhood is characterized by fractures and skeletal deformities. At least four genetic syndromes account for the variable presentations in OI. Serum alkaline phosphatase activity is normal or elevated in all forms. OI type 1 is the most common variety and is characterized by osteoporosis and excessive bone fragility, distinctly blue sclerae and presenile conductive hearing loss in adolescents and adults. In OI, studies of collagen synthesized by cultured skin fibroblasts show abnormalities in the type 1 collagen with either a reduction or a structural abnormality.

5. J **Sexual abuse**

Sexual abuse in children is most commonly from other family members and the incidence among stepfathers is about five times higher than in biological fathers. Other medical abnormalities include genital infection, genital or anal trauma, recurrent urethritis, enuresis, encopresis (involuntary passing or incontinence of faeces) and inappropriate sexual behaviour like mimicking a sexual act. A child suspected of suffering abuse must be thoroughly examined by a specialist and the social worker and the police may need to be involved.

Aetiological factors in developmental delay and mental retardation

A   Birth asphyxia
B   Crohn's disease
C   Down's syndrome
D   Duchenne muscular dystrophy
E   Fetal alcohol syndrome
F   Fragile X syndrome
G   Hypothyroidism
H   Noonan's syndrome
I   Normal variant
J   Phenylketonuria
K   Sequelae to bacterial meningitis

For each patient described below, choose the SINGLE most likely diagnosis from the above list of options. Each option may be used once, more than once, or not at all.

1. A 16-month-old girl is referred to the community paediatrician as the infant's mother is concerned that the child is not walking well. She is able to stand and walk with one hand held. On examination, there is nothing unusual to find.

2. An 11-year-old boy is doing poorly in school and has been referred for a paediatric opinion. On examination, he has slightly large ears, large jaw, hyperextensible joints and unusually large testes. His elder brother and uncle also have similar features.

3. A 7-year-old girl is doing well in school after a spell in hospital for suspected meningitis. However, her parents think that she is not progressing well through the developmental milestones and is having temper tantrums.

4. A newborn boy was found to be hypotonic during the neonatal check-up. On examination, he has a flat occiput, oblique palpebral fissures, clinodactyly, a single palmar crease and a pansystolic murmur over the left sternal edge.

5. A 3-year-old boy has difficulty in standing up, climbing stairs and running. On examination, his calves are enlarged.

Answers to **4.25**

1. **I   Normal variant**

    By 18 months, if she is still unable to walk independently then she will
    fall outside the normal range. For all milestones there is quite a wide
    normal range.

2. **F   Fragile X syndrome**

    This syndrome is due to a chromosome break involving the long arm of
    the X chromosome (band q 27–28) and is associated with mental
    retardation with or without macro-orchidism in males. The assessment
    of the mentally retarded male is incomplete without testicular
    measurement and a chromosomal study for this X-chromosome marker.

3. **K   Sequelae to bacterial meningitis**

    The long-term sequelae of meningitis at any age can be disastrous. It can
    vary from none to severe physical and mental handicap. The common
    sequelae are deafness (sensorineural), mental retardation, seizures, delay
    in the acquisition of language, visual impairment and behavioural
    problems.

4. **C   Down's syndrome**

    The presence of an extra 21 chromosome results in the best-recognized
    and most frequent human chromosomal syndrome. The important
    clinical features are mental retardation, hypotonia, a flat occiput,
    oblique palpebral fissures, epicanthal folds, speckled irides (Brushfield
    spots), a protruding tongue, congenital heart disease (septal defects), a
    simian crease (single palmar crease), short broad hands, hypoplasia of
    the middle phalanx of the 5th finger (clinodactyly) and a high-arched
    palate.

5. **D   Duchenne muscular dystrophy**

    This is the most common hereditary neuromuscular disease and is
    inherited as an X-linked recessive trait. The abnormal gene is at the X
    p21 loci. Early gross motor skills are usually achieved at the appropriate
    ages or may be mildly delayed. Weakness is usually noted by the 3rd
    year of life and most boys are confined to a wheelchair by 12 years.
    Enlargement of the calves (pseudohypertrophy) and wasting of the thigh
    muscles are classic features. Cardiomyopathy and intellectual
    impairment are constant features of this disease. Death usually occurs by
    18–20 years and is caused by respiratory failure, intractable congestive
    cardiac failure or pneumonia.

Psychiatry

Diagnosis of neurotic disorders

A Acute stress reaction
B Adjustment disorder
C Agoraphobia
D Anxious personality disorder
E Atrial tachycardia
F Depersonalization
G Generalized anxiety disorder
H Hyperthyroidism
I Panic disorder
J Phaeochromocytoma
K Post-traumatic stress disorder

For each patient below, choose the SINGLE most likely diagnosis from the above list of options. Each option may be used once, more than once, or not at all.

1. A 35-year-old woman presents with a 3-month history of weight loss, palpitations and sleep disturbance. Her appetite is very good and she finds the weather warm and intolerable.

2. A previously fit 30-year-old lady complains of unpredictable attacks of palpitations, sweating and chest pain. She fears that she may die during these episodes and states that her mother suffered from a similar complaint.

3. A 45-year-old recently divorced housewife has a 5-month history of nervousness, poor concentration, difficulty in relaxing and lightheadedness. Her symptoms are persistent and she worries how she will cope. Her GP found no abnormality on physical examination.

4. A 62-year-old female survivor of a train crash is admitted to an A&E observation ward shortly afterwards. She is disorientated, dazed and does not appear to understand simple instructions. She is extremely anxious and agitated, but her symptoms settle within 24 hours and she is discharged home.

5. A 38-year-old hypertensive male complains of attacks of anxiety, palpitations and headache. He denies any specific worries. He is found to have an abnormal glucose tolerance.

Answers to 5.1

The WHO defines neurotic disorders as mental disorders without any demonstrable organic cause, in which the patient may have considerable insight and usually does not confuse his morbid subjective experiences with external reality. Behaviour can be significantly affected but usually remains within socially acceptable limits. Physical illness such as hyperthyroidism, phaeochromocytoma, parathyroid disease, angina pectoris and atrial tachycardia may present with symptoms similar to panic and anxiety disorders.

1. H Hyperthyroidism

There are sufficient symptoms and signs here to suggest an organic cause. In particular, loss of weight in association with a good appetite and heat intolerance brings in hyperthyroidism for consideration.

2. I Panic disorder

A panic disorder is characterized by recurrent, unpredictable attacks of severe anxiety. There is almost invariably a fear of dying, losing control or going mad. There is comparative freedom from anxiety symptoms between attacks. It is slightly more common in women, commonest in the age group 25–44 years, and there is evidence of familial transmission. Panic disorder can occur with or without agoraphobia.

3. G Generalized anxiety disorder

Anxiety is generalized, persistent and not restricted to any particular environmental circumstances. Symptoms include apprehension, motor tension and autonomic overactivity. The condition is commoner in women, often related to chronic environmental stress, and the course is often fluctuating and chronic.

4. A Acute stress reaction

An acute stress reaction is characterized by an immediate, clear temporal connection between the impact of an exceptional stressor and the onset of symptoms. The onset is immediate or within a few minutes. There is often an initial dazed state with subsequent symptoms showing a mixed and changing pattern. Symptoms are usually rapidly resolving and are minimal after 3 days. Note the contrast with post-traumatic stress disorder where there is a delayed or protracted response to a stressful situation of an exceptionally stressful nature.

5. J Phaeochromocytoma

Phaeochromocytoma is suggested by the paroxysms of pallor, perspiration, palpitations, hypertension and hyperglycaemia, which are a result of catecholamine excess. It is often difficult to distinguish from a panic disorder.

Investigation of disturbed behaviour

A Computerized tomography (CT) scan of the head
B Electroencephalogram (EEG)
C Full blood count
D Liver function tests
E Magnetic resonance imaging (MRI) scan of the head
F Serum calcium
G Synacthen test
H Thyroid function
I Urea and electrolytes
J Urinalysis
K Urine drug screen

For each presentation below, choose the SINGLE most discriminating investigation from the above list of options. Each option may be used once, more than once, or not at all.

1. A dishevelled 19-year-old man found acting strangely outside a nightclub is brought to the A&E department by the police. The man is convinced that a group of men are plotting to kill him and that he heard them discussing this. His blood alcohol level is zero.

2. A 14-year-old boy presents with a 6-month history of recurrent episodes of confusion. Witnessed by his mother, they are described as lasting about 15 minutes during which he wanders aimlessly, picks at his clothing, and his speech is vague and confused. There is a history of a childhood head injury. He complains of a 'rising' feeling in his abdomen before these episodes.

3. A middle-aged female consults her GP with concerns that she is being spied upon by one of her neighbours. Her doctor notices that she has put on weight and that her voice is hoarse.

4. An 18-year-old girl presents with a 2-month history of weight loss, lethargy and low mood. Over the last 24 hours she has become increasingly confused and is dizzy on standing.

5. A 54-year-old postmenopausal woman complains of feeling weak and tired. She also suffers from attacks of loin pain and constipation. Her friends have noticed that she is unusually irritable and depressed in mood. Her weight is stable.

Answers to 5.2

1. **K Urine drug screen**

   The history is strongly suggestive of substance abuse. This is particularly prevalent in young males. The symptoms are of persecutory delusions and 3rd person auditory hallucinations, which would be compatible with an amphetamine psychosis. This can present with identical symptoms to paranoid schizophrenia. The nightclub is also a clue as illicit substances, particularly stimulants and hallucinogens are often consumed at such premises.

2. **B Electroencephalogram (EEG)**

   Consciousness is impaired in complex partial seizures of temporal lobe onset. Automatisms are common and include symptoms such as lip smacking, chewing, swallowing, searching, fumbling, wandering, being resistive, undressing and vocalization. Patients may also have autonomic and psychic symptoms such as visual/auditory/olfactory/gustatory hallucinations and depersonalization, depression, amnesia, ecstasy, fear and déjà vu. An EEG may help to confirm the diagnosis; a head CT or MRI scan may be required.

3. **H Thyroid function**

   Hypothyroidism may present with a variety of psychiatric symptoms such as confusion, disorientation, depression, hallucinations and persecutory, hypochondriacal and grandiose delusions. This concept of 'myxoedematous madness' was originally documented by Asher in 1949.

4. **G Synacthen test**

   The history is suggestive of adrenal hypofunction (Addison's disease). Common features include lethargy, anorexia, nausea, vomiting, weight loss, postural hypotension and loss of body hair in females. Less often hypoglycaemia and depression may be present. The short Synacthen test is the screening test for adrenocortical insufficiency.

5. **F Serum calcium**

   Her symptoms are suggestive of hypercalcaemia, the commonest causes of this being malignant disease and primary hyperparathyroidism. The saying 'stones, bones, psychic groans and abdominal moans' sums up the symptoms nicely (stones = renal calculi; bones = bony pains; psychic moans = tiredness, lassitude, poor concentration, personality changes; abdominal moans = pain, nausea, vomiting, rarely peptic ulceration and pancreatitis). Primary hyperparathyroidism is most often seen among postmenopausal women but can occur in both sexes at any age.

Treatment of mood disorders

A Atypical antipsychotics
B Benzodiazepines
C Carbamazepine
D Cognitive analytical therapy
E Cognitive behavioural therapy
F Electroconvulsive therapy (ECT)
G Lamotrigine
H Psychodynamic psychotherapy
I Selective serotonin reuptake inhibitor (SSRI)
J Sodium valproate
K Tricyclic antidepressant (TCA)

For each problem below, choose the SINGLE most appropriate treatment from the above list of options. Each option may be used once, more than once, or not at all.

1. A 70-year-old retired cleaner is admitted to hospital following an overdose of 50 paracetamol tablets. She complains of a 2-month history of low mood, lethargy and poor concentration. She refuses admission to hospital but agrees to stay with her daughter. It is not felt appropriate to detain her under the Mental Health Act. What treatment would you choose after she has recovered from her overdose?

2. A 30-year-old journalist is admitted to the psychiatric ward. She presents with a severely depressed mood, significant weight loss, refusal to eat or drink, recurrent thoughts of self-harm, agitation and early morning wakening. She is also convinced that her internal organs are rotting away.

3. A 45-year-old schoolteacher complains of low mood, reduced energy, poor concentration and anxiety symptoms. He is adamant that he does not want treatment with tablets but is happy to consider other options.

4. A 22-year-old unemployed woman is treated for a moderate depressive episode with fluoxetine. Four weeks after starting treatment, she is still suffering with nausea, dizziness and headache, which she finds intolerable, and asks if she can try an alternative treatment.

5. A 50-year-old labourer with a known bipolar affective disorder has been well on lithium prophylaxis for a number of years. However, he has gained a significant amount of weight and is keen to stop his lithium. He is hypersensitive to carbamazepine and wishes to know if there are any other treatment options.

Answers to 5.3

1. **I   Selective serotonin reuptake inhibitor (SSRI)**

   Parasuicide (deliberate self-harm) should always be taken seriously and a thorough psychosocial assessment carried out. This is particularly the case within the elderly population where the demographic correlates of parasuicide and actual suicide are similar. In this case, admission under the Mental Health Act was not felt to be appropriate but the symptoms were compatible with depression. An SSRI would be the most appropriate treatment, as it is safer in overdose and may be better tolerated in the elderly than the tricyclics.

2. **F   Electroconvulsive therapy (ECT)**

   The history suggests a severe depressive episode with psychotic symptoms (hypochondriacal delusions). This is potentially life threatening due to her refusal to eat or drink and the persistent thoughts of self-harm. ECT is the most appropriate course of action. Other indications for ECT include: poor response or intolerance to medication, stupor, previous response to ECT, severe postpartum depression and severe suicidal risk.

3. **E   Cognitive behavioural therapy**

   He is a candidate for psychological therapy. Primary care trials have suggested that cognitive behavioural therapy (CBT) is an effective treatment for depression. For more severe illness, interpersonal therapy is probably better.

4. **K   Tricyclic antidepressant (TCA)**

   Gastrointestinal symptoms, headache and dizziness are well recognized as the side effects of the SSRIs. Such symptoms are to be expected when starting a drug or escalating the dosage, but should settle within 10–14 days. In this case, she is intolerant to the drug and has two options: reduce the present dosage or change to another antidepressant. Given the symptoms described are classic effects of the SSRIs, it may be most appropriate to change to an antidepressant from another group.

5. **J   Sodium valproate**

   Lithium, carbamazepine and sodium valproate are the three most well recognized agents used as mood stabilizers. Sodium valproate has very recently been licensed for this purpose in the UK. Carbamazepine and sodium valproate are perhaps more useful than lithium in the treatment and prophylaxis of rapid-cycling mood disorder.

Epidemiology of important psychiatric disorders in the UK

A   <1%
B   1%
C   3 to 6%
D   10%
E   20%
F   25%
G   35%
H   40 to 50%
I   60%
J   70%
K   90%

For each statement below, choose the SINGLE most likely answer from the above list of options. Each option may be used once, more than once, or not at all.

1. The lifetime risk of schizophrenia in the general population.

2. The lifetime risk of a unipolar affective disorder in the general population.

3. The lifetime risk of schizophrenia in a sibling of an individual who is known to suffer with schizophrenia.

4. Population prevalence of depression diagnosed by general practitioners.

5. The lifetime risk of a bipolar affective disorder in the general population.

Answers to **5.4**

Prevalence is the number of people affected with a disorder at a given time. Incidence is the number of new cases of a disorder over a defined time period. Lifetime risk is the chance of having an episode of the illness during the course of one's lifetime.

1. **B   1%**

    It is important to know that schizophrenia occurs equally in men and women, although women tend to present at a slightly later age. The annual incidence of schizophrenia is 2 to 4 per 10 000 people. The point prevalence is 0.1 to 0.5% of the population.

2. **C   3 to 6%**

    Between 3 and 6% of the population will suffer with an episode of unipolar affective disorder at some point in their lives (Epidemiological Catchment Area study). Other studies have suggested much higher rates (National Comorbidity Survey = 17%). The lower lifetime prevalence identified in the ECA study may have been due to a different diagnostic schedule being used (cf. National Comorbidity Survey). It is well recognized that the prevalence is approximately twice as high in women.

3. **D   10%**

    The lifetime risk of schizophrenia increases with genetic proximity to an affected family member. The parent of an affected child has a 5% lifetime risk, whereas the sibling of an affected individual has a 10% lifetime risk of developing the illness. The child of two affected parents has a 46% risk.

4. **C   3 to 6%**

    Of these, 10% are referred to psychiatrists (i.e. 3 in 1000) and one-third of these are admitted to a psychiatric inpatient unit (i.e. 1 in 1000).

5. **B   1%**

    This again is approximately 1%, affecting males and females equally. Familial transmission is evident. A first-degree relative of an individual suffering from a bipolar affective disorder has a 7.8% risk of developing the illness and approximately 11.4% risk of developing a unipolar affective disorder.

Epidemiology of suicide

A   4 per 100 000 population
B   11 per 100 000 population
C   2 per 10 000 population
D   0.5%
E   1%
F   5 to 10%
G   10 to 15%
H   25 to 45%
I   50%
J   75%
K   >90%

For each statement below, choose the SINGLE most likely answer from the above list of options. Each option may be used once, more than once, or not at all.

1. Suicide as a percentage of all deaths.

2. The suicide rate among men in England and Wales.

3. The percentage of completed suicides with a history of a psychiatric illness.

4. The percentage of completed suicides with a history of deliberate self-harm.

5. The risk of eventual suicide in an individual who suffers from schizophrenia, depression or the alcohol dependence syndrome.

Answers to 5.5

1. E   1%

There are approximately 5000 deaths per year from suicide in England and Wales. However, it is likely that this is an underestimate as verdicts of accidental death or an open verdict may be reached if there is any doubt about the cause of death.

2. B   11 per 100 000 population

The rates are approximately 11 per 100 000 population for men and 4 per 100 000 for women in England and Wales. Rates are higher for males at all ages. In young men, it is the second commonest cause of death after accidents. Suicide rates have started to decrease but the highest risk group is still young men. Note that these are official rates and remember that suicide is under-reported for a variety of reasons.

3. K   >90%

Over 90% of those who complete suicide have a psychiatric illness. Virtually all psychiatric disorders increase the risk of suicide, the highest risk groups being those who suffer from schizophrenia, depression and alcohol addiction. Other risk factors include adverse life events, unemployment or retirement, certain professions (e.g. vets, pharmacists, farmers, dentists, doctors), elderly age, male sex, social isolation and physical ill health.

4. I   50%

Approximately 50% of those who complete suicide have a history of previous deliberate self-harm (DSH). Of those who carry out DSH, 1% will complete suicide by the end of 1 year, and 10% will do so eventually. Among individuals who have carried out DSH, their risk of suicide in the following year is 100 times higher than the general population.

5. G   10 to 15%

Lifetime risk of suicide in an individual who suffers from depression or alcohol dependence is approximately 15%. Among those with schizophrenia, the lifetime risk is approximately 10%. The risk of suicide is also higher than in the general population for those with other psychiatric disorders such as drug abuse, organic disorders, personality disorders and neurotic disorders.

Diagnosis of psychotic disorders

A   Acute schizophrenia-like psychotic disorder
B   Delusional disorder
C   Hebephrenic schizophrenia
D   Induced delusional disorder
E   Paranoid schizophrenia
F   Schizoaffective disorder – depressive type
G   Schizoaffective disorder – manic type
H   Schizoaffective disorder – mixed type
I   Schizotypal disorder
J   Simple schizophrenia
K   Undifferentiated schizophrenia

For each presentation below, choose the SINGLE most likely diagnosis from the above list of options. Each option may be used once, more than once, or not at all.

1. A 40-year-old woman is arrested for causing a public disturbance outside the house of her local vicar. She has been pursuing him for over 8 years and is convinced of his love for her. She believes that he communicates especially to her when he gives his sermons.

2. Since leaving university 3 months ago, a 22-year-old man has become increasingly withdrawn and perplexed. He says he is bothered by voices discussing him amongst themselves. On the way to the hospital, the family's car stopped at some traffic lights. The lights turned green and he knew this was a sign that judgement day had arrived.

3. A 32-year-old lady is admitted to the psychiatric unit in a disturbed state. She has had multiple previous admissions with a similar presentation. For the past month she has felt that alien forces have been controlling her body and are inserting thoughts into her head. She is noticeably excited and irritable in mood.

4. A 45-year-old married man is charged with assaulting his wife. He is convinced that she has been unfaithful to him but provides no basis for this. He has been persistently searching through her private belongings.

5. A 65-year-old man has lived a reclusive and eccentric lifestyle for many years. He isolates himself and his speech is vague and overelaborate but is not overtly incoherent. He tends to be suspicious about the motives of others and appears cold and aloof in manner. There have not been definite schizophrenic symptoms at any time.

Answers to 5.6

1. B   Delusional disorder

Delusional disorders are characterized by a single delusion, or a set of related delusions, which are usually persistent and may be life-long. The onset is often in middle age. The delusional belief must have been present for at least 3 months in order to make this diagnosis and must be personal rather than subcultural. There should be no evidence of brain disease and no history of schizophrenic symptoms. Erotomania or de Clerambault's syndrome is characterized by an unfounded belief that he/she is loved from afar by another person.

2. E   Paranoid schizophrenia

The schizophrenic disorders are characterized by distortions of thinking and perception with inappropriate or blunted affect. To make a diagnosis symptoms must have been present for most of the time during a period of 1 month or more. Symptoms that have special importance for the diagnosis include thought echo/insertion/withdrawal/broadcast; delusions of control/passivity/delusional perception; running commentary or third person hallucinations and persistent delusions.

3. G   Schizoaffective disorder – manic type

In a schizoaffective disorder, schizophrenic and affective (mood) symptoms are prominent within the same episode of illness, either simultaneously or within a few days of each other. Their relationship to schizophrenic and mood disorders is unclear. For a diagnosis of the manic type, there must be a prominent elevation of mood, or a less obvious elevation of mood plus irritability or excitement. One or two typical schizophrenic symptoms must also be present.

4. B   Delusional disorder

Morbid jealousy, or the Othello syndrome, is another subtype of a delusional disorder. The distinction between morbid and normal jealousy is often difficult as both are part of the same spectrum. Delusional jealousy can be symptomatic of a delusional disorder, schizophrenia, alcohol dependence syndrome or a paranoid personality disorder. Usually the patient is a male over 40 years of age.

5. I   Schizotypal disorder

This is a disorder characterized by eccentric behaviour and abnormalities of thinking and affect that resemble those seen in schizophrenia but with no definite schizophrenic symptoms. The schizotypal disorder tends to be a chronic, fluctuating condition.

Diagnosis of dementia

A   Alzheimer's disease
B   Huntington's disease
C   Lewy body dementia
D   Neurosyphilis
E   New variant Creutzfeldt–Jakob disease
F   Normal pressure hydrocephalus
G   Parkinson's disease
H   Pick's disease
I   Pseudodementia
J   Vascular dementia
K   Wilson's disease

For each patient below, choose the SINGLE most likely diagnosis from the above list of options. Each option may be used once, more than once, or not at all.

1. A 78-year-old retired miner presents with a 2-year history of progressive memory loss, which fluctuates considerably from day to day. He describes seeing clear visions of his ex-workmates and swears that they were there in the same room with him. He has had a number of recent falls and appears sensitive to psychotropic medication.

2. A 70-year-old retired teacher has become increasingly forgetful over the last 6 months. Friends have noticed that her short-term memory is very variable. She complains of a low mood, which lifts as the day goes on, and has disturbed sleep and appetite.

3. A 30-year-old student presents with a 6-month history of depressive symptoms, anxiety and social withdrawal. His friends have noticed that he has become increasingly irritable, forgetful and more impatient than before.

4. An 82-year-old ex-shop assistant attends the memory clinic with her son and daughter. Her children are concerned that over the past 3 years her memory has gradually been failing. She forgets her chores but is using lists to prompt herself. She is having difficulty in handling money and her self-care skills have also deteriorated significantly.

5. A 62-year-old shop assistant is taken to the GP by his concerned wife. She has noticed that over the past few years his personality has changed subtly such that he is slightly disinhibited. His decision-making is often irrational and he can be embarrassing when guests visit their home. He has also become fixed on certain routines.

Answers to **5.7**

1. **C Lewy body dementia**

   The central feature needed for a diagnosis of Lewy body dementia (LBD) is progressive cognitive decline, which interferes with normal occupational or social functioning. Also, there are three core features: fluctuating cognition (with variations in alertness and attention), visual hallucinations (usually well formed) and spontaneous motor features of parkinsonism. Two of these are needed for a diagnosis of probable LBD, one for possible LBD. Recurrent falls, syncope, neuroleptic sensitivity, systematized delusions and other hallucinations are all supportive of the diagnosis. LBD may account for 20% of dementias in the elderly.

2. **I Pseudodementia**

   Depressive pseudodementia, or cognitive change in depression, is an atypical presentation of a depressive disorder. Depression in old age often presents with cognitive impairment but this usually resolves after treatment. Features that suggest pseudodementia (rather than dementia) include: history of depression, depressed mood, diurnal variation of mood, other biological symptoms and exaggerated or intermittent symptom presentation.

3. **E New variant Creutzfeldt–Jakob disease**

   New variant Creutzfeldt–Jakob disease (CJD) typically presents in the younger age group (19 to 39 years). Presenting symptoms are usually 'psychiatric' i.e. depressive symptoms, anxiety, withdrawal and personality changes. Mild stimuli may be unpleasant (dysaesthesiae) and this may affect the face or limbs. The disease course is insidious and death may occur in 7 to 24 months.

4. **A Alzheimer's disease**

   Alzheimer's dementia (AD) is the commonest cause of dementia (50–70% of cases) and is characterized by an insidious onset and a slow deterioration in the absence of other systemic or brain disease/neurological signs. It is an example of cortical dementia with impairment of memory, language, and visuospatial and perceptual function. Risk factors include increasing age (biggest factor), family history, Down's syndrome and a head injury. Diagnosis is largely clinical.

5. **H Pick's disease**

   A high proportion of frontal lobe dementias (or Pick's disease) are of pre-senile onset (<65 years). The onset is insidious and usually involves changes in personality, behaviour, mood and language. Commonly, loss of social skills, disinhibition, poor judgement and a 'shallowness' of affect are present. Speech can become less spontaneous. Memory impairment tends to occur later in the disease process.

Management of eating disorders

A Appetite suppressants
B Atypical antipsychotic agent
C Cognitive behavioural or interpersonal therapy
D Day hospital placement
E Family therapy
F Inpatient treatment in specialist unit
G Psychodynamic psychotherapy
H Psychosurgery
I Selective serotonin reuptake inhibitor (SSRI)
J Self-help manual or group
K Weight monitoring and nutritional education in primary care

For each scenario below, choose the SINGLE most appropriate
management from the above list of options. Each option may be used
once, more than once, or not at all.

1. A young woman presents to her GP with symptoms suggestive of an
    eating disorder. She does not satisfy the ICD-10 criteria for anorexia
    nervosa but her menstrual periods have become irregular, her body mass
    index is 19 and she has some overvalued ideas regarding her body
    shape. What is the most appropriate first course of action?

2. A 16-year-old girl presents with symptoms compatible with anorexia
    nervosa. The psychiatrist seeing her in the outpatient department notes
    that the interaction within the family is disturbed and rigid. What would
    be an appropriate treatment on an outpatient basis?

3. A 20-year-old female student presents to her GP and states that she has a
    morbid fear of fatness. She is preoccupied with eating and food and has
    episodes of gross overeating interspersed with efforts to try and lose
    weight. She tries to counter the effects of food by dieting and self-
    induced vomiting. Her weight is within normal limits and her menstrual
    cycle is regular. What is the first course of action?

4. A young woman with a diagnosis of bulimia nervosa is receiving
    treatment in a specialist unit. She finds the psychotherapeutic input
    particularly beneficial. What most likely psychotherapy is she receiving?

5. A 17-year-old schoolgirl with a diagnosis of bulimia nervosa is very
    distressed by the frequency and severity of her episodes of binge eating
    and vomiting. She refuses psychotherapeutic input but is amenable to
    drug treatment and monitoring by her GP. What is an appropriate
    pharmacological agent to help with her symptoms?

Answers to **5.8**

1. **K   Weight monitoring and nutritional education in primary care**

    The principle of stepped-care in anorexia nervosa is that with increasing severity of the illness the patient moves from simple to more skilled intensive treatments. The first step on the ladder is for the GP to monitor weight and to give general nutritional education in the primary care setting.

2. **E   Family therapy**

    Family therapy and family counselling are equally effective in anorexia nervosa. Family interaction is often felt to be disturbed or dysfunctional in anorexia nervosa. Minuchin described this as the 'psychosomatic family' showing rigidity, lack of conflict resolution, over-protectiveness and enmeshment. In family therapy, the whole family is seen, interactions observed and interventions made. However, in family counselling, the parents are seen together, the patient seen separately and advice is given (no observations or interventions). In both types of therapy, the parents are encouraged to take control of their daughter's eating.

3. **J   Self-help manual or group**

    These three core symptoms (morbid fear of fatness, preoccupation with eating and attempts to counteract the fattening effects of food) are suggestive of bulimia nervosa. Stepped-care is also an approach used in treating bulimia nervosa beginning with input at the primary care level. This may involve a self-help manual/advice or a self-help group.

4. **C   Cognitive behavioural or interpersonal therapy**

    Cognitive behavioural (CBT) and interpersonal (IPT) therapies are the most beneficial of the 'talking treatments' in bulimia nervosa. Behavioural therapy has also been used but has a lower remission rate. Group therapy may be beneficial.

5. **I   Selective serotonin reuptake inhibitor (SSRI)**

    The Bulimia Nervosa Collaborative Study Group demonstrated the benefit of fluoxetine in reducing the frequency of binge eating and vomiting. They found that fluoxetine was most effective when used in a higher dose than in depression (60 mg daily versus 20 mg daily). This is, however, controversial as the optimum dose and treatment duration are unknown.

Adverse effects of psychotropic medication

A   Acute dystonia
B   Akathisia
C   Anticholinergic side effects
D   Discontinuation syndrome
E   Hypertensive crisis
F   Neuroleptic malignant syndrome
G   Neurotoxicity
H   Parkinsonism
I   Relapse of depressive illness
J   Serotonin syndrome
K   Tardive dyskinesia

For each scenario below, choose the SINGLE most appropriate adverse reaction from the above list of options. Each option may be used once, more than once, or not at all.

1. A 22-year-old student has a diagnosis of an acute psychotic disorder. He is started on oral haloperidol and within a few days becomes very unwell. He is feverish, has muscle stiffness and is intermittently dizzy and confused.

2. A 25-year-old secretary suffers with paranoid schizophrenia and she is prescribed risperidone. She has been feeling restless and agitated recently and finds it difficult to sit still.

3. A 40-year-old housewife has been treated with fluoxetine for a depressive illness with little benefit and the decision is made to change her to another antidepressant. Two weeks after stopping fluoxetine, phenelzine (a monoamine oxidase inhibitor) is commenced. Within a couple of days she complains of headache, shaking and stiffness, and has a tonic–clonic epileptic seizure.

4. A 45-year-old office-worker has been successfully treated with paroxetine for the first episode of a depressive illness. After 1 year of remission, a joint decision is made to gradually reduce and stop his medication. Approximately 3 days later, he complains of irritability, anxiety, sleep disturbance, crying spells, nausea and fatigue.

5. A 31-year-old artist has a diagnosis of a bipolar affective disorder and is on maintenance lithium therapy. Due to a period of sustained agitation he is started on haloperidol. A week later, he is admitted to the local hospital with vomiting, unsteady gait, slurred speech and confusion. The lithium level is 0.65 mm/L.

Answers to 5.9

1. **F   Neuroleptic malignant syndrome**

    This is an idiosyncratic reaction, the core symptoms being hyperpyrexia, rigidity, autonomic instability and fluctuating confusion/level of consciousness. This can be caused by any neuroleptic but haloperidol and depot fluphenazine are most commonly implicated. The aetiology is unknown. It often occurs soon after starting or increasing the drug. Creatine kinase (CK) is elevated. It is more prevalent in young males.

2. **B   Akathisia**

    Akathisia is possibly the most common side effect of antipsychotic medication affecting as many as 50% of patients. It consists of motor restlessness and subjective agitation. Individuals are intolerant of inactivity and there is shifting of the legs with tapping of the feet. It is dose-related and there is an association with violence and suicide.

3. **J   Serotonin syndrome**

    The serotonin syndrome occurs as a result of a drug interaction between monoamine oxidase inhibitors (MAOI) and opiates, clomipramine, imipramine or selective serotonin reuptake inhibitors (SSRI). Three main groups of symptoms occur: neurological (myoclonus/headache/ tremor/rigidity/seizures); mental state changes (irritability/confusion/ agitation/coma); and other symptoms (e.g. hyperpyrexia/cardiac arrhythmias). Combinations of SSRI and MAOI should be avoided. At least 2 weeks should be allowed before changing from an SSRI to a MAOI and 5 weeks if switching from fluoxetine to a MAOI.

4. **D   Discontinuation syndrome**

    SSRI discontinuation syndrome is commonest with paroxetine which has a short half-life and no active metabolite. It is least frequent with fluoxetine, which has a long half-life. The most frequent symptoms include dizziness, nausea, vomiting, fatigue, lethargy, flu-like symptoms, sleep disturbance, anxiety, irritability and crying. Symptoms usually emerge within 1 to 3 days.

5. **G   Neurotoxicity**

    Lithium neurotoxicity can occur at therapeutic blood levels and its risk is increased by intercurrent illness, salt depletion and dehydration. It is also potentiated by other drugs including phenothiazines, haloperidol, carbamazepine and calcium channel blockers. If prolonged, it can be irreversible and haemodialysis may be necessary. Suggestive signs include vomiting, ataxia, slurred speech and confusion.

Diagnosis of sleep disorders

A Hypersomnia
B Insomnia
C Klein–Levine syndrome
D Narcolepsy
E Nocturnal paroxysmal dystonia
F Periodic limb movement disorder
G Sleep disorder secondary to depressive illness
H Sleep paralysis
I Sleep terrors (night terrors)
J Sleep–wake schedule disorder
K Sleepwalking (somnambulism)

For each patient below, choose the SINGLE most likely diagnosis from the above list of options. Each option may be used once, more than once, or not at all.

1. A mother brings her 8-year-old son to the GP's surgery. She states that he is waking at night, about 2 hours after getting off to sleep, in a very distressed state. He thrashes about the bed and appears very fearful and sweaty. These episodes last about 5 minutes and afterwards he has little recall of what has happened.

2. A 30-year-old woman has a 10-year history of unusual symptoms. She complains of irresistible episodes of daytime sleepiness, collapse and seeing unusual visions just when dropping off to sleep. She also has attacks of being paralysed just before she wakes up in the mornings. She thinks her uncle suffered with similar problems.

3. A 22-year-old man sees his GP with complaints of excessive sleepiness. He sleeps for up to 20 hours a day and has the desire to eat constantly but feels thirsty. His girlfriend is also worried about his excessive sex drive. He complains of feeling low in mood and of having unusual visual experiences.

4. The parents of a 12-year-old girl are concerned about her episodes of nocturnal wandering. She has a long history of rising from the bed at night and has actually wandered out into the street. She has no recollection of this but notices that she is sometimes confused when she wakes up in the mornings.

5. A 51-year-old female shift-worker consults her GP for advice on sleep hygiene. She finds it difficult to establish a sleep routine, often falling asleep at work and finding it hard to get to sleep when she goes to bed. This is interfering with her ability to carry out her job effectively.

Answers to **5.10**

1. **I   Sleep terrors (night terrors)**

   For a definite diagnosis, there needs to have been at least one episode of night-time wakening during which the patient typically appears anxious, panicky with body movement/thrashing and autonomic hyperactivity. Episodes are commonest during childhood, last 1 to 10 minutes and typically occur in the first third of nocturnal sleep. There is unresponsiveness to arousal and recall of the event is minimal. A physical disorder must be excluded.

2. **D   Narcolepsy**

   Narcolepsy comprises a tetrad of hypersomnia, cataplexy (sudden loss of muscle tone and collapse), sleep paralysis (frightening feeling of being unable to move when waking or falling asleep) and hypnagogic/ hypnopompic (visual images that persist into the half-waking state before awakening) hallucinations. Only 25% of those affected have the full tetrad of symptoms. This affects 1 in 10 000 of the population and the onset is usually between 15 to 35 years of age. There is a genetic component. First-degree relatives of those affected have a 40 times greater risk than the general population.

3. **C   Klein–Levine syndrome**

   This is a non-familial disorder with the aetiology possibly involving the hypothalamus. It may be triggered by injury or infection and symptoms are usually intermittent but recurring. It affects young men and the main symptoms include hypersomnia, increased body temperature, compulsive overeating, hypersexuality, polydipsia, hallucinations and mood changes. Treatment may not be needed but stimulants can be useful.

4. **K   Sleepwalking (somnambulism)**

   A definite diagnosis is suggested by the presence of episodes of rising from bed and walking about, the sufferer being resistant to being woken up by others, no recollection of the episode, possibly short periods of confusion on wakening and no evidence of a physical disorder. This usually occurs during the first third of the night, is commoner in children and there may be a family history. Diagnosis is clinical and can be confirmed by a polysomnogram.

5. **J   Sleep–wake schedule disorder**

   The individual's sleep pattern is out of synchrony with that which is normal for a particular society. Insomnia during the major sleep period and hypersomnia during the waking period are experienced most days for at least 1 month. This results in interference with activities of daily living or distress. Working shifts and time-zone changes may be risk factors.

Classification of psychiatric disorders into ICD-10 categories (International Classification of Diseases, 10th revision)

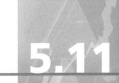

A Behavioural and emotional disorders
B Behavioural syndromes associated with physiological disturbances
C Disorders of adult personality and behaviour
D Disorders of psychological development
E Mental and behavioural disorders due to psychoactive substance use
F Mental retardation
G Mood (affective) disorders
H Neurotic, stress-related and somatoform disorders
I Organic, including symptomatic mental disorders
J Schizophrenia, schizotypal and delusional disorders
K Unspecified mental disorder

For each patient below, choose the SINGLE most likely diagnostic category from the above list of options. Each option may be used once, more than once, or not at all.

1. A 14-year-old boy is assessed by the educational psychologist and is found to have a global reduction in his level of intellectual functioning. This is thought to be due to childhood viral encephalitis.

2. A 7-year-old boy is taken by his parents to his GP. The boy is extremely active, cannot concentrate or sit still for any length of time and often places himself in positions of danger such as running out in front of cars.

3. A 9-year-old boy is assessed by the community paediatrician following parental concerns regarding his school progress. He is very able academically but he is disruptive in class, has no friends and is being bullied. He finds it very difficult to play cooperatively in team activities. He lacks empathy and displays repetitive behaviours.

4. A 12-year-old girl is referred to a psychologist for help with her fear of dogs. She gets extremely anxious if she sees or hears a dog even if this is on the television. She avoids areas of her neighbourhood where she thinks she will come across dogs.

5. An 80-year-old lady is admitted to the old age psychiatric ward with a 2-week history of fluctuating confusion. She is intermittently drowsy, irritable, agitated and has sleep disturbance. She is disorientated in time and reports seeing naked men coming into her room.

Answers to **5.11**

1. F   Mental retardation

This category comprises mild, moderate, severe and profound mental retardation (learning difficulty). It is essentially a condition of arrested/incomplete development of the mind, especially characterized by impairment of skills manifest during the developmental period and which contribute to the overall level of intelligence including cognitive, language, motor and social abilities.

2. A   Behavioural and emotional disorders

This ICD-10 category comprises hyperkinetic, conduct and emotional disorders with childhood onset, disorders of social functioning and tic disorders. The symptoms described are suggestive of a hyperkinetic disorder which is a group of disorders characterized by: onset before the age of 6, overactivity, impaired attention, pervasiveness over different situations and persistence over time.

3. D   Disorders of psychological development

This category includes specific developmental disorders of speech and language, scholastic skills, motor function and pervasive developmental disorders. The history is suggestive of Asperger's syndrome, which is a type of pervasive developmental disorder (PDD). Other PDDs include conditions such as autism and Rett's syndrome. They are characterized by qualitative abnormalities in reciprocal social interaction and communication patterns and by restricted, stereotyped, repetitive repertoires of activities and interests. These difficulties are usually present from infancy.

4. H   Neurotic, stress-related and somatoform disorders

This category comprises phobic anxiety disorders (including agoraphobia, social and specific phobias), other anxiety disorders (including panic disorder and generalized anxiety disorder), obsessive compulsive disorder, reactions to severe stress and adjustment disorders (including post-traumatic stress disorder), dissociative and somatoform disorders. The symptoms here are suggestive of a specific phobia restricted to a very particular situation, e.g. certain animals, heights, flying or going to the dentist.

5. I   Organic, including symptomatic mental disorders

This category includes the dementias, delirium, and other mental, personality and behavioural disorders due to brain disease, damage and dysfunction. Delirium associated with the use of alcohol or other psychoactive substances should not be classified in this section.

Diagnosis of alcohol-related disorders

A   Acute alcohol intoxication
B   Alcohol dependence syndrome
C   Alcoholic hallucinosis
D   Alcohol-induced hypoglycaemia
E   Alcohol-related dementia
F   Alcohol withdrawal state
G   Alcohol withdrawal state with delirium
H   Harmful use of alcohol
I   Korsakoff's psychosis
J   Pathological intoxication with alcohol
K   Wernicke's encephalopathy

For each patient below, choose the SINGLE most likely diagnosis from the above list of options. Each option may be used once, more than once, or not at all.

1. A 45-year-old stockbroker with a long history of alcohol-related problems is admitted to the medical ward in a confused state. His wife reports that recently he has also been unsteady on his legs. On examination, he has an ocular palsy and a polyneuropathy.

2. A 38-year-old hairdresser consults her general practitioner with concerns about her alcohol use. She states that she has difficulty in controlling her alcohol intake and feels compelled to drink. She is drinking more than she used to in order to achieve the same effect and gets tremulous and sweaty if she tries to reduce the amount that she drinks.

3. A 35-year-old pharmaceutical representative presents to her GP in a distressed state. She admits to a long-standing heavy alcohol intake but is more concerned regarding the recent strange experiences. She is hearing music playing in the office at work and derogatory voices commenting on her drinking habits. On occasions, the voices would tell her to 'finish it all'.

4. A 70-year-old retired man is admitted to the old age psychiatry ward with a history of impaired recent memory. On examination, he is noted to be alert but gives a rambling and highly improbable account of his life prior to the hospital admission. He also has a peripheral neuropathy.

5. A 25-year-old teacher visits her GP primarily because of the concerns that her friends have about her when they are having a night out in town. After consumption of a small amount of alcohol she becomes boisterous, aggressive and often gets into arguments. This is out of character for her and recently she narrowly escaped being arrested by the police.

Answers to 5.12

1. **K   Wernicke's encephalopathy**

   Wernicke's encephalopathy is characterized by the classic triad of confusion, ocular palsy and ataxia. The commonest cause is thiamine deficiency from malnutrition due to chronic alcoholism. The onset of symptoms is often sudden. The patient is fully conscious but may find it hard to concentrate and answer questions.

2. **B   Alcohol dependence syndrome**

   The alcohol dependence syndrome requires three or more of the following symptoms to be present at some point during the past year – a strong desire to drink, difficulty controlling the onset, termination or level of alcohol use, and the presence of a physiological withdrawal state when alcohol use has been reduced or stopped. There is also evidence of tolerance.

3. **C   Alcoholic hallucinosis**

   In alcoholic hallucinosis (a psychotic disorder), hallucinations occur in clear consciousness. These experiences can be a continuation of hallucinations during a withdrawal state or can start afresh in someone who is still drinking. Experiences are usually auditory and may start as ill-formed, but develop into 2nd or 3rd person hallucinations. Persecutory delusions may result. The vast majority of sufferers will recover if abstinence is achieved and maintained.

4. **I   Korsakoff's psychosis**

   This is a late consequence of alcoholism and is characterized by impaired recent memory, retrograde amnesia, peripheral neuropathy and confabulation. Confabulation is the tendency, when asked about past events and experiences, to produce implausible, rambling accounts of unlikely happenings. There is no insight into the sometimes ridiculous stories. The pathology is indistinguishable from Wernicke's encephalopathy and the aetiology is again thiamine deficiency.

5. **J   Pathological intoxication with alcohol**

   Pathological intoxication is also known as 'mania à potu' or a pathological reaction to alcohol. This is not recognized to occur with other psychoactive drugs. Soon after consumption of the amounts of alcohol that would not produce intoxication in the majority of people, there is a sudden onset of aggressive or violent behaviour. This tends to be out of character for the person when sober. The episode is often followed by fatigue, heavy sleep and subsequent amnesia.

Diagnosis of psychiatric disorders presenting with physical symptoms

A Depersonalization derealization syndrome
B Dissociative anaesthesia
C Dissociative convulsion
D Dissociative fugue
E Dissociative motor disorder
F Dissociative stupor
G Ganser's syndrome
H Hypochondriacal disorder
I Neurasthenia
J Somatization disorder
K Somatoform autonomic dysfunction

For each patient below, choose the SINGLE most likely diagnosis from the above list of options. Each option may be used once, more than once, or not at all.

1. A 25-year-old woman presents with a 6-week history of 'funny turns' starting at about the same time as when the long-term relationship with her partner ended. A friend who witnessed these attacks states that she collapses to the floor, shakes all over, her arms thrash about and she does not respond to verbal prompts.

2. A 44-year-old lady has been off work for the past 2 months and feeling weak and exhausted with the slightest physical effort. She cannot sleep, her muscles ache and she finds it impossible to relax. No abnormal physical findings are evident.

3. A 48-year-old lady is seen in the general medical clinic at her local hospital. Over the last 20 years, she has complained of multiple physical symptoms, the most recent of these being intermittent chest pains. She has had all the necessary investigations and no physical finding has been found to account for her pains. She has seen numerous specialists.

4. A 13-year-old boy is taken to see his GP by his worried parents. He has been complaining that he cannot move his left leg properly and that this causes him to limp when he walks. His doctor cannot find a physical cause to explain his symptoms.

5. A 40-year-old man consults his GP on a regular basis with concerns about his physical health. Specifically, he believes that he has stomach cancer and he complains of indigestion and weight loss. He has been thoroughly investigated and declared to be in excellent health.

Answers to **5.13**

1. **C   Dissociative convulsion**

    Dissociative (or conversion) disorders are characterized by a loss of the normal integration between memories of the past, awareness of identity and immediate sensations and control of bodily movements. They are psychogenic in origin and linked with traumatic life events, difficult relationships or insoluble problems. The resulting unpleasant effect is then transformed into physical symptoms, as 'seizures' in this case.

2. **I   Neurasthenia**

    This is synonymous with the chronic fatigue syndrome. There are two main types: increased fatigue after mental effort, and lethargy after minimal physical exertion. Also present must be two of the following symptoms: muscle aches and pains, dizziness, indigestion, tension headaches, disturbed sleep, irritability and difficulty relaxing. A depressive illness or anxiety disorder should be ruled out.

3. **J   Somatization disorder**

    Somatization disorder (often familial) consists of at least a 2-year history of multiple and variable physical symptoms for which no satisfactory physical cause has been found, ongoing refusal to accept reassurance regarding negative test findings, and some degree of impairment in family or social functioning because of symptoms and related behaviours. Typically, patients (mostly females) have had contact with numerous doctors and have many volumes of hospital notes.

4. **E   Dissociative motor disorder**

    Dissociative motor disorders can be of several types: loss of ability to move a limb or any type of ataxia, apraxia, akinesia, aphonia, dysarthria or paralysis. The symptoms may not be compatible with any anatomical or physiological principles. The resulting loss of function and disability helps the patient escape from psychological distress or conflict.

5. **H   Hypochondriacal disorder**

    Hypochondriacal disorder is characterized by a persistent belief that there is at least one serious physical illness underlying the symptoms (even though all investigations have confirmed no physical cause) or an ongoing preoccupation with a presumed deformity or physical abnormality. Reassurance from many different doctors is not accepted. There is no familial component and it is equally prevalent in men and women.

Substance abuse

A   Benzodiazepine abuse
B   Benzodiazepine withdrawal
C   Cocaine abuse
D   Cocaine withdrawal
E   Opioid abuse
F   Opioid withdrawal
G   LSD abuse
H   LSD withdrawal
I   Ecstasy abuse
J   Ecstasy withdrawal
K   Amfetamine (amphetamine) withdrawal

For each presentation below, choose the SINGLE most likely cause from
the above list of options. Each option can be used once, more than once,
or not at all.

1. A 36-year-old man is admitted to a medical ward with cellulitis of his
    forearm. Six hours after his admission he develops nausea and diarrhoea
    and he becomes agitated and restless. He also has rhinorrhoea and
    increased lacrimation. On examination, his pupils are dilated.

2. A 16-year-old college student is brought to the A&E department by his
    friends after he had collapsed at a party. They report that he was dancing
    all night and could have taken some drugs. His body temperature is
    41°C and the skin and mucous membranes appear dry. He has also had
    a convulsion in the ambulance.

3. A 16-year-old girl is found by the police on the top of a ten-storey
    building. When interviewed she says she believes that she can fly. She is
    elated and talks of hearing colours and feeling that the room around her
    has moving walls and ceiling.

4. A 41-year-old drug dealer has been in police custody for 2 hours when
    he is observed to be talking to himself. He begins to scratch himself and
    appears frightened. He is seen shouting in his cell, 'spiders, get off me'.

5. A 52-year-old man complains of anxiety, disturbed sleep, tiredness and
    trembling of his hands. He was aware of these symptoms a few days
    after his recent hospitalization for a chest infection.

Answers to 5.14

1. **F   Opioid withdrawal**

   Heroin is the most commonly used opioid. Its main effect is euphoria
   which is initially intense. Regular users may develop chronic malaise,
   anorexia, pin-point pupils and constipation. Dependence occurs within
   weeks if regularly used. Stopping opioid use leads to an unpleasant
   withdrawal syndrome referred to as 'cold turkey'. It begins within
   4–12 hours after the last dose and peak effects are within 24–48 hours.
   The symptoms include insomnia, sweating, vomiting, diarrhoea, dilated
   pupils, runny nose and eyes, yawning and tachycardia.

2. **I   Ecstasy use**

   Ecstasy (3,4-methylenedioxymethamphetamine – MDMA) is an
   amphetamine and possesses both stimulant and hallucinogenic
   properties. It is widely used at parties and in night clubs and the effects
   last about 4–6 hours. It produces a feeling of euphoria and intimacy
   towards others. Adverse reactions are hyperpyrexia and acute renal
   failure due to dehydration. This is more common in users who have
   been dancing for long hours in crowded, hot places without drinking
   water.

3. **G   LSD abuse**

   Lysergic acid diethylamine (LSD) is chemically related to
   5-hydroxytryptophan, an important neurotransmitter. It is a
   hallucinogen and its effects peak 2 hours after consumption. It causes
   changes in the sense of time and place, heightened perception of sounds
   and colour and movement of stationary objects. It can also cause
   synaesthesia in which a stimulus in one sensory modality is experienced
   in another, e.g. hearing colours. Delusions such as believing that one
   can fly can lead to serious accidents.

4. **C   Cocaine abuse**

   Cocaine is a stimulant derived from the leaves of the coca shrub. Acute
   effects include euphoria, agitation and dilated pupils. High doses can
   result in auditory, visual and tactile hallucinations (cocaine bug).
   Chronic use leads to tolerance and drug withdrawal causes anxiety,
   irritation and an intense craving for the drug.

5. **B   Benzodiazepine withdrawal**

   Benzodiazepines are widely prescribed and produce physical
   dependence. Abrupt discontinuation of the drug during hospitalization
   for an unrelated illness can cause withdrawal symptoms which are
   related to the half-life of the drug used. Symptoms include rebound
   anxiety, insomnia, agitation, tremor, malaise and weakness.

Trauma and Orthopaedics

Anatomical structures damaged in wrist trauma

A Brachioradialis
B Flexor carpi radialis
C Flexor carpi ulnaris
D Flexor digitorum profundus
E Flexor digitorum superficialis
F Flexor pollicis longus
G Median nerve
H Palmaris longus
I Pronator quadratus
J Radial nerve
K Ulnar nerve

For each scenario below, choose the SINGLE structure most likely to be affected from the above list of options. Each option may be used once, more than once, or not at all.

1. A patient sustained an incised wound over the volar aspect of his wrist. The examining doctor asks him to flex his middle finger while holding his other fingers in extension. Which muscle/tendon is he testing?

2. A patient fell onto broken glass and sustained a puncture wound over the volar aspect of his right wrist. Thumb abduction is weak and he complains of loss of sensation over the lateral three and a half digits. Which structure has been damaged?

3. A patient fell onto a metal spike and sustained a penetrating injury to the volar aspect of his right wrist. Examination reveals a claw hand. Which structure has been damaged?

4. A patient slashed his own wrist with a razor blade and sustained a transverse incised wound over the volar aspect of his wrist. The wound was explored and one of the wrist tendons was found to have been severed. Repair of that tendon was felt to be unnecessary. Which is this tendon that has little effect on hand and wrist function?

5. A patient is asked to abduct his fingers while the examining doctor places his thumb on the ulnar side of his wrist, feeling for the tensing of a tendon. Which muscle/tendon is being tested?

Answers to **6.1**

1. **E**   Flexor digitorum superficialis

This is the superficialis test. Flexion at the proximal interphalangeal joint of a finger can be achieved both by the superficialis and the profundus tendon. Because the profundus tendons act in unison (quadregia effect), holding the other fingers in extension will neutralize the effect of the profundus tendon on the finger being tested. Flexion at the proximal interphalangeal is then solely due to the action of the superficialis.

2. **G**   Median nerve

Loss of sensation suggests nerve damage. The distribution is characteristic for the median nerve. The median nerve is the motor supply to all of the small muscles of the thenar eminence, except for the adductor which is supplied by the ulnar nerve.

3. **K**   Ulnar nerve

The clawing deformity is a result of the paralysis of the interossei and the medial two lumbrical muscles, which flex the fingers at the metacarpophalangeal joints with the distal joints extended. When these muscles are paralysed, the unopposed action of the long flexors and extensors of the ring and little fingers produce hyperextension at the metacarpophalangeal joints and flexion of the distal phalangeal joints. The ulnar nerve may be injured by penetrating wounds at any point in its course and in fractures, dislocations and arthritis of the elbow and wrist.

4. **H**   Palmaris longus

This is a weak flexor and is absent in 10–15% of the population. The main use of this presumed vestigial tendon is for reconstruction of other tendon pathologies and its absence can cause problems. The other similar donor tendon is the plantaris tendon. Such self-inflicted injuries are common and doctors dealing with such injuries must be competent in carrying out an adequate examination and have a high index of suspicion, as partial injuries are commonly missed.

5. **C**   Flexor carpi ulnaris

The abductor digiti minimi has its origin at the pisiform bone at the insertion of the tendon of the flexor carpi ulnaris. Its action is to abduct the little finger. The flexor carpi ulnaris inserts at the pisiform bone and acts synergistically to fix the point of origin during the action of the abductor digiti minimi.

Soft tissue and bony injuries

A   Achilles tendon rupture
B   Fractured calcaneum
C   Injury to digital branch of ulnar nerve
D   Malunited Colles' fracture
E   Median nerve injury
F   Rupture of deltoid ligament
G   Rupture of extensor pollicis longus
H   Rupture of subscapularis
I   Rupture of supraspinatus tendon
J   Talofibular ligament injury
K   Un-united Colles' fracture

For each patient below, choose the SINGLE most likely diagnosis from the above list of options. Each option may be used once, more than once, or not at all.

1. A 45-year-old man develops a sudden pain in his left heel while playing badminton. He limps into the A&E department. The duty doctor examines him in the prone position. When his calf muscles are gently squeezed the foot fails to plantar-flex and remains still.

2. A 65-year-old lady reports to the A&E department with inability to effectively use her right thumb. She was treated 2 months ago for a right Colles' fracture.

3. A 50-year-old farmer after intensive physiotherapy to his right shoulder reports to the fracture clinic. He had sustained an anterior dislocation of his shoulder 3 months ago which was reduced promptly. Now he cannot pick up any object above his shoulder. Attempted abduction of his shoulder results in a characteristic shrug, but passive abduction is still possible.

4. A 21-year-old lady wearing high-heeled shoes twists her ankle on a kerb and limps into A&E with a swollen and painful right ankle. Inversion of the foot in equinus position is extremely painful. X-rays of the foot and ankle are normal.

5. A 73-year-old man fell backwards in his green house and cut his left hand with glass. He has a wound in the middle of his palm with a spurting vessel. He has paraesthesiae over the palmar aspect of his left middle and index fingers.

Answers to **6.2**

1. A   Achilles tendon rupture

Simmond's test/Thompson's test is used to assess the integrity of the Achilles tendon. With the patient prone, the calf is squeezed; if the tendon is intact the foot is seen to plantar-flex; if the tendon is ruptured the foot remains still.

2. G   Rupture of extensor pollicis longus

Rupture of extensor pollicis longus occasionally occurs a few weeks after a Colles' fracture. This attrition rupture occurs where the tendon loops around the Lister's tubercle (the dorsal tubercle of the radius).

3. I   Rupture of supraspinatus tendon

Any tear of the rotator cuff usually involves the supraspinatus tendon. Most cuff tears run through an already damaged area of tissue often associated with repetitive minor trauma or subacromial impingement. Shoulder dislocation is commonly associated with damage to the rotator cuff in patients over 50 years of age. Supraspinatus is responsible for the first 30 degrees of abduction at the shoulder joint. Abnormal shoulder shrugging is due to compensatory scapulothoracic movement in an effort to improve shoulder abduction.

4. J   Talofibular ligament injury

The talofibular ligament, which is part of the lateral ligament complex of the ankle, is often ruptured in an ankle sprain. Passive inversion of the foot is painful and routine X-rays of the ankle are normal.

5. E   Median nerve injury

Altered sensation to the middle and index fingers after a laceration to the hand is due to a direct injury to the digital branches of the median nerve.

Spinal injuries

A   Analgesia and early physiotherapy
B   An indwelling urinary catheter
C   Carefully walk the patient with support
D   Intermittent self-catheterization
E   Log-roll with four helpers
F   Log-roll with two helpers
G   Magnetic resonance image (MRI) scan
H   Suprapubic catheterization
I   Transfer on a spinal board
J   Turn patient every 6 hours
K   Turn patient every 2 hours

For each patient below, choose the SINGLE most appropriate management from the above list of options. Each option may be used once, more than once, or not at all.

1. A 32-year-old lady motorist is injured in a 50-mph road traffic accident. She complains of pain in her back. The paramedics have to decide upon the safest way to transfer her to the ambulance.

2. An elderly lady falls down the stairs of her residential home and is complaining of back pain. The doctor assessing the patient decides upon the safest way to assess the patient's spine.

3. A roof tiler falls off the roof of a house. An X-ray taken in the resuscitation room shows a fracture dislocation of T12 over L1. The bulbocavernous reflex is absent. His anal sphincters are patulous on rectal examination and he has no useful function below the level of his injury. The doctor decides upon the best way to manage the urinary tract.

4. A 40-year-old building site worker with a traumatic paraplegia is just being brought into one of the orthopaedic wards awaiting transfer to a spinal centre. It will be at least another 6 hours before he is transferred. The ward sister is worried about the risk of pressure sores.

5. A 30-year-old business executive applies a sudden brake to her car to avoid an irate pedestrian. This ends in a low-energy rear-end collision with a car coming behind her. She is thrown forwards and the head jerked backwards. She walks into the A&E department a day later with pain and stiffness in her neck. There are no neurological signs and the cervical spine X-ray is normal.

Answers to **6.3**

1.   I   Transfer on a spinal board

Patients with suspected spinal injuries should be moved as carefully as possible to minimize intervertebral movement. Transferring the patient on a spinal board can achieve this. It is important to note that the spinal board is only a device for transfer of the patient to hospital, and once the patient is on an assessment trolley the board should be carefully removed. These devices can lead to the development of pressure sores in individuals with sensory loss.

2.   E   Log-roll with four helpers

Log-rolling the patient requires four helpers and aims to minimize the intervertebral movement. One individual is in charge of the neck and cervical spine. Two persons control the thorax and abdomen and one person looks after the legs. The examining doctor should be free to perform the examination with reasonable assurance for the safety of the patient.

3.   B   An indwelling urinary catheter

The high-energy nature of a fracture dislocation at the thoracolumbar junction will often result in an injury to the spinal cord. Urine production continues but the patients will often develop painless retention. In the initial period an indwelling urinary catheter is the treatment of choice. There is a risk of infection with long term indwelling urethral or suprapubic catheters and most patients learn to self-catheterize as part of their rehabilitation.

4.   K   Turn patient every 2 hours

The anaesthetic skin of a traumatic paraplegic patient may develop significant pressure sores within a few hours. Every 2 hours the patient is either manually rolled on to alternate sides to avoid pressure or special turning beds are used for the same purpose. Stretching exercises are employed when spasticity may lead to contracture formation but they do not play a role in early management.

5.   A   Analgesia and early physiotherapy

'Whiplash injury' is commonly used to describe a soft tissue injury to the neck when it is suddenly jerked into hyperextension, although the actual mechanism of injury often involves many patterns of movement at the time of impact. There is often a delay in presentation; patients usually complain of pain and stiffness in the neck and sometimes they have ill-defined symptoms like dizziness, headache and paraesthesiae in the arms. There are usually no physical signs and X-rays show only postural changes due to spasm. MRI may show some altered signals in significant soft tissue injuries but is not usually needed in the management of low-energy trauma to the neck with a delayed presentation.

Diagnosis of knee trauma

A   Anterior cruciate ligament injury
B   Lateral collateral ligament injury
C   Lateral meniscus injury
D   Medial collateral ligament injury
E   Medial meniscus injury
F   Osteochondral fracture
G   Patella fracture
H   Posterior cruciate ligament injury
I   Rupture of the patellar ligament
J   Rupture of the quadriceps tendon
K   Triad of O'Donahue

For each patient below, choose the SINGLE most likely diagnosis from the above list of options. Each option may be used once, more than once, or not at all.

1. A 20-year-old football player presents with a hyperextension injury to his right knee sustained in a tackle during a football match. He heard a 'pop' at the time of injury. The knee became swollen immediately and he was unable to continue playing.

2. A 17-year-old football player injures his right knee in a tackle and it swells up immediately. An X-ray of his knee reveals lipohaemarthrosis but there is no sign of a significant fracture. The knee is aspirated and 100 mL of blood is obtained with fat globules floating on the surface of the blood.

3. Following an injury, a 22-year-old rugby player is unable to extend his knee. Examination reveals a palpable gap above the patella and a lateral X-ray of the knee looks normal apart from some soft tissue fullness proximal to the patella.

4. A 24-year-old rugby player receives a blow to the lateral aspect of his left knee during a tackle. There is increased laxity on valgus stressing of the knee but the anterior drawer or Lachman test is normal (with the knee semi-flexed, the tibia will not yield when pushed forwards).

5. A 24-year-old football player sustains a twisting injury to his right knee. He is unable to fully extend his right knee and on examination there is an effusion and tenderness over the medial joint line.

Answers to **6.4**

1.   A   Anterior cruciate ligament injury

The anterior cruciate ligament prevents anterior glide of the tibia upon the femur, which may be ruptured by a twisting movement or by a tackle which forces the proximal tibia forwards. Around 70% of patients describe hearing a snapping or popping sound at the time of injury. Immediate swelling of the knee following injury is suggestive of bleeding into the joint (haemarthrosis). Patients will often have a restricted range of movement in the knee due to the haemarthrosis and removal of this will also help to relieve pain.

2.   F   Osteochondral fracture

Marrow fat enters the knee joint when there is an intra-articular fracture. A fat-fluid level within the suprapatellar bursa (lipohaemarthrosis) is indicative of an intra-articular fracture, even if not seen on the X-ray.

3.   J   Rupture of the quadriceps tendon

A palpable, sometimes visible, dent above the patella is characteristic of the rupture of the quadriceps tendon. The patella is usually situated in a relatively normal position after a quadriceps rupture due to the intact patella retinaculae. This is in contrast to the patella lying 'high' with rupture of the patellar tendon.

4.   D   Medial collateral ligament injury

Although isolated tears of the medial collateral ligament are uncommon, a blow to the lateral aspect of the knee will result in valgus stress and damage the medial collateral ligament MCL. A positive anterior drawer test (the tibia will yield when pressed forwards) is indicative of anterior cruciate ligament (ACL) injury. In the context of a medial collateral ligament injury an injury complex involving the MCL, ACL and the medial meniscus must be considered (triad of O'Donahue).

5.   E   Medial meniscus injury

A meniscal tear is usually caused by a twisting injury to the knee, when it is semiflexed and weight-bearing. A springy lock to full extension (part of the displaced meniscus prevents full extension) together with sudden unlocking (reduction of the displaced meniscus) are important symptoms though tenderness in the joint line may be the only sign. Magnetic resonance imaging (MRI) may be used to confirm the diagnosis. Alternatively early arthroscopy for locked knees can be used to diagnose and treat the cause simultaneously.

Diagnosis of nerve trauma

A Axillary nerve
B Brachial plexus
C Common peroneal nerve
D Femoral nerve
E Lateral cutaneous nerve of thigh
F Median nerve
G Radial nerve
H Sciatic nerve
I Sural nerve
J Tibial nerve
K Ulnar nerve

For each patient below, choose the SINGLE most likely diagnosis from the above list of options. Each option may be used once, more than once, or not at all.

1. A 40-year-old patient has sustained an anterior dislocation of his right shoulder. There is loss of sensation over the 'regimental badge' area of the shoulder.

2. A 35-year-old patient presents with a spiral fracture of the shaft of the right humerus. Examination reveals a right wrist drop.

3. A 60-year-old patient sustains a posterior dislocation of his right hip in a road traffic accident. He now has foot drop on the same side.

4. A 20-year-old pedestrian is hit by a car in his lower leg. X-rays reveal a fracture of the proximal fibula. He also has foot drop in the affected leg.

5. A 25-year-old patient sustains a glass cut to the back of his right heel at work. Examination confirms severance of the right Achilles tendon. He also has numbness over the lateral border of the foot.

Answers to **6.5**

1. **A** **Axillary nerve**

An axillary nerve (C5, 6) injury is a well-known complication of anterior shoulder dislocation and fractures of the proximal humerus, as the nerve winds around the neck of the humerus. Anaesthesia over the 'regimental patch' (area overlying the deltoid), which is exclusively supplied by the axillary nerve, is a good indication of injury to this nerve. Most cases resolve over a 3-month period but deltoid wasting will be evident in long standing cases.

2. **G** **Radial nerve**

The radial nerve (C5, 6, 7, 8) curves around the spiral groove of the shaft of the humerus before dividing just below the elbow into the posterior interosseous nerve (supplies extensor musculature of the forearm) and the superficial radial nerve (supplies sensation). Radial nerve palsy is most commonly due to fracture of the humerus or prolonged pressure on the arm (e.g. Saturday-night palsy whilst intoxicated by alcohol). Clinical features include wrist drop and paralysis of the wrist extensors. Weakness of the triceps occurs with lesions high in the arm. Sensory loss is minimal but usually extends over the first dorsal interosseous muscle on the dorsum of the hand and along the radial border of the wrist.

3. **H** **Sciatic nerve**

A sciatic nerve (L4, 5; S1, 2, 3) injury must always be considered in posterior dislocation of the hip. Where a posterior wall fracture is present there will have been a large transfer of energy around the hip joint and the nerve is at particular risk. The patient will be in considerable pain with posterior dislocation of the hip and the lower limb will be short, adducted and internally rotated. As with all of these injuries, care must be taken prior to anaesthesia to document neurological deficit because this is often poorly assessed when the patient is in pain and examination is difficult.

4. **C** **Common peroneal nerve**

'Bumper-height', direct trauma can damage the common peroneal nerve. Both dorsiflexion (deep peroneal branch) and eversion (superficial peroneal branch) of the foot will be affected. There is sensory loss over the first web space (deep peroneal nerve), the dorsum of the foot and the front and side of the lower leg (superficial peroneal nerve).

5. **I** **Sural nerve**

The sural nerve runs alongside the Achilles tendon and supplies sensation to the lateral border of the foot. It is particularly at risk during operative repair of fibula fractures and from rupture of the Achilles tendon.

Diagnosis of vascular injury accompanying skeletal trauma

A   Compression of anterior or posterior tibial artery
B   Compression of dorsalis pedis artery
C   Contusion of axillary artery
D   Contusion of brachial artery
E   Contusion of femoral artery
F   Contusion of subclavian artery
G   Laceration of an intercostal artery
H   Rupture of the thoracic aorta
I   Thrombosis of brachial artery
J   Thrombosis of popliteal artery
K   Thrombosis of radial artery

For each patient below, choose the SINGLE most likely diagnosis from the above list of options. Each option may be used once, more than once, or not at all.

1.   A 30-year-old man presents in shock with chest and pelvic injuries following a road traffic accident. Plain X-rays reveal fractures of the sternum, left clavicle, and several ribs on the left side. There is evidence of mediastinal widening and he requires continuous fluid support to maintain his blood pressure.

2.   An 8-year-old boy presents with an injury to his left elbow after falling off a tree. Examination reveals swelling and deformity to the left elbow with an absence of the radial pulse. X-ray shows a supracondylar fracture of the left humerus with substantial deformity.

3.   A 25-year-old man suffers a fracture dislocation of his right ankle while playing rugby. Examination reveals absent distal pulses of the right foot.

4.   A 35-year-old man is brought to the A&E department after a motorcycle accident in which his hip is forcefully extended and abducted. His right lower limb pulses are diminished.

5.   A 25-year-old builder presents after falling off a roof and sustaining a fracture to the right tibial shaft. His right pedal pulses are absent, and his right foot is cold.

Answers to **6.6**

1. **H** Rupture of the thoracic aorta

The presence of rib fractures in association with shoulder girdle injuries indicates a high-energy injury. Most visceral injuries seen are due to rapid deceleration and are frequently fatal at the scene. Severe deceleration injuries should be suspected with the fractures of the sternum, first rib and shoulder girdle. Rupture of the thoracic aorta (usually between the left subclavian artery and ligamentum arteriosum) and subsequent circulatory shock is uncommon, but should be suspected when the chest X-ray shows mediastinal widening and often blunting of the contour of the aortic knuckle. An arch aortogram is the investigation of choice to investigate a leak.

2. **D** Contusion of brachial artery

Supracondylar fractures are one of the most serious fractures in childhood because they are associated with an interruption to blood supply to the forearm, if the brachial artery is kinked, contused or severed at the anterior aspect of the proximal fragment of the humerus. If untreated the ensuing ischaemia may lead to muscle atrophy in the forearm (Volkmann's ischaemic contracture). Usually, with traction and correction of the deformity the pulse returns.

3. **B** Compression of dorsalis pedis artery

Fracture dislocation of the ankle is commonly associated with absence of the foot pulses due to kinking of the vessels. Prompt reduction should be undertaken in the emergency department.

4. **E** Contusion of femoral artery

Anterior dislocation of the hip is rare but can occur with violent abduction in road traffic accidents. The dislocated hip can compress the femoral artery, which lies anteriorly, and compromise its flow. Reduction should be performed promptly. Other complications of anterior dislocation include aseptic necrosis of the femoral head and osteoarthrosis.

5. **A** Compression of anterior or posterior tibial artery

A displaced fracture of the tibial shaft can cause injuries to the anterior or posterior tibial artery but most commonly these vessels are kinked at the fracture site. If left untreated this can compromise the circulation in the foot and ankle and lead to irretrievable tissue damage. Absent pulses are a surgical emergency and if reduction of the fracture does not restore the pulses consideration should be given to an urgent arteriogram.

Diagnosis of head trauma

A   Basal skull fracture
B   Cerebral contusion
C   Concussion
D   Depressed skull fracture
E   Diffuse axonal injury
F   Extradural haematoma
G   Intracerebral haemorrhage
H   Post-concussional syndrome
I   Subarachnoid haemorrhage
J   Subdural haematoma
K   Uncal herniation

For each patient below, choose the SINGLE most likely diagnosis from the above list of options. Each option may be used once, more than once, or not at all.

1. A 20-year-old man sustains a head injury in a road traffic accident. He remains deeply comatosed after initial resuscitation. He has no other significant injury and the computed tomography (CT) of his head is normal.

2. A 46-year-old woman who presented with a severe head injury develops a dilated pupil on the right side and weakness on the left side.

3. A 20-year-old man was punched in the right temporal region of his head. He became unconscious initially but regained full consciousness after a few minutes. An hour later, he deteriorated suddenly and became unrousable.

4. A 25-year-old man has been involved in a fight and was kicked repeatedly in his head. On arrival in the A&E department his Glasgow Coma Scale is 8. He has bruising behind his left ear and leakage of a clear fluid from the same ear.

5. A 39-year-old man with a severe head injury has a computed tomography (CT) scan that suggests a collection of blood in a crescent-shaped pattern, conforming to the convexity of the cerebral hemisphere.

Answers to **6.7**

1.   E   Diffuse axonal injury

Diffuse axonal injury occurs with severe head injuries causing distortion and tearing of axonal tracts in the cerebral hemispheres and brainstem on impact. Tiny neuronal lesions (retraction balls) can be seen microscopically in the brain. Initially there is impaired consciousness which is transient in mild cases. Prolonged coma is associated with severe disability and increased risk of mortality.

2.   K   Uncal herniation

The uncus is the most medial portion of the cerebral hemisphere which is often the first part of the brain to herniate through the tentorial notch, with raised intracranial pressure from an expanding mass. As the uncus is forced medially and downward, the ipsilateral 3rd cranial nerve is compressed producing pupillary dilatation and other signs of a 3rd nerve palsy. As herniation progresses, the pyramidal tract becomes involved producing a contralateral hemiplegia. With intracranial pressure (ICP) monitoring it is possible to assess the effects of treatment on the ICP in order to try to minimize the risk of herniation.

3.   F   Extradural haematoma

Extradural or epidural haematoma is usually due to injury to the middle meningeal artery associated with a fracture in the temporal bone. The initial loss of consciousness is from cerebral concussion. After a brief interval the patient regains consciousness and appears to have made a full recovery. However, during this interval blood begins to accumulate between the fracture site and the underlying dura leading to a rise in the ICP. This can then cause a mechanical distortion of the brain and impair cerebral perfusion. Prompt evacuation of blood is the treatment of choice.

4.   A   Basal skull fracture

The diagnosis of basal skull fracture is mainly clinical as fractures are rarely seen on plain skull X-rays. Signs of basal skull fracture include haemotympanum, cerebrospinal fluid otorrhoea or rhinorrhoea, retromastoid (Battle's sign) or periorbital ecchymosis ('raccoon eyes') and a 7th nerve palsy. The petrous temporal bone is the commonest site of basal skull fracture.

5.   J   Subdural haematoma

The appearance on the computed tomography (CT) is classically that of an acute subdural haematoma which is four times more common than an extradural haematoma. The blood accumulates between the dura and the arachnoid following tears of the bridging veins or cortical lacerations. The interval between injury and clinical presentation may vary between a few minutes to several weeks.

Diagnosis of thoracic trauma

A Blunt oesophageal rupture
B Cardiac tamponade
C Flail chest
D Massive haemothorax
E Myocardial contusion
F Open pneumothorax
G Pulmonary contusion
H Simple pneumothorax
I Tension pneumothorax
J Traumatic aortic rupture
K Traumatic diaphragmatic rupture

For each scenario below, choose the SINGLE most likely diagnosis from the above list of options. Each option may be used once, more than once or not at all.

1. A 20-year-old man is stabbed in the left side of his chest. On examination in the A&E department, he has a blood pressure of 90/60 mmHg, pulse rate of 140 beats per minute, a respiratory rate of 38 breaths per minute, distended neck veins, tracheal deviation to the right and a tympanitic percussion note, with absent breath sounds over the left side of the chest.

2. A 25-year-old man is stabbed in the left side of his chest. He is brought to the A&E department with a blood pressure of 65/40 mmHg, pulse rate of 140 beats per minute, distended neck veins and muffled heart sounds.

3. An 18-year-old man is brought to the emergency unit after having fallen 20 feet from a tree, landing on the right side of his chest. He exhibits paradoxical movements on the right side of his chest wall with inspiration and expiration. Chest X-ray reveals fractures of his right 6th to 8th ribs at two places.

4. A 60-year-old man is brought to the emergency department following a head-on collision in a motor vehicle accident. He feels well in himself and is haemodynamically stable. His chest X-ray, however, reveals a widened mediastinum, obliteration of the aortic knob, tracheal deviation to the right and depression of the left main bronchus.

5. A 20-year-old man received a gun shot wound to the right side of his chest. A chest drain is inserted on the same side and an initial drainage of 1500 mL of blood is obtained.

Answers to **6.8**

1.   **I**   Tension pneumothorax

The scenario gives the classic signs of a tension pneumothorax. The increased pressure impedes venous return causing a decrease in cardiac output and hence hypotension. It is a life-threatening condition. Needle decompression should be done immediately. With highly suggestive signs as in this case, aspiration of air should be started and no time should be wasted in confirming the diagnosis by X-ray.

2.   **B**   Cardiac tamponade

With a history and evidence of thoracic injury, this so-called Beck's triad of distended neck veins, muffled heart sounds and hypotension is diagnostic of a cardiac tamponade. However, the neck veins may be collapsed if there is hypovolaemia due to concomitant bleeding from another site.

3.   **C**   Flail chest

A flail chest is created when two or more consecutive ribs are each fractured in at least two sites. This causes paradoxical movements with the inward movement of the fragment on inspiration and a failure of the normal mechanism of ventilation.

4.   **J**   Traumatic aortic rupture

This is classically caused by a deceleration injury. Many patients with such an injury die at the scene of the accident. Those who survive have the haematoma contained by an intact adventitial layer of the aorta. They are often misleadingly asymptomatic.

5.   **D**   Massive haemothorax

An initial drainage of over 1500 mL of blood is by definition a massive haemothorax. The likelihood of the patient requiring thoracotomy to stop the bleeding is high.

Trauma to the spine and spinal cord

A   Anterior spinal cord injury
B   Brown–Séquard injury
C   C6 spinal cord injury
D   C7 spinal cord injury
E   Central spinal cord injury
F   Chance fracture
G   Conus medularis injury
H   Hangman's fracture
I   Jefferson's fracture
J   Neurogenic shock
K   Spinal shock

For each scenario below, choose the SINGLE most likely diagnosis from the above list of options. Each option may be used once, more than once, or not at all.

1.   A 20-year-old man fell 15 feet off a ladder, landing on the top of his head and sustaining an injury to his neck. There are no abnormal neurological signs but the X-ray of the cervical spine reveals 'over-hanging of the lateral masses' of C1.

2.   A 30-year-old man sustained a cervical cord lesion. He is able to flex but not extend his elbow. He has sensory function in the radial aspect of his hand but not in the ulnar three fingers. How would you describe the level of his injury?

3.   A 30-year-old patient sustained a significant spinal cord injury. During the first 24 hours after the injury he had a complete loss of the deep tendon reflexes and the anal reflex.

4.   A 67-year-old man, known to suffer from cervical spondylosis, has had a fall and sustained a hyperextension injury to his neck. He has an incomplete cervical spinal cord injury; the motor dysfunction of the hands and arms is disproportionately worse than that of the lower extremities.

5.   A 20-year-old man has been stabbed in his neck. He has loss of motor function and position sense on one side of his body and has sensory loss on the other side of his body.

Answers to **6.9**

1. **I** **Jefferson's fracture**

Jefferson's fracture is a blow-out fracture of C1 from a direct downward force on the skull. A typical lateral view of the cervical spine may reveal an increased space (over 3 mm) between the odontoid peg and the arch of C1 and an increased prevertebral soft tissue shadow. Classically, 'overhanging of lateral masses' (asymmetry of the alignment of the lateral mass of C1 on C2), is seen in the open mouth 'peg' view. Typically, patients are neurologically intact.

2. **C** **C6 spinal cord injury**

The neurological level of a spinal cord injury is defined by the lowest functional level. Flexion of the elbow is a function of the biceps which is innervated by C5, 6, whereas extension of the elbow is a function of the triceps which is innervated by C7, 8. C6 also supplies sensation of the skin over the outer third of the hand.

3. **K** **Spinal shock**

The 'shock' to the injured cord may make it appear completely functionless but some recovery usually begins after 24 hours. It has been described as a concussion of the spinal cord. The cord-mediated reflexes are lost and the full extent of neurological injury cannot be determined until the 'shock' is over.

4. **E** **Central spinal cord injury**

Central spinal cord injury is rare but is important to recognize, as it is the reverse of the normal pattern. The patient may be erroneously regarded as malingering and the diagnosis missed. This normally occurs in a hyperextension injury in a patient with a narrowed canal, either congenitally, for example in spinal stenosis, or as a result of degenerative changes. The lesion is in the central portion of the cord. Because the more proximal innervation is placed centrally within the cord, the upper limbs are more affected than the lower limbs.

5. **B** **Brown–Séquard injury**

Brown–Séquard injury is a hemisection of the cord caused usually by a penetrating injury. A classic picture (spastic monoparesis and loss of or impaired position and vibration sense on the same side and loss or diminution of pain and temperature sense on the opposite side) is rare. Sensation to touch is often preserved because of the decussation of the mixed fibres. Contralateral pain and temperature loss occur because these fibres cross one or two levels above the root level. Motor decussation occurs higher up and so all levels are affected on the ipsilateral side below the injury.

Results of traumatic injury

A   Axillary nerve injury
B   Colles' fracture
C   Compartment syndrome
D   Deep vein thrombosis
E   Fractured neck of femur
F   Fracture of scaphoid
G   Fracture of trapezium
H   Musculocutaneous nerve injury
I   Posterior dislocation of hip
J   Rupture of anterior leg muscles
K   Suprascapular nerve injury

For each scenario below, choose the SINGLE most likely diagnosis from the above list of options. Each option may be used once, more than once, or not at all.

1. A 25-year-old young male is seen in the A&E department 2 days after he had a fall on to his outstretched right hand. Now he has tenderness and fullness of the anatomical snuff-box of the right wrist.

2. A 70-year-old lady has a fall in the high street and is brought to the A&E department with a dislocated right shoulder. The doctor examining her finds an area of numbness of the skin over the deltoid.

3. An 80-year-old frail lady who lives alone is found on the floor of her kitchen and is brought to the A&E department by the ambulance crew. After initial resuscitation, she is found to have a shortened and externally rotated left leg, which is painful on movement.

4. A 50-year-old woman slips on ice and reports to the A&E department with a dinner-fork deformity of her right wrist, which is painful and which she supports with her other hand.

5. A 23-year-old footballer is admitted to the ward with a fracture of his right tibia and fibula immobilized in an above-knee backslab. Three hours later, he complains of severe pain in his right leg and passive movements of his toes make it worse. The foot pulses are now barely palpable.

Answers to **6.10**

1. F Fracture of scaphoid

The scaphoid bone fracture is the most common fracture involving the carpal bones. It is typically common in the young male and is very often dismissed as a sprain thus delaying treatment. Clinical examination should demonstrate tenderness in the anatomical snuff-box.

2. A Axillary nerve injury

Anterior dislocation of the shoulder is the commonest of all large joint dislocations. This is usually caused by a fall on the hand. The lateral outline of the shoulder is flattened in a thin individual. The arm must always be examined for nerve and vessel injury.

3. E Fractured neck of femur

A fractured neck of femur is more commonly seen in the eighth or ninth decade of life. There is usually a history of a fall. The patient lies with the limb in external rotation and the leg can appear shortened. Minimally displaced intracapsular fractures will often not show this typical deformity. Loss of the ability to raise the straight leg is one of the most sensitive indicators of pathology in the hip.

4. B Colles' fracture

A Colles' fracture is the most common of all fractures in older people and postmenopausal women. The typical appearance is of a 'dinner-fork' deformity with prominence on the dorsum of the wrist and dorsal displacement of the hand.

5. C Compartment syndrome

The compartment syndrome is a clinical entity and occurs as a result of increased pressure within a compartment limited by the fascia, caused by muscle injury with consequent oedema. The commonest causes are an electrical or violent injury to the leg. Loss of sensation, pain and decreased pulses indicate the presence of a compartment syndrome. The most important diagnostic factor is a history of significant pain not improved with ordinary analgesia. Passive stretching of the ischaemic muscles within the compartment leads to a dramatic increase in pain in the calf and this should not be ignored.

Investigations of musculoskeletal injuries

A   Arteriogram
B   Arthrogram of the wrist
C   Computerized tomography (CT) scan
D   Doppler scan
E   INR (International normalized ratio)
F   Myelogram
G   Nerve conduction studies
H   Platelet count
I   Technetium 99m bone scan
J   X-ray of affected leg
K   X-ray of the knee

For each patient below, choose the SINGLE best investigation from the above list of options. Each option may be used once, more than once, or not at all.

1. A 26-year-old bricklayer is seen twice in 3 weeks in the fracture clinic with a clinically suspected scaphoid fracture. On both occasions X-rays fail to show any bony injury. The surgeon decides to investigate further.

2. A 30-year-old lady had inter-locking nailing for a fracture of her left tibia and fibula. Postoperatively she developed foot-drop, which has not resolved in 6 weeks.

3. A 50-year-old postman, who is on warfarin for valvular heart disease, is admitted to the ward with a fracture of the tibia and fibula. After 6 hours he develops the compartment syndrome in that leg. As the orthopaedic registrar becomes aware of this he immediately checks for the blood results on the computer.

4. A 25-year-old motorcyclist crashes head-on into an oncoming car and lands on the nearby embankment. He is now in the resuscitation room. He is complaining of severe pain in the base of his cervical spine. Routine cervical spine X-rays are inconclusive.

5. An 80-year-old lady is recovering after a hemiarthroplasty of her left hip. On the seventh day she develops swelling and tenderness of her left calf.

Answers to **6.11**

1.   **I** Technetium-99m bone scan

When a clinical diagnosis of fracture of the scaphoid is not confirmed by X-rays, it is initially treated as a fracture, with immobilization in plaster. Repeat X-rays should be done approximately 2 weeks later. If these fail to show a fracture, a technetium-99m bone scan is a sensitive test to detect increased activity around an undisplaced fracture.

2.   **G** Nerve conduction studies

A foot-drop developing postoperatively after a locked intra-medullary nail insertion to the tibia suggests an injury to the common peroneal nerve, by either a locking screw or by pressure on the nerve at the time of surgery. It is reasonable to wait for a few weeks in such situations. A nerve conduction or EMG study would be used to assess whether this is neuropraxia or serious damage to the nerve.

3.   **E** INR (International normalized ratio)

Surgical decompression may be required to salvage the nerves and vessels in the compartment syndrome. When planning any surgery on patients with suspected clotting difficulties it is essential to check the INR and adjust it downwards using fresh frozen plasma or vitamin K before the surgical intervention.

4.   **C** Computerized tomography (CT) scan

Although the majority of cervical spine fractures can be detected by standard X-rays (anteroposterior, lateral and open-mouth views), some fractures of the atlas and cervicodorsal junction (C7 and T1) can only be detected by CT scan or tomography.

5.   **D** Doppler scan

Duplex Doppler scanning of the deep veins is accepted as the ideal non-invasive investigation to diagnose venous thromboses. It avoids the small risk of anaphylaxis associated with intravenous contrast media.

Management of musculoskeletal injuries (1)

A   Bivalve the plaster
B   Dynamic hip screw fixation
C   Hemiarthroplasty
D   Neighbour strapping
E   No action needed
F   Occlusive antiseptic dressing and splinting
G   Open reduction and internal fixation
H   Reduce and apply plaster
I   Skeletal traction
J   Suture the wound
K   Wound debridement with internal or external fixation

For each patient below, choose the SINGLE most appropriate course of action from the above list of options. Each option may be used once, more than once, or not at all.

1.   A 19-year-old girl is hit by a car while crossing the road. Her main injury is a fracture of the right tibia and fibula with an open wound.

2.   A 35-year-old man presents with a closed, stable fracture of the proximal phalanx of the ring finger sustained during a game of cricket.

3.   A 70-year-old woman is admitted after falling on her elbow. An X-ray shows a minimally displaced supracondylar fracture of the humerus.

4.   A 65-year-old woman is brought to the A&E department after she fell on her outstretched hands. She complains of pain in her right wrist and examination reveals a 'dinner-fork' deformity.

5.   An 80-year-old normally fit and independent woman is admitted with a displaced subcapital fracture of the neck of the left femur, sustained through a fall 24 hours before admission.

Answers to 6.12

1. **K** **Wound debridement with internal or external fixation**

Fractures following road traffic accidents are frequently contaminated and commuted. An open fracture of the tibia must be cleaned, debrided and stabilized in position either by internal or external fixation. Surgery should be performed as soon as possible (ideally within 6 hours).

2. **D** **Neighbour strapping**

Stable fractures of the proximal phalanx allow at least 30% of active range of movement in the adjacent joints without displacing the fracture fragments. These fractures can usually be treated with strapping adjacent fingers (neighbour strapping) with good results. Care should be taken to check for rotational disorders.

3. **G** **Open reduction and internal fixation**

A supracondylar fracture in adults almost always requires internal fixation because the proximity of the fracture to the joint leads to a tendency for movement to occur at the fracture site. This leads to an increased probability of non-union. It is an important fracture in childhood because of possible complications such as vascular damage (contused or severed brachial artery), compartment syndrome, Volkmann's ischaemic contracture (muscle necrosis from disruption of the microcirculation), median nerve damage and malunion.

4. **H** **Reduce and apply plaster**

A Colles' fracture is a fracture of the distal metaphysis of the radius within 2.5 cm of the wrist joint, with dorsal and radial displacement of the distal radial segment. A displaced Colles' fracture produces the classic 'dinner-fork deformity'. Once reduced, a plaster can be applied from just distal to the elbow to just proximal to the metacarpophalangeal joints to allow free finger movement.

5. **C** **Hemiarthroplasty**

Hemiarthroplasty (replace femoral head with a Thompson or Austin–Moore prosthesis and leave the acetabulum intact) is carried out for displaced intracapsular fractures of the proximal femur in older patients. It allows for early mobilization and avoids the high risk of complications of internal fixation (reserved for younger patients) such as avascular necrosis or nonunion. There is a risk of the metallic femoral head eroding into the floor of the acetabulum in which case a total hip replacement may be indicated. Femoral neck fractures in the elderly or frail subjects are often best treated with hemiarthroplasty where the patient will tolerate anaesthesia.

Management of musculoskeletal injuries (2)

A   Apply plaster of Paris
B   Bivalve the plaster and padding completely
C   Check distal pulses
D   Manipulation of fracture
E   Neighbour strapping
F   Occlusive antiseptic dressing and splinting
G   Open reduction and internal fixation
H   Release the plaster partly
I   Support with a sling
J   Wound debridement and stabilization of bone
K   X-ray of elbow

For each patient below, choose the SINGLE most appropriate initial management from the above list of options. Each option may be used once, more than once, or not at all.

1. A 35-year-old woman falls out of a tree on to her left shoulder. When examined, she kept the left arm clasped to her chest and a soft, tender swelling was seen over the middle of her left clavicle.

2. An 8-year-old boy falls off a climbing frame and is brought to the A&E department with a swollen and deformed left elbow.

3. The on-call orthopaedic duty doctor is called to the A&E department to see a 5-year-old boy, who has sustained a minimally angulated fracture of the ring-finger metacarpal.

4. The orthopaedic nurse calls the duty doctor to see a 10-year-old boy who has returned from theatre. He is complaining of pins and needles in his right hand. He is in an above-elbow plaster of Paris cast, following manipulation of a displaced greenstick fracture of his radius and ulna.

5. A 3-year-old child falls from a slide and sustains a minimally angulated greenstick fracture of the distal radial metaphysis.

Answers to **6.13**

1. I Support with a sling

A fracture of the clavicle causes pain if the arm is moved, hence `the arm clasped to the chest' posture. The arm should be supported with a sling for 3 weeks until the pain subsides. Thereafter, active exercise sould be encouraged to regain full mobility.

2. C Check distal pulses

Supracondylar fractures of the distal humerus is the commonest injury around the elbow in children. The great danger of this fracture is injury to the brachial artery, so it is important to feel the distal pulses (radial or ulnar) and check the circulation.

3. F Neighbour strapping

Metacarpal fractures in the middle and ring fingers are often well stabilized because of the intermetacarpal ligaments. Usually neighbour strapping is sufficient to treat these fractures.

4. A Bivalve the plaster completely

Plaster immobilization though safe, can lead to complications. The development of pins and needles or numbness in a limb after such a procedure is usually due to a tight cast. If elevation fails to relieve the symptoms the plaster must be bivalved throughout its length, through all the padding down to skin.

5. A Apply plaster of Paris

Minimally angulated fractures in young children will remodel and correct minor deformities as the child grows. The appropriate management of this injury is to protect the fracture in a below-elbow plaster for 3 weeks.

Childhood hip problems

A Congenital coxa vara
B Developmental dysplasia of the hip
C Juvenile rheumatoid arthritis (Still's disease)
D Osteoarthritis
E Perthes' disease
F Poliomyelitis
G Pyogenic arthritis
H Reiter's syndrome
I Slipped upper femoral epiphysis
J Transient synovitis
K Tuberculous arthritis of the hip

For each patient below, choose the SINGLE most likely diagnosis from the above list of options. Each option may be used once, more than once, or not at all.

1. A 7-year old boy presents with a 1-month history of intermittent limp and pain in his right groin. He is generally well and has a normal erythrocyte sedimentation rate (ESR) and white blood count (WBC). Movements in his right hip are slightly restricted and X-rays reveal an area of increased density within the capital epiphysis.

2. A 14-year old boy presents with a 2-month history of pain in his right hip. He is obese and walks with a painful limp. His right leg is externally rotated and slightly shorter than the unaffected side. The ESR and WBC are normal, and so is the anteroposterior X-ray view of his right hip. The lateral view, however, reveals the characteristic abnormality.

3. A 6-year old boy presents with a single episode of pain in his right hip. He walks with a limp and movements of his right hip are restricted. The ESR, WBC and X-rays are all normal and the child is clinically well. His symptoms resolve completely within 4 weeks.

4. A 26-month-old girl is noted to have a waddling gait. Her parents complain that applying napkins has been difficult with her. At birth, she was delivered by breech. An X-ray of her left hip reveals disruption of the Shenton's line.

5. A 4-year old boy presents with a 2-day history of a high temperature and pain in his left hip, with marked restriction in the range of movements. He looks ill and his ESR and WBC are grossly elevated. An X-ray of his left hip is normal.

Answers to **6.14**

1. **E Perthes' disease**

    Perthes' disease is characterized by avascular necrosis of the femoral
    head. The disease typically presents in children aged between 4 and
    8 years with boys being four times more commonly affected than girls.
    The child is generally well with normal inflammatory indices. X-rays
    taken in the early stage of the disease are often normal.

2. **I Slipped upper femoral epiphysis**

    This condition classically affects pubertal boys and about half are
    overweight. Apart from the 30% of cases where trauma may be a
    contributory factor, there is a gradual onset of symptoms.
    Anteroposterior (AP) views of the hip may be normal but look for a
    double shadow in the femoral neck (metaphyseal bleach of Steele). A
    lateral view is essential for detection of the slip – the femoral epiphysis
    appears to be displaced posteriorly. Significant shortening is
    uncommon, with a normal AP X-ray. This is usually associated with
    large slips.

3. **J Transient synovitis**

    This condition affects children between 6 and 12 years of age, and more
    commonly boys than girls. The child is generally well and inflammatory
    indices are normal. X-rays are essentially normal though on rare
    occasions may reveal an increased joint space. Ultrasound may reveal
    fluid in the joint. The condition is benign and resolves spontaneously
    within 3 to 6 weeks.

4. **B Developmental dysplasia of the hip**

    This condition is six times more common in females than males, and it
    usually affects the left hip. About 25% of cases are bilateral. Breech
    presentation and family history are predisposing factors. All newborns
    are screened clinically for this condition. Asymmetry of the lower limbs
    and a waddling gait are common in those who present late. There is
    often a restriction in hip abduction and parents may complain about
    difficulty in changing napkins. Shenton's line or arch is used to test
    radiographically the relationship of the head and neck of the femur with
    the acetabulum. It is a radiological description of the line formed when
    the inferior border of the superior pubic ramus is followed laterally and
    then curves along the medial border of the femoral neck.

5. **G Pyogenic arthritis**

    This is a very serious condition and even a slight delay in diagnosis and
    treatment may result in rapid, irreversible destruction of the joint. The
    infection is blood-borne and staphyloccocus is often the responsible
    organism. Ultrasound scan will reveal a joint effusion.

Lower back pain

A   Ankylosing spondylitis
B   Metastatic lesions of the spine
C   Multiple myeloma
D   Osteoarthrosis
E   Osteoporosis
F   Prolapsed intervertebral disc
G   Pyogenic infection of the spine
H   Rheumatoid arthritis
I   Spinal stenosis
J   Spondylolisthesis
K   Tuberculosis of the spine

For each patient below, choose the SINGLE most likely diagnosis from the above list of options. Each option may be used once, more than once, or not at all.

1. A 25-year-old man stooped to lift a box up from the floor when he experienced pain in his lower back. He complains of pain radiating to his right foot and he also has numbness in the same foot. On examination, there is weakness in plantar flexion of his right foot, loss of sensation on the outer border of his right foot and a diminished ankle jerk on the right side. Straight leg raising is grossly restricted on the right side. X-rays of his lumbar spine are normal.

2. A 50-year-old man has a long history of backache and morning stiffness. He has numbness and pain in his legs on walking, especially when he is walking down a slope. He is a non-smoker and has good pedal pulses bilaterally.

3. A 25-year-old man has a few years' history of backache. Examination reveals gross restriction in spinal movements. His chest expansion is also reduced. His erythrocyte sedimentation rate (ESR) is 80. X-rays of the spine reveal ossification of the interspinous ligaments.

4. A 60-year-old woman has been experiencing constant backache for 3 months. X-rays of her lumbar spine reveal poor bone density. Her ESR is elevated at 110 and her urine is positive for Bence Jones protein.

5. A 50-year-old man with a history of chronic ill health, night sweats, episodic pyrexia and backache has an angular deformity in his spine. X-rays of his spine reveal multiple collapsed vertebral bodies and a paraspinal soft tissue shadow at the lower thoracic level.

Answers to **6.15**

1. **F Prolapsed intervertebral disc**

    This patient has a prolapsed disc at L5/S1 level affecting the S1 nerve
    root on the right side. This is often caused by a flexion injury tearing the
    annulus fibrosus, allowing the contents of the nucleus pulposus to
    herniate through. X-rays are often normal, or may show narrowing of
    the disc space. Magnetic resonance imaging (MRI) is diagnostic.

2. **I Spinal stenosis**

    This patient has neurogenic claudication caused by a small diameter
    spinal canal. Differential diagnosis includes vascular claudication. In
    contrast to vascular claudication the symptoms are worse on walking
    down a slope, as extension of the spine causes further decrease in the
    diameter of the spinal canal. The claudication distance is also more
    variable in spinal stenosis.

3. **A Ankylosing spondylitis**

    This condition affects mainly young males. There is a strong genetic
    element with 90% of patients carrying the HLA B27 antigen. Chest
    expansion is reduced due to the ankylosis of the costovertebral joints.
    The classic X-ray appearance is described as showing a bamboo spine.

4. **C Multiple myeloma**

    This is an important cause of secondary osteoporosis and must be borne
    in mind when a patient presents with a constant backache and is found
    to have a high ESR. The condition must also be borne in mind if a
    patient presents with a pathological fracture. The patient is usually
    middle-aged or elderly and often presents with a history of general
    malaise and constant, rather than mechanical, pain. The ESR is often
    elevated and other investigations to be considered include an MRI scan
    (lytic lesions are poorly seen on a bone scan) and blood investigations
    to check calcium levels.

5. **K Tuberculosis of the spine**

    The spine is the commonest site for skeletal tuberculosis. This is a rare
    disease but the incidence of tuberculosis has been rising in recent years.
    The entire spine should be X-rayed as multiple sites may be involved. A
    paraspinal soft tissue shadow suggests oedema or a paravertebral
    abscess.

Trauma to the abdominal organs 6.16

A Aortic injury
B Bladder injury
C Bowel perforation
D Duodenal injury
E Hepatic injury
F Pancreatic injury
G Renal injury
H Rupture of the diaphragm
I Splenic injury
J Testicular injury
K Urethral injury

For each patient below, choose the SINGLE most likely diagnosis from the above list of options. Each option may be used once, more than once or not at all.

1. A 25-year-old man sustains a stab wound below his right nipple. He is hypotensive. His chest X-ray is normal and, apart from the wound, there is no clinical sign of chest injury.

2. A 35-year-old man had fallen 15 feet off a ladder, landing on to his left side. X-rays revealed fractures of his left 8th and 9th ribs laterally. He was prescribed analgesia and discharged from the hospital. He returns to the department today, 10 days after the incident, with pain in his left shoulder tip and hypotension.

3. A 40-year-old man sustained a pelvic fracture. He has blood at the urethral meatus and extensive scrotal and perineal bruising. Rectal examination reveals a high-riding prostate.

4. A 20-year-old man sustained blunt trauma to his abdomen. A nasogastric tube was sited. A chest X-ray revealed elevation of the left diaphragm with the end of the nasogastric tube in the left hemithorax.

5. A heavy metal beam fell onto the back of a 25-year-old man at work. X-rays of his lumbar spine show fractures in the transverse processes of L2 and L3 on the left side. He also has haematuria.

Answers to **6.16**

1.   E   Hepatic injury

   The dome of the diaphragm may rise to the 4th intercostal space. Hence any penetrating wound beneath the nipple line may result in intra-abdominal trauma.

2.   I   Splenic injury

   Delayed rupture of the spleen occurs in approximately 5% of blunt trauma to the spleen. The initial injury results in intraparenchymal haemorrhage contained by the capsule, or a small amount of extracapsular bleeding contained by peritoneal folds or omentum. With the liquefaction and breakdown of the haematoma, osmotic pressure increases, drawing water into it. This results in an increase in volume and pressure, leading to rupture and haemorrhage.

3.   K   Urethral injury

   This is a classic description of a urethral injury associated with pelvic fracture. In patients with such a presentation a urinary catheter must never be passed unless urethral injury has been ruled out by a retrograde cystourethrogram. Passage of a urinary catheter may convert a partial urethral tear into a complete tear and introduce infection.

4.   H   Rupture of the diaphragm

   This injury is easily missed as the chest X-ray signs are often non-specific. However, the appearance of a nasogastric tube in the chest cavity is diagnostic. Right-sided diaphragmatic rupture is rare and diagnosis is often delayed.

5.   G   Renal injury

   Upper lumbar spine transverse process fracture in itself requires only symptomatic treatment, but an associated renal trauma must be carefully looked for.

Diagnosis of lower leg syndromes/symptoms

A   Acute compartment syndrome
B   Chronic compartment syndrome
C   Gastrocnemius muscle tear
D   Lumbar radiculopathy
E   Rupture of Achilles tendon
F   Shin splint
G   Stress fracture
H   Tarsal tunnel syndrome
I   Thrombophlebitis
J   Tibialis posterior dysfunction
K   Vascular claudication

For each patient below, choose the SINGLE most likely diagnosis from the above list of options. Each option may be used once, more than once, or not at all.

1.   While pushing a car the patient felt a sudden pop in the back of his heel. On examination his calf is bruised, plantar flexion of the foot is weak and he has difficulty walking.

2.   An athlete developed pain and tenderness over the muscles in the anterior compartment of both of his lower legs after an early season training session in long-distance running.

3.   A patient presents with pain in his right lower leg. He has a restricted straight leg raising test and a diminished ankle jerk on the same side.

4.   A patient sustained a closed fracture of his right tibia in a road traffic accident. His lower leg is grossly swollen and passive stretching of the muscle in the anterior compartment causes excruciating pain.

5.   A long-distance runner complains of pain in his right lower leg. There is a well-localized area of tenderness over the proximal third of his tibia. X-rays are normal but a bone scan reveals increased uptake in the same area.

Answers to **6.17**

1. C Gastrocnemius muscle tear

The mode of injury is attempted plantar flexion against resistance. Characteristically, a sudden pain in the upper calf is felt by the patient. Importantly, plantar flexion is preserved but is weak, suggesting integrity of the Achilles tendon. An ultrasound scan is a useful tool to differentiate the two injuries.

2. F Shin splint

The term 'shin splint' is often used loosely to describe a wide variety of lower leg overuse syndromes. True shin splint is myositis or tendinitis of the muscles in the anterior and/or lateral compartments of the lower leg. It often happens in early season training, before the muscles are adapted to the volume and intensity of the training regime.

3. D Lumbar radiculopathy

In any clinical assessment always beware of referred symptoms, where the primary lesion is elsewhere. The pain down the legs, diminished ankle reflex and restricted leg raising all suggest a lesion in the lower lumbar region involving principally the L5/S1 segments.

4. A Acute compartment syndrome

There are four compartments in the lower leg. They are the anterior, peroneal, superficial posterior and deep posterior compartments. Each compartment is bound by a semirigid fascia. Tissue oedema as a result of trauma causes an increase in the interstitial pressure which can in turn lead to a decrease in arterial flow. If the pressure is not relieved by fasciotomy, irreversible muscle necrosis and nerve damage may result. A marked increase in pain on passive stretching of the muscle of the compartment is a characteristic feature.

5. G Stress fracture

Early X-rays are often normal. X-rays 2 weeks from the onset of symptoms may reveal callus formation. Management would initially include a period of rest from any exacerbating activities. Investigation is only usually undertaken for non-professional athletes after a failure of conservative treatment. If confirmed on a bone scan most stress fractures will heal with simple rest of the affected part.

Diagnosis of elbow trauma

A   Anterior capsular strain
B   Bicipital tendinitis
C   Cubital tunnel syndrome
D   Elbow dislocation
E   Lateral epicondylitis
F   Medial epicondylitis
G   Olecranon bursitis
H   Osteochondritis dissecans
I   Panner's disease
J   Triceps tendinitis
K   Ulnar collateral ligament injury

For each patient below, choose the SINGLE most likely diagnosis from the above list of options. Each option may be used once, more than once, or not at all.

1. A golfer developed pain over the medial aspect of his right elbow. On examination, there is tenderness over the common flexorpronator origin of the elbow.

2. A tennis player developed pain over the lateral aspect of his right elbow. On examination, there is tenderness over the common extensor origin of the elbow at the lateral epicondyle. Resisted extension of the fingers worsens the pain.

3. A factory worker whose work involves repetitive flexing and extending of the elbow joint has developed posterior elbow pain. The pain is increased on extension of his elbow against resistance. The X-ray reveals a traction spur at the olecranon, which corresponds to the site of maximal tenderness on examination.

4. A young throwing athlete developed pain in his elbow. X-rays reveal defects in the capitellum and loose bodies.

5. A 30-year-old carpet-layer developed a round, fluctuant swelling over the dorsal aspect of his elbow.

Answers to **6.18**

1. **F** Medial epicondylitis

Also called golfer's elbow. This is an overuse injury involving the origin of the flexorpronator group of muscles. Such a problem is not confined to golfers; any activity that subjects the forearm muscles to repetitive stress can cause it.

2. **E** Lateral epicondylitis

Also called tennis elbow. It is a very common condition and not only confined to tennis players. It is an overuse injury affecting the common extensor origin (lateral epicondyle) and is usually self-limiting. Management includes local steroid injections, splinting and surgery as a last resort. At operation, a small amount of inflammatory tissue is often found beneath the tendon origins.

3. **J** Triceps tendinitis

This is also an overuse injury, secondary to repetitive extension of the elbow. The point of maximal tenderness is around the insertion of the triceps tendon at the olecranon.

4. **H** Osteochondritis dissecans

Throwing sports subject the elbow to a significant valgus force resulting in medial collateral tension, lateral joint compression and posterior impingement. Osteochondritis dissecans is most often found in adolescent athletes competing in gymnastics and various throwing sports. The proposed aetiology is that the repetitive valgus force overloads the lateral joint and that this leads to fragmentation of the capitellum. Panner's disease (also called Koehler's disease: osteochondrosis of the navicular bone) is similar but is usually found in younger children and fragmentation of the cartilage is not usually seen.

5. **G** Olecranon bursitis

This is often caused by repetitive minor injuries to the olecranon bursa although it can also be a result of an acute injury. It can also be caused by infection, or may develop secondary to other conditions such as rheumatoid arthritis.

Glasgow Coma Score

A	0
B	1
C	3
D	5
E	7
F	8
G	9
H	11
I	13
J	15
K	16

For each question below, choose the SINGLE most likely score from the above list of options. Each option may be used once, more than once, or not at all.

1. What is the minimum score in a patient's Glasgow Coma Score (GCS)?

2. What is the maximum score in a patient who is in a coma?

3. Following a head injury the patient is groaning, his eyes remain closed on painful stimulation and he exhibits an extensor response to pain. What is his Glasgow Coma Score?

4. Following a head injury the patient opens his eyes to verbal command, withdraws to painful stimulation on his right side but there is no response to pain on his left side, and he utters incomprehensible sounds. What is his Glasgow Coma Score?

5. A patient has a dense right-sided hemiplegia and expressive dysphasia. His comprehension is not impaired. He opens his eyes spontaneously and obeys command. What is his Glasgow Coma Score?

Answers to **6.19**

1. C   3

The Glasgow Coma Score, rather strangely, starts at 3. The maximum score is 15. In patients with head injury, the initial GCS correlates with the severity of injury and predicts the probability of eventual neurological recovery. In patients with an initial score of 3 or 4, about 80% of them will die or remain in a vegetative state. If the initial score is over 11, only about 6% will die or remain in a vegetative state.

The Glasgow Coma Score:

Eye opening	Spontaneously	4
(E)	To verbal command	3
	To pain	2
	No response	1
Best motor response	Obeys command	6
(M)	Localizes pain	5
	Normal flexion (withdrawal)	4
	Abnormal flexion (decorticate)	3
	Extension (decerebrate)	2
	None (flaccid)	1
Verbal Response	Orientated	5
(V)	Confused	4
	Inappropriate words	3
	Incomprehensible sounds	2
	None	1

2. F   8

Coma is defined by a GCS of 8 or less.

3. D   5

The GCS for this patient is E1M2V2, a total score of 5.

4. G   9

The GCS for this patient is E3M4V2, a total score of 9. In each of the three categories the *best* response is recorded – hence M4 (right side) instead of M1 (left side).

5. J   15

In any rule there are always some exceptions. Obviously his level of consciousness is unimpaired despite his speech problem. His GCS is 15.

Ears, Nose and Eyes

Causes of hearing loss

A Acoustic neuroma
B Barotrauma
C Cholesteatoma
D Glue ear (serous otitis media)
E Ménière's disease
F Noise exposure
G Otitis externa
H Otitis media
I Otosclerosis
J Ototoxicity
K Presbycousis

For each of the following presentations choose the SINGLE most likely cause from the options above. You may use each option once, more than once, or not at all.

1. A 24-year-old student attends a rock concert and the following morning presents with deafness and ringing in his ears.

2. A 64-year-old man presents with progressive hearing loss in his right ear over the last 6 months. He has also noticed a foul-smelling discharge from the ear and, in the last 2 weeks, there has been drooping of the right side of his face.

3. An 18-year-old woman develops pain, fever and hearing loss in her left ear. For 1 week she has had a viral upper respiratory illness.

4. A 36-year-old man developed a viral upper respiratory illness while on a skiing holiday. On the return flight he noticed a feeling of pressure in his left ear, which became more painful and was associated with deafness. The pain has now settled but the deafness remains.

5. A 35-year-old woman complains of a 1-year history of increasing deafness. She is now in the mid-trimester of pregnancy and has noticed a marked deterioration in her hearing.

Answers to 7.1

1. F   Noise exposure

Acute acoustic trauma is the most likely diagnosis when hearing loss and tinnitus follow an episode of intense noise exposure. There may be a history of a single very intense exposure, such as attendance at a rock concert, or more usually the episode which triggers the symptoms is simply the latest episode in a long sequence, e.g. repeated attendance at loud concerts or discos, or repeated use of power tools. The hearing loss and tinnitus may resolve over a week or so, but many cases are associated with permanent damage and incurable symptoms.

2. C   Cholesteatoma

A foul-smelling discharge is a sign of anaerobic infection and usually indicates chronic otitis media with perforation, which may be associated with cholesteatoma. The discharge from a cholesteatoma usually has a characteristic and easily recognizable smell. A cholesteatoma causes an erosive infection in the middle ear and mastoid, which may extend into surrounding structures such as the facial nerve (as in this case), the labyrinth, or meninges.

3. H   Otitis media

Acute otitis media is often secondary to an upper respiratory infection and presents as severe, prolonged earache with pyrexia. The eardrum is often reddened in appearance. In some cases, pus may discharge through a perforation before antibiotic treatment is started.

4. B   Barotrauma

Upper respiratory tract infections cause oedema of the Eustachian tube which may then become blocked. The blockage may be difficult to clear. The middle ear becomes partly filled by a serous exudate which causes a sensation of blockage in the ear and conductive deafness; it also becomes difficult to equalize the residual air pressure in the middle ear with the surrounding air pressure. If the surrounding pressure changes quickly, as in flying or diving, a significant pressure difference builds up across the eardrum which is painful and occasionally may be associated with rupture of the drum, or transmission of pressure effects to the inner ear causing permanent sensorineural hearing loss.

5. I   Otosclerosis

Otosclerosis is due to the replacement of normal bone by vascular, spongy bone around the oval window. It affects young adults, is associated with a family history in 50% of cases and, classically, worsens during pregnancy. Definitive treatment is by surgical replacement of the stapes bone.

Epistaxis

A Anticoagulation therapy
B Environment (high altitude)
C Hypertension
D Nasopharyngeal tumour
E Osler–Weber–Rendu– syndrome
F Septal perforation
G Septoplasty
H Shock
I Silver nitrate cautery trauma
J Sinusitis
K Wegener's granulomatosis

For each of the clinical pictures below choose the SINGLE most appropriate cause from the above list. You may choose each option once, more than once, or not at all.

1. A 65-year-old man presents with recurrent epistaxis and has a recent history of pulmonary thromboembolism.

2. A 45-year-old woman presents with severe epistaxis. She has red spots on her lips with telangiectasia on the face and nose.

3. A 52-year-old man presents with epistaxis, nasal obstruction and right-sided otalgia. He has also noticed a right-sided swelling in his neck for the past month.

4. A 35-year-old man presents with a history of frequent epistaxis, excessive crusting inside the nose, and a frequent need to clear his nose by blowing or picking.

5. A 48-year-old man presents with left-sided epistaxis and crusting of his nose. Blood tests demonstrate a raised cANCA (cytoplasmic antineutrophil cytoplasmic antibodies).

Answers to **7.2**

1. A Anticoagulation therapy

As this patient has a history of pulmonary thromboembolism he is probably being treated with warfarin. Anticoagulation therapy, if not well regulated, can lead to epistaxis, especially in the elderly.

2. E Osler–Weber–Rendu syndrome

This is an autosomal dominant disorder in which the vessel walls lack contractile elements and mucosal telangiectasia are present throughout the respiratory and gastrointestinal systems. It often requires laser coagulation treatment of the vessels or grafting of the nasal cavity.

3. D Nasopharyngeal tumour

These can often present with epistaxis, nasal obstruction, a lump in the neck and referred otalgia. Sometimes they can lead to serous otitis media due to Eustachian tube blockage. If there is nerve involvement this can also lead to facial, palatal and pharyngeal loss of sensation. Other possible symptoms include Horner's syndrome and vocal cord, pharyngeal, palatal, shoulder and tongue paralysis. Diagnosis is made by nasopharyngoscopy and biopsy. Treatment depends on the tumour type but includes radiotherapy and/or chemotherapy to the primary tumour and surgery to the involved nodes in the neck.

4. F Septal perforation

Most septal perforations are due to trauma, either habitual picking of the nose, or surgical trauma. Once a perforation appears in the septum, it will not heal and it is very difficult to repair surgically. The edges of the perforation tend to get covered in crusts which build up to block the nose, and break away with repeated bleeding. Treatment is usually by avoiding further trauma and using emollient creams.

5. K Wegener's granulomatosis

This can present with epistaxis, nasal congestion, discharge, crusting and a friable, ulcerated mucosa over the septum. There may be otic, respiratory and renal symptoms. Diagnosis is made specifically by finding increased cANCA (cytoplasmic antineutrophil cytoplasmic antibodies) in most cases and p (perinuclear) ANCA may be present in some cases. Biopsy can be definitive. Treatment is with cyclophosphamide.

Diseases of the ear

A Cholesteatoma
B Chondromalacia
C Furuncle
D Meningitis
E Myringitis
F Nasopharyngeal tumour
G Otitis externa
H Otitis media
I Otosclerosis
J Sinusitis
K Wegener's granulomatosis

For each of the following presentations choose the SINGLE most likely option from the above list. You may use each option once, more than once, or not at all.

1. A 45-year-old man presents with a history of repeated ear infections, progressive conductive hearing loss and an attic crust.

2. A 20-year-old woman with no previous history of ear complaints presents with a 2-day history of severe pain in the right ear. The ear is extremely tender to examine.

3. A 55-year-old man presents with unilateral right-sided otalgia with signs of otitis media. There is a history of recurrent epistaxis during the past 3 months.

4. A 19-year-old man, with a known history of otitis media, presents with headache, lethargy, sweating and shivering.

5. A 48-year-old woman presents with bilateral, conductive deafness of gradual onset and mild tinnitus. On examination, a flamingo tinge is seen through the tympanic membranes.

Answers to **7.3**

1.   A   Cholesteatoma

This presentation suggests a cholesteatoma. There are two types, congenital and acquired. Symptoms may arise from the disease or its complications. There is usually an associated infection producing a discharge which is often foul and creamy. Deafness results due to ossicular erosion or toxins due to the chronic inflammation. Diagnosis is by micro-otoscopy which may show a retraction pocket, or an attic crust. Pure tone audiometry may show conductive and/or sensory neural hearing loss. Finally, radiology (plain X-ray, CT or MRI scanning) may show the lesion and its extent. Treatment depends on the extent of the disease. Simple suction clearance may control early disease.

2.   C   Furuncle

A furuncle is an acute staphylococcal infection of a hair follicle, producing an extremely painful localized swelling or boil. It is often very difficult to visualize the actual boil, as the whole ear is too tender to allow adequate examination, and the swelling can be very small in comparison to the amount of pain. Treatment is by inserting wicks and with antistaphylococcal antibiotics.

3.   F   Nasopharyngeal tumour

Obstruction of the Eustachian tube by a nasopharyngeal tumour can lead to a unilateral otitis media and otalgia. Other symptoms include epistaxis, nasal congestion and crusting. All cases of persistent unilateral otitis media in elderly patients should be considered to be potentially neoplastic and excluded by examination of the nasopharynx.

4.   D   Meningitis

This is just one of the intracranial complications of untreated otitis media. Others include extradural abscess, brain abscess, subdural empyema, lateral sinus thrombosis, focal otic encephalitis and otic hydrocephalus.

5.   I   Otosclerosis

This is an autosomal dominant disease which presents with conductive deafness, tinnitus and sometimes mild vertigo. The tympanic membrane looks normal in most cases though in some patients a diagnostic `flamingo tinge', caused by hyperaemia of the promontory, can be seen, often referred to as the Schwartz sign. Otosclerosis can be treated with a hearing aid or with a stapedectomy. It is important to counsel the patients before the surgical option as it can lead to a `dead' ear.

Abnormalities of the external eye

A   Arcus senilis
B   Blepharitis
C   Dendritic ulcer
D   Ectropion
E   Entropion
F   Lagophthalmos
G   Pinguecula
H   Pterygium
I   Ptosis
J   Stye
K   Xanthelasma

For each of the following presentations choose the SINGLE most likely abnormality from the options above. You may use each option once, more than once, or not at all.

1. A 35-year-old woman complains of a burning, gritty sensation in both eyes. Examination reveals slight redness and some scaling of the eyelid margins.

2. An 82-year-old man has persistent watering of his left eye and continually needs to wipe it with a tissue. On close inspection, the left lower eyelid appears to be turned inwards.

3. A 63-year-old woman complains of an abnormal discoloration of her left eye. There is a yellow nodule on the nasal side of the conjunctiva which is encroaching on the cornea.

4. A 26-year-old man has an intensely painful right eye. He has marked photophobia and watering of the eye. Application of 1% fluorescein drops reveals a linear, branching-shaped area on the cornea.

5. On routine examination of a 34-year-old man an abnormality of his right upper eyelid is noted. The lid is lower than the left at rest and does not rise when he looks upwards.

Answers to **7.4**

Recognition of abnormalities of the external eye is important since they commonly present in general practice and emergency departments. It is important to be familiar with the correct terminology to facilitate clear communication with specialist colleagues.

1. **B   Blepharitis**

Inflammation of the eyelid margin is termed blepharitis. A more localized inflammation with a swelling would suggest either a stye – a staphylococcal infection of an eyelash follicle – or a chalazion (retention of the secretion from a meibomian gland together with infection).

2. **E   Entropion**

Examination of the eyelids may reveal in-turning of an eyelid (entropion) where the eyelashes irritate the conjunctiva, or eversion of the eyelid (ectropion) which may include the tear duct punctum. Both are commoner in elderly people where there is laxity of the skin and subcutaneous tissues. A facial nerve palsy is another cause of an ectropion. Surgery may be indicated to prevent exposure keratopathy in the case of ectropion or continued irritation from an entropion.

3. **H   Pterygium**

This is a benign leash of vessels and fibrous tissue which spreads across the eye. It is thought to be caused by exposure to UV radiation. It is only of importance if it encroaches on the central cornea and interferes with vision. The treatment is by surgical excision.

4. **C   Dendritic ulcer**

Dendritic ulcers are caused by Herpes simplex infection. There may be a previous history of herpetic infection elsewhere, e.g. cold sores. Occasionally, factors such as stress, sunlight or concurrent illness may trigger reactivation of the disease. It is important to recognize the distinctive pattern of the ulcer. Treatment with steroid eyedrops can cause catastrophic deterioration and must be avoided.

5. **I   Ptosis**

Drooping of the eyelid (ptosis) may be senile, congenital, mechanical or neurological. It can be due to a 3rd nerve palsy or Horner's syndrome. The term lagophthalmos is applied when there is incomplete closure of the eyelid over the eyeball.

Initial management of eye trauma

A Amethocaine eye drops
B Antibiotic and mydriatic eye drops with eye pad
C Enucleation of the globe
D Evisceration of the globe
E Mydriatic eye drops and eye pad
F No action needed
G Pad both eyes and reassure
H Pad both eyes with no pressure and refer urgently to ophthalmology
I Prolonged irrigation
J Refer to ophthalmology for fracture reduction
K Remove foreign body and give antibiotic eye drops

For each presentation below, choose the SINGLE most appropriate initial management from the above list of options. You may use each option once, more than once, or not at all.

1. A 40-year-old mountain cyclist fell off his bicycle into a fence. He has a 3-cm splinter of wood protruding from his left eye.

2. A 24-year-old lady has used a sun-bed without protective goggles. She has an intensely painful, watering right eye with no evidence of corneal abrasion or foreign body.

3. A 32-year-old mother has a red, painful eye following an injury from her young child's fingers. Application of 1% fluorescein reveals a corneal abrasion.

4. A 42-year-old steelworker has been using an angle grinder. He has a small splinter of steel on his left cornea. X-ray of the orbit reveals no other injuries.

5. A 30-year-old man has double vision following an injury to his right eye while playing squash. There is a small area of sensory loss over his right lower eyelid.

Answers to 7.5

1.   H   Pad both eyes with no pressure and refer urgently to ophthalmology

Large foreign bodies should not be removed. They should be padded without any pressure to support the object and the patient transferred for an urgent ophthalmology opinion. The unaffected eye is also padded to prevent damage due to conjugate movement. Small foreign bodies can be removed providing adequate examination has been performed to exclude other foreign bodies by everting the eyelids and considering X-ray or ultrasound examination of the globe.

2.   E   Mydriatic eye drops and eye pad

The use of sun-beds or arc welding without adequate protection against ultraviolet light can damage the corneal epithelium. Mydriatics (to dilate the pupil and rest the eye) and padding of the eye help relieve the pain. Review again after 24 hours and consider referral to an ophthalmologist.

3.   B   Antibiotic and mydriatic eye drops with eye pad

Corneal abrasions from an injury due to a young child's fingers is a common reason for attendance at emergency departments. Antibiotic prophylaxis is needed while the abrasion heals. One per cent fluorescein eye drops and ultraviolet light will demonstrate the lesion. Review after 24 hours with a view to a specialist referral if there is concern.

4.   K   Remove foreign body and give antibiotic eye drops

Symptoms include pain, watering and photophobia. Small foreign bodies can be removed under topical anaesthetic, providing adequate examination has been performed to exclude other foreign bodies by everting the eyelids and, if indicated, by X-ray or ultrasound examination of the globe. An antibiotic ointment is instilled and the eye padded until the epithelium is healed. Review in 24 hours.

5.   J   Refer to ophthalmology for fracture reduction

A blow-out fracture of the orbit is suspected when there has been an injury from a squash ball, and when lid swelling, diplopia, epistaxis and infraorbital nerve anaesthesia are also present. The diplopia is due to tethering of the orbital contents in the fractured orbit floor. Involvement of the inferior orbital nerve leads to loss of sensation over the lower eyelid. Treatment options include conservative management, fracture reduction and squint correction. However, a hyphaema (effusion of blood into the anterior chamber) is a more common consequence of a squash ball injury.

Causes of acute reduction or loss of vision

A   Acute glaucoma
B   Acute iritis
C   Amaurosis fugax
D   Central retinal artery occlusion
E   Central retinal vein occlusion
F   Giant cell arteritis
G   Migraine
H   Optic neuritis
I   Papilloedema
J   Proliferative diabetic retinopathy
K   Vitreous haemorrhage

For each of the following presentations choose the SINGLE most likely cause from the options above. You may use each option once, more than once, or not at all.

1. A 75-year-old man presents with sudden, marked deterioration of vision in his left eye. He also has vague malaise, weight loss, pain in the jaw, especially when chewing, and discomfort when brushing his hair. Examination of the eye is normal. He has tenderness over the arteries in his scalp.

2. A 60-year-old man with a history of hypertension has sudden loss of vision in his right eye, which occurred over a matter of seconds. Examination reveals a prominent red fovea and an afferent pupillary defect (absent or diminished direct light response).

3. A 55-year-old man with a history of type 1 diabetes mellitus has sudden loss of vision in his left eye. There is an absent red reflex and fundoscopy proves impossible because of an opaque haze.

4. A 19-year-old woman complains of marked deterioration in the vision of her right eye over the last 3 days with pain on eye movement. On testing, she has a visual acuity of 6/60 on the right and 6/6 on the left. There is an afferent pupillary defect.

5. A 70-year-old man with type 2 diabetes mellitus presents the day after an annual review to his GP. He complains of nausea, vomiting and severe pain in his left eye. He has a fixed mid-dilated pupil and the cornea looks 'hazy'.

Answers to **7.6**

1. F Giant cell arteritis

Ischaemic optic neuropathy occurs when the optic nerve is deprived of its blood supply due to inflammation or atherosclerosis of the posterior ciliary arteries. The presence of malaise, jaw claudication and scalp tenderness would suggest giant cell arteritis. Corticosteroids should be started immediately to avoid irreversible blindness.

2. D Central retinal artery occlusion

The sudden, painless loss of vision, pallor of the retina and a 'cherry red spot' (the avascular fovea is thinner than the surrounding retina thus exposing the underlying choroidal circulation) indicates an occlusion of the central retinal artery. The commonest cause is an embolus from an atheromatous artery. Intermittent massage of the eye, if attempted within 6 hours, may force an embolus into a distal branch of the vessel.

3. K Vitreous haemorrhage

Preretinal and vitreous haemorrhages are associated with new vessel formation (neovascularization) in proliferative diabetic retinopathy. The fragile vessels are pulled forwards and are ruptured as the posterior vitreous fascia detaches. A vitreous haemorrhage may present as loss of vision in one eye or as a floating shadow in the field of vision. Fundoscopy reveals an absent red reflex and a featureless haze. Referral to an ophthalmologist is required as a matter of urgency.

4. H Optic neuritis

Optic neuritis is an inflammation or demyelination of the optic nerve. Ocular pain is common and is exacerbated by eye movement. The usual field defect is a central scotoma with loss of colour vision. There is an afferent pupillary defect whereby the direct light response is sluggish or absent. Most patients have good recovery of their eyesight but about two-thirds develop other signs of multiple sclerosis within 5 years.

5. A Acute glaucoma

At an annual review, a diabetic would normally have their pupils dilated with tropicamide and there is a risk of precipitating acute glaucoma especially in the elderly, those with a family history and where a shallow anterior chamber is present. Symptoms of acute glaucoma include sudden loss of vision, severe pain and occasionally vomiting. Examination shows ciliary injection, corneal oedema, a fixed and semidilated oval pupil, and a shallow anterior chamber. This is an overstated risk, perpetuating the myth and resulting in a reluctance among physicians to dilate and examine the fundi.

Assessment of trauma to the eye

A Blow-out fracture of the orbit
B Corneal abrasion
C Hyphaema
D Lens dislocation
E Radiation burn
F Retinal detachment
G Retrobulbar haemorrhage
H Ruptured globe
I Traumatic iritis
J Traumatic mydriasis
K Vitreous haemorrhage

For each patient below, choose the SINGLE most likely diagnosis from the above list of options. Each option may be used once, more than once, or not at all.

1. A 35-year-old man is stabbed in his right eye with a knife. On examination, he has an irregular pupil, a soft globe and a marked subconjunctival haemorrhage.

2. After a blow to his eye, a 19-year-old short-sighted man has had flashing lights and floaters for 1 week and now notices a shadow at the edge of his visual field.

3. A 23-year-old woman develops a fixed, dilated pupil after being hit in her eye. She is mentally alert and there are no other neurological signs.

4. A 45-year-old man has been hit in his eye. On examination, there is a collection of blood in the anterior chamber of the eye.

5. A 16-year-old boy has been poked in the eye. Fluorescein-staining reveals an area of increased uptake.

Answers to **7.7**

1.   H   Ruptured globe

The history and clinical signs are typical of a ruptured globe. The eye must be examined very carefully and gently. Pressure must not be applied to the globe as it may cause extrusion of the contents.

2.   F   Retinal detachment

With a retinal detachment the patient may also complain of a curtain-like shadow in the peripheral vision. Central vision may not be involved until the detachment affects the macula.

3.   J   Traumatic mydriasis

Uncal herniation from an intracranial mass lesion must always be considered when a patient presents with a fixed and dilated pupil, but this is extremely unlikely in the absence of impaired consciousness. Traumatic mydriasis is an efferent pupillary defect. The pupil is dilated and is not responsive to direct or consensual light. It is usually the result of a traumatic sphincter tear in the iris. The patient must be referred to an ophthalmologist as she may have a hyphaema.

4.   C   Hyphaema

Blood in the anterior chamber is, by definition, a hyphaema. No specific treatment is required but other pathologies must be sought, as it is an indication of significant injury. There is a significant risk of a recurrence. Referral as an urgent case is required.

5.   B   Corneal abrasion

A corneal abrasion is a very common condition. The eye is often intensely painful but healing occurs very rapidly, with most of the symptoms subsiding in about 2 days.

Causes of a red eye

A   Acute angle closure glaucoma
B   Allergic conjunctivitis
C   Bacterial conjunctivitis
D   Corneal ulcer
E   Episcleritis
F   Foreign body (corneal or conjunctival)
G   Inflamed pingueculum/pterygium
H   Iritis (anterior uveitis)
I   Scleritis
J   Subconjunctival haemorrhage
K   Viral conjunctivitis

For each of the following presentations, choose the SINGLE most likely cause from the options above. You may use each option once, more than once, or not at all.

1. A 58-year-old woman presents with nausea, vomiting and severe pain in her right eye with blurred vision. She reports seeing coloured haloes around lights. She has had similar episodes before which are relieved by sleep. On examination, the right eye has reduced vision, is markedly injected, the corneal reflection is dull and the pupil is mid-dilated and non-reactive. The left eye appears normal.

2. A 25-year-old man has a 1-day history of redness of the left eye with mild discomfort. There is a past history of ophthalmic herpes zoster. There is no visual loss or discharge from the eye. Examination shows an area of sectorial redness and engorged episcleral blood vessels.

3. A 26-year-old girl has a 2-day history of a red left eye with a foreign body sensation. She has a discharge and the eyelids are sticky in the mornings with a gritty feeling. Her vision is normal. There is a crusty purulent discharge on the lashes of her left eye.

4. A 17-year-old girl recovering from an upper respiratory tract infection presents with a 3-day history of a gritty sensation, with watery eyes and a sensitivity to light. The eyelids are swollen and the right preauricular lymph node is palpable and tender.

5. A 65-year-old man presents to the A&E department with sudden onset of severe redness of his right eye associated with a mild discomfort. This occurred after attempting to move a heavy table. He has well-controlled hypertension and is otherwise well. Examination shows normal vision, a large well-defined area of redness extending from the corneal margin.

Answers to **7.8**

1. **A   Acute angle closure glaucoma**

The history of nausea, vomiting, coloured haloes and a severely painful red eye, with a mid-dilated pupil suggests acute angle closure glaucoma. Hypermetropia (long-sight) is a predisposing factor. The acute attack is precipitated by a mechanical blockage of the drainage structures in the anterior chamber by iris tissue when the pupil dilates in dim light (e.g. cinema), or by systemic anticholinergics (antihistamines, anti-psychotics). Attacks are initially aborted by sleep-induced miosis of the pupil.

2. **E   Episcleritis**

Episcleritis is a mild inflammation of the episcleral tissues and the overlying conjunctiva. Typically, it has an acute onset with redness and mild discomfort. It is a recurrent, benign, self-limiting condition and may be nodular or diffuse. The episcleral vessels (large, radial and beneath the conjunctival vessels) are congested, and blanch with topical 2.5% phenylephrine. The majority of cases are idiopathic but collagen vascular disease, rheumatoid arthritis, gout, syphilis and herpes zoster can also be associated with episcleritis.

3. **C   Bacterial conjunctivitis**

Bacterial conjunctivitis is a common and usually self-limiting acute condition characterized by a purulent discharge with sticky eyelids typically worse in the morning, and associated with a foreign body sensation. Both eyes are often involved, but usually one eye is affected before the other. Conjunctival hyperaemia is maximal in the fornices.

4. **K   Viral conjunctivitis**

This presents acutely with watering, redness, discomfort and photophobia. Preauricular lymphadenopathy is frequent and typical. It is bilateral in 60% of cases. Adenoviral infections are the commonest and 10 of the 31 known serotypes have been implicated. It is highly contagious for the first 2 weeks and spontaneously resolves in a fortnight. Keratitis can occur in 30–80% depending on the serotype and should be suspected if there is persistent discomfort and photophobia.

5. **J   Subconjunctival haemorrhage**

This is characterized by blood under the conjunctiva which can sometimes result in a large haematoma with no visible sclera or posterior limit. The vast majority are idiopathic, but other causes include straining, trauma, hypertension, bleeding disorders or a conjunctival neoplasm (lymphoma) with a secondary haemorrhage.

Systemic diseases and the eye

A Ankylosing spondylitis (AS) with iritis (anterior uveitis)
B Cluster headache
C Diabetes mellitus
D Giant cell arteritis (temporal arteritis)
E Graves' disease
F Hypertension
G Migraine
H Reiter's syndrome
I Rheumatoid arthritis and scleritis
J Sjögren's syndrome
K Stevens–Johnson syndrome

For each patient below, choose the SINGLE most likely diagnosis from the
above list of options. Each option may be used once, more than once, or
not at all.

1. A 65-year-old woman presents with sudden loss of vision in her right
    eye and a severe right-sided temporal headache. She also feels unwell
    and lethargic with painful, stiff shoulders. There is light perception only
    in her right eye with a mild, cloudy swelling of the optic nerve head. Her
    ESR is 80 mm/h.

2. A 25-year-old woman presents with painful and discharging red eyes,
    fever, generalized rash, oral lesions and arthralgia. She has been treated
    with codeine phosphate for a painful sports injury. The skin lesions have
    red-centred vesicles surrounded by a pale, oedematous ring, resembling
    a 'target'.

3. A 25-year-old man presents with bilateral, non-sticky, red eyes, arthralgia
    mainly affecting his lower limbs, pain and tenderness of the lower back
    and dysuria. He has had a mild gastrointestinal infection.

4. A 30-year-old man presents with a painful, red left eye. Examination
    shows mildly reduced vision and redness. The left pupil is smaller than
    the right and the right eye appears normal. He has a long-standing
    history of low back pain and stiffness.

5. A 40-year-old woman has increasing pain and redness of her right eye
    which shows a widespread inflammation of the anterior segment. The
    vascular pattern is distorted and oedematous. Phenylephrine (2.5%)
    does not blanch the vessels. She also has a history of worsening pain
    and swelling of the small joints of her hands and feet.

Answers to **7.9**

1. **D** Giant cell arteritis

This typically affects patients over 60 years of age. Females are affected more than males. The medium and large muscular arteries are thickened by inflammatory cells. Ischaemic optic neuropathy, from occlusion of the posterior ciliary arteries, gives rise to the features as seen in this case. Characteristically, patients have a high ESR. The risk of blindness in the other eye is 66% in the first week and treatment should be instituted immediately with high dose steroids.

2. **K** Stevens–Johnson syndrome

The target lesions are diagnostic of erythema multiforme, which is referred to as Stevens–Johnson syndrome when the mucosa is also involved. This is an acute, but usually self-limiting condition affecting the skin and mucosa. Many agents can precipitate it including drugs and infectious agents such as herpes simplex and Mycoplasma. However, in as much as 50% of cases no cause is identified.

3. **H** Reiter's syndrome

The triad of conjunctivitis, urethritis and arthritis constitutes Reiter's syndrome. It predominantly affects men (20:1), occurring after an enteric or venereal infection or a non-specific urethritis. The arthritis usually occurs 2 weeks after the infection. Conjunctivitis is mild, bilateral, may be mucopurulent, and resolves spontaneously. Acute anterior uveitis may occur later in up to 30%. HLA B27 is positive in nearly 70% of patients.

4. **A** Ankylosing spondylitis (AS) with iritis (anterior uveitis)

The ocular symptoms and findings described here are typical of acute iritis. Slit lamp examination will show flare and cells in the normally quiet anterior chamber. The back pain in a young male along with acute iritis is suggestive of AS. Around 95% of patients are HLA B27-positive. About 30% of men with acute iritis will have AS.

5. **I** Rheumatoid arthritis and scleritis.

Scleritis produces a deep boring pain and is a much more serious condition than episcleritis, which is virtually pain-free. A drop of 2.5% phenylephrine blanches the congested episcleral vessels in episcleritis but not the deeper vessels of the sclera and thus helps to differentiate the two conditions. Rheumatoid arthritis is the most common cause of scleritis.

Medicolegal Issues

Medical ethics and the law

A   Call police
B   Implement Mental Health Act
C   Implement Public Health Act
D   Respect patient's wishes
E   Respect wishes of the next of kin
F   Seek a court order
G   Seek a judicial review
H   Seek a psychiatric review
I   Treat under common law
J   Withhold resuscitation in the event of cardiac arrest
K   Withhold treatment

For each presentation below, choose the SINGLE most appropriate action from the above list of options. Each option may be used once, more than once, or not at all.

1. A 45-year-old man presents with weight loss and night sweats. He has a history of alcohol abuse and has had frequent hospital admissions. Acid-fast bacilli have been found in his sputum but he refuses treatment and threatens to self-discharge.

2. An 18-year-old girl attends the A&E department after taking an overdose of tablets including paracetamol but refuses to have her blood taken for toxicology. She also refuses any treatment. She appears to appreciate the consequences of this decision.

3. A 30-year-old woman refuses a blood transfusion despite suffering a life-threatening postpartum haemorrhage. She is a devout Jehovah's Witness.

4. An 82-year-old woman with severe dementia is admitted with bronchopneumonia following a dense stroke. Her family insists that she should be resuscitated in the event of a cardiac arrest.

5. The family of a 45-year-old man would like to withdraw all treatment for him. He has been in a persistent vegetative state for the last 18 months following a motorcycle accident.

Answers to **8.1**

1. C Implement Public Health Act

This patient has open tuberculosis of the respiratory tract which poses a serious risk of infection to others. The consultant in communicable disease control or in Public Health needs to be informed. Often patients change their minds and heed medical advice. It may be necessary to obtain a magistrate's order for admission, detention and compulsory examination under the Public Health Act although compulsory treatment is not allowed.

2. D Respect patient's wishes

Every adult has a right and must have the capacity to decide whether to accept or decline treatment, even if refusal leads to permanent injury or death. In this case, the patient has capacity understand the nature of the proposed treatment, the principal benefits and risks, and the consequences of refusing treatment. Hence her wishes should be respected. Where the patient lacks capacity (long term mental incapacity or temporary incapacity from unconsciousness, pain, shock or the effects of drugs), doctors have a duty to act in the patient's best interests or in accordance to an advanced directive, if available. The court should be applied to for assistance when in doubt, especially in cases of reduced capacity.

3. D Respect patient's wishes

This patient has a right to refuse treatment (blood transfusion) because of her religious beliefs which make the refusal reasonable. Failure to respect the patient's wishes may lead to charges of assault.

4. J Withhold resuscitation in the event of cardiac arrest

Although the views of the health team, patient, relatives and close friends are useful in making the decision of 'do not resuscitate', the ultimate responsibility of making the decision lies with the consultant or the general practitioner. It is appropriate in this case because resuscitation is unlikely to be successful. Even if resuscitation is successful, it will be followed by a quality of life which is not in the best interests of the patient.

5. F Seek court order

Airedale NHS Trust v Bland [1993] AC 789 decided that the withdrawal of treatment would not be contrary to the criminal law. The withdrawal of nutrition and hydration was an omission rather than an act, and being kept alive was not in the best interests of the patient. Although there are now guidelines for the withdrawal of treatment in persistent vegetative state (from the British Medical Association and the Royal College of Physicians), the health authority should still seek a declaration from the courts to allow withdrawal of treatment.

Regulations regarding fitness to drive

A Breach patient confidentiality and inform the Driving and Vehicle Licensing Agency (DVLA)
B Driving licence subject to regular review
C Inform police
D No action needed
E Reapply for driving licence
F Refer for driving assessment
G Stop driving for life
H Stop driving for 1 month
I Stop driving for 6 months
J Stop driving for 1 week
K Stop driving until symptom-free

For each problem below, choose the SINGLE most appropriate course of action from the above list of options. Each option may be used once, more than once, or not at all.

1. A 69-year-old woman plans to continue driving her car after the age of 70 years as her independence can then be maintained. She is generally fit and well except for a few simple falls over the last 3 months.

2. A 55-year-old man is about to be discharged after a small cerebrovascular accident from which he has made a full recovery. He had been admitted with sudden onset of right-sided weakness but this was associated with a tonic–clonic seizure lasting 20 minutes. He would like to resume driving his car as soon as possible.

3. A 75-year-old man with moderate dementia would like to continue driving his car. His family is worried about his safety although he remains independent with his activities of daily living.

4. An 80-year-old man has just had a permanent pacemaker inserted for prolonged pauses detected on 24-hour ECG monitoring.

5. A 35-year-old woman with well-controlled epilepsy is due to stop her antiepileptic treatment under medical supervision. She last had a seizure 10 years ago and is presently able to drive her car.

Answers to **8.2**

1.   E   Reapply for driving licence

It is the responsibility of drivers themselves to inform the Driving and Vehicle Licensing Agency (DVLA) and to reapply for their driving licence when they reach 70 years of age if they are planning to continue to drive. Subject to a declaration of medical fitness to drive, a licence is reissued for 3 years.

2.   H   Stop driving for 1 month

Driving may resume 1 month after a cerebrovascular event (which includes a thrombotic or haemorrhagic stroke, transient ischaemic attack, amaurosis fugax) if there has been satisfactory clinical recovery. Epileptic attacks occurring within 24 hours of the event may be treated as being provoked and so the epilepsy regulations do not apply. Otherwise a solitary fit would mean 1 year off driving. There is no need to notify the DVLA unless there is some residual neurological deficit 1 month after the event.

3.   F   Refer for driving assessment

Formal on-road testing (or even simulation) is useful to assess driving performance. Problems with performing multiple tasks, concentration, visual inattention, reaction time, memory and confidence may be identified. An assessment of activities of daily living may be a useful predictor of competence behind the wheel. Subjects with severe dementia who refuse to give up driving despite exhaustive attempts to dissuade them may be reported to the DVLA as they pose a danger to themselves and to the public.

4.   J   Stop driving for 1 week

Following pacemaker implants, driving may be resumed after 1 week providing that there is no other disqualifying condition.

5.   I   Stop driving for 6 months

This patient should be warned that there is a 40% risk of a seizure in the first year of withdrawal of medication compared with those who have continued on treatment. She may resume driving 6 months later providing she remains well. The epilepsy regulations will apply should she have a recurrence of fits. Some patients may opt to continue with the medication (particularly if it is well-tolerated) if their fitness to drive is an important issue.

Death certificates and cremations

8.3

A   Ask the patient's GP to issue a death certificate
B   Ask your consultant to issue a death certificate
C   Collect the fee and keep a record
D   Consult the doctor who issued the death certificate and view the body
E   Cremate with the pacemaker box in situ
F   Do not cremate
G   Do not issue a death certificate
H   Issue the death certificate and ask for a hospital postmortem
I   Obtain consent from relatives
J   Refer to the coroner
K   Requires no action

For each scenario below, choose the SINGLE most appropriate action from the above list of options. Each option may be used once, more than once, or not at all.

1. A 65-year-old woman was admitted with a left lower lobar pneumonia 5 days ago. She was making good progress with treatment but died suddenly last night. The medical team is unclear about the nature of the terminal event.

2. A 72-year-old man with a known abdominal aortic aneurysm was admitted with back pain. He collapsed 4 hours later and died. The doctor suspects that his aortic aneurysm had ruptured but is not sure if death was caused by a cardiorespiratory event.

3. A doctor is asked to fill in part 1 of a cremation form for a woman who was under his care during her final illness, but who died when another team was on call. So, a different doctor issued the death certificate.

4. A 92-year-old man with sinoatrial disease and a permanent pacemaker dies in hospital from intractable heart failure. The relatives wish to have him cremated.

5. The pathologist performing a postmortem on a patient with an amoebic liver abscess wishes to retain and preserve the liver for educational purposes.

Answers to **8.3**

1. **H**   Issue the death certificate and ask for a hospital postmortem

The death certificate can be issued with pneumonia as the cause of death. The relatives should be asked for their consent for a postmortem as the actual cause of the sudden death is not clear. In most cases, the consent is readily obtained but if they decline then their wishes should be respected. They should not be subjected to any pressure, least of all the implication that a postmortem can be arranged without their consent by referring the matter to the coroner.

2. **J**   Refer to the coroner

Death occurring within 24 hours of admission to hospital or after an operation must be referred to the coroner, who may not ask for a postmortem if he is happy with the doctor's impression about the cause of death. Other circumstances when a death must be referred to the coroner include when foul play is suspected, when death is due to occupational disease or if it occurs within 1 year of an assault. A coroner's postmortem does not require consent from the relatives.

3. **D**   Consult the doctor who issued the death certificate and view the body

The part 1 of a cremation form is completed by the doctor who looked after the patient during their last illness, even though he may not have been present at the time of the death and may not have issued the death certificate. However, he must consult and discuss with the doctor who did issue the death certificate, consult the patient's case notes and identify the deceased so that he has all the correct details before filling in the cremation form.

4. **C**   Collect the fee and keep a record

The death certificate can be issued as the cause of death is clear, and the patient can be cremated. The pacemaker must be removed before the cremation since there is a risk of explosion. The doctor will get a fee both for the cremation certificate and for removing the pacemaker. A record of the fees should be kept for income tax purposes.

5. **I**   Obtain consent from relatives

The problem of postmortem tissue retention for research and teaching purposes has attracted a lot of unfavourable publicity for the medical profession. Tissues cannot be taken from a coroner's postmortem. A hospital postmortem can be performed with the consent of relatives, but they should be given full information if any tissues are to be retained for research or teaching purposes.

The Mental Health Act 1983

8.4

A Section 1
B Section 2
C Section 3
D Section 3(2)
E Section 3(4)
F Section 4
G Section 5(2)
H Section 5(4)
I Section 6
J Section 7
K Section 8

For each description below, choose the SINGLE most appropriate Section of the Mental Health Act from the above list of options. Each option may be used once, more than once, or not at all.

1. This Section is designated as the doctor's holding power, and facilitates emergency detention of the patient (who is already an inpatient) in hospital. Duration is up to 72 hours and the signatory is the doctor in charge of the patient's care or the nominated deputy.

2. This Section is designated as the nurse's holding power and facilitates emergency detention of the patient (who is already an inpatient receiving treatment for a psychiatric disorder) in hospital for 6 hours until the patient is assessed by a doctor.

3. This Section is for emergency admission. One doctor and the nearest relative/approved social worker are the signatories. Its duration is up to 72 hours. Grounds for detention include the presence of mental disorder, and it being necessary for the interests of the patient's health, safety or the protection of others that the patient requires urgent hospitalization for assessment.

4. The purpose of this Section is admission for assessment. Grounds for admission include mental disorder, and it is necessary for the patient's health, safety or protection of others that requires hospitalization for assessment. Two doctors and the nearest relative/approved social worker are the signatories and Section duration is for up to 28 days.

5. This Section facilitates admission for treatment and lasts 6 months in the first instance. This is then renewable for a further 6 months and subsequently yearly. Grounds for detention include the presence of mental illness, mental impairment, severe mental impairment or psychopathic disorder.

Answers to **8.4**

Sections 5(2), 5(4), 4, 2 and 3 are the most important Sections to be aware of. Sections 3(2) and 3(4) do not make up part of the Mental Health Act.

1. **G   Section 5(2)**

   This may be applied to any hospital inpatient where a mental disorder is suspected. This includes inpatients on medical and surgical wards. The signatory should be the consultant in charge of the patient's care even if this is an orthopaedic surgeon (or his/her nominated deputy which is usually the junior doctor on-call). It is good practice to inform the consultant in charge of the patient's care or the on-call consultant if Section 5(2) is being considered.

2. **H   Section 5(4)**

   The patient must suffer from a mental disorder and detention must be in the interests of the patient's health, safety or for the protection of others. There must be a need for immediate restraint and it must be when the doctor is not immediately available.

3. **F   Section 4**

   This is infrequently used and is considered bad practice. Section 4 should only be used when the matter is of urgent necessity and there is not enough time to get a second medical recommendation. It should only be used in a genuine emergency and not for convenience. There must be evidence of an immediate risk of mental or physical harm to the patient or others, and/or danger of serious harm to property and/or the need for physical restraint of the patient.

4. **B   Section 2**

   Section 2 is designated for assessment and/or treatment. Section 2 (as opposed to Section 3) should be considered when the diagnosis is unclear, when there is a need for inpatient assessment to formulate a treatment plan, or when the patient has not previously been admitted to hospital and has not been in regular contact with specialist psychiatric services.

5. **C   Section 3**

   Grounds for admission for treatment include the presence of mental illness, mental impairment, severe mental impairment or psychopathic disorder. If the diagnosis is of a psychopathic disorder or mental impairment, then treatment must be likely to alleviate or prevent deterioration of the condition. Treatment must be necessary for the patient's health, safety or for protection of others and it cannot be provided unless the patient is detained.

Index